See What Others Have to Say About
The Complete Idiot's Guide to T'ai Chi and QiGong,
Acclaimed Primer and Reference Used by
Top T'ai Chi, QiGong, and Health Professionals

Visionary! If you only buy one book on T'ai Chi, *then this is the book*. This book is all you ever needed to know to change your life. I have taught T'ai Chi for several decades myself, yet I have now read Bill's book from cover to cover *seven times*, and *still* get something new from it each time.

—Dr. Michael Steward Sr., D.MA, Ph.D., MA, Senior Coach for Team USA, Inductee of the World Sports Medicine and World Martial Arts Hall of Fame

… living an extremely unhealthy life style … taking numerous medications for arthritis, depression, and pain … then one day while browsing in the library I discovered a book … *The Complete Idiot's Guide to T'ai Chi and QiGong*. I was so impressed that I ordered Bill's videos …. Now that I am practicing T'ai Chi and QiGong daily I am off most of my medications. People keep telling me I look "different" and that I look happy. Well, I am happy and I feel great! … Thank you! Thank you! Thank you!

—Dave Long, Washington

I had the privilege of studying T'ai Chi with this book's author, Bill Douglas. As a practicing physician, there are certainly times where stress can seem to be the norm. I found T'ai Chi to be profoundly beneficial in reducing stress, increasing mental clarity, and improving my emotional as well as physical health. Where else can you find such a highly effective tool to achieve these worthwhile goals without fancy equipment or complicated formulas? If T'ai Chi can help with stress in an ER room where lives often hang in the balance, imagine what it can do for everyone else!

—John D. Hernandez, M.D., Integrative Medicine

Sometimes Chinese culture can be difficult to explain. Sifu Bill Douglas successfully uses American culture to explain the art of T'ai Chi Chuan. He simplifies difficult concepts, making them easier to understand. This book takes the best parts of T'ai Chi and makes them understandable [to Westerners] without requiring a grounding in Chinese culture and history.

—Sifu Yijiao Hong, USA All-Tai Chi Grand Champion and USA Team member; Certified Int'l. Coach and Judge, Int'l Wushu Federation.

Douglas has achieved for QiGong what Apple did for the computer. He's brought it to the people … great place to start for beginners … teachers may also find this an excellent manual "on how to explain these concepts to the general public …."

—R. Poccia, Stress Management Instructor, Beyond Anonymous, San Francisco

It has been a year since I began practicing T'ai Chi under the teaching of the author of this book, Bill Douglas and his associate instructor Erik Feagans. This span of time certainly allows me to evaluate the result of this gentle "martial art," not only as stress management therapy but, more impressively, with regard to its effect on my physical health.

Suffering for years from chronic neck pain consequent to a whiplash injury, and also suffering from a limited motion of the right shoulder, I approached the T'ai Chi course with some skepticism. The course was initiated after unsuccessful sessions of physical therapy, including mobilization, ultrasounds, heat application, etc. After two months of T'ai Chi, the pain in the cervical region disappeared while the range of motion of my right shoulder returned completely to normal. This achievement remained unchanged during the past winter up until now.

I would not hesitate to recommend T'ai Chi to individuals suffering from the same ailments as well as to mature persons who are seeking to maintain or improve their health and to remain free of chronic pain due to the aging process.

—Loredana Brizio-Molteni, M.D., F.A.C.S.

After leaving my very first T'ai Chi class with the author of this book, I remember driving home and it was as if someone had opened up every one of my senses. It was an overwhelming sense of happiness that swept over me. It was at that very moment I knew T'ai Chi is something I want in my life forever.

—Lisa Shikles, Shawnee, Kansas

Because of my practice of T'ai Chi and QiGong, my barometer for detecting "dis-ease" within myself earlier, allows me to prevent serious infection and speed up healing. I feel T'ai Chi is a wonderful part of a revolution in health care, whereby each of us takes much more responsibility for our own health and healing.

—Susan Norman, C.I.M.T.

… I found you by accident while looking for an alternative to back surgery … with three ruptured discs in my lower back … I read your book from cover to cover … I am also now over half way through your second tape, and my range of motion is better than it has been in years. I have also managed to lose a few pounds … Recently I went to my regular medical doctor … he told me he was very pleased with my range of moti and my attitude … He was so intrigued by my description of your program that he has borrowed my book and the tapes I have finish

—Mark Herndon, Georgia

Since beginning Bill Douglas's T'ai Chi program, I have taught the exercises I learned for the past five years in our Pain Management multidisciplinary program at Research Medical Center. My clients have found improved breathing, larger mobility, better posture, improved balance and coordination, flexibility, increased endurance and strength, and relaxation.

—Berni Wheeler, Occupational Therapist

I have found so many health benefits since beginning Bill Douglas's T'ai Chi program, which I began during a nervous breakdown with panic, chest pains, fatigue, and chronic migraines. I saw Bill's T'ai Chi and QiGong program information and I gave it a try. I felt sudden and immediate benefits. My chest pain started to go away, my heavy fatigue went away, my nervousness calmed. My migraines are now nonexistent, as is the severe hay fever I'd had since childhood. And if that isn't enough, I have also lost my craving for fatty foods I once used to soothe my stress, and am now losing weight.

—Tina Webb, Shawnee, Kansas

As a physical therapist assistant, I believe that these techniques that are taught by Bill through his book and tapes will become one of the essential tools to be utilized in medical facilities as an adjunct to standard therapy.

Not a day goes by when I am not able to help an individual find pain control using Bill's QiGong techniques, and many find increased balance and coordination, even after a small taste of Tai Chi seeing automatic difference. Personally, tests show me with a 90 percent improvement in overall balance and in one test a 105 percent improvement in balance since beginning Tai Chi.

—Joyce Rupp, Physical Therapist Assistant, Hays, Kansas

During a time of high stress levels at work I began to have heavy Parkinson's type tremors. At a psychiatrist's recommendation I began taking Xanax, but the anxiety still continued. After my very first T'ai Chi class with this book's author, I was so calm I forgot to take my Xanax that afternoon. Before this I'd anxiously looked forward to each dose. … I've told my therapist to tell other patients about T'ai Chi.

—Tarren Rains, Edwardsville, Kansas

From the perspective of a health psychologist serving patients who are coping with chronic illness and stressful life events, I see the gentle mindfulness exercises of T'ai Chi and QiGong relaxation therapy as potentially useful for a broad spectrum of people. The author of this book, Bill Douglas, explains the complexities of T'ai Chi and QiGong in the form of an invitation, easing his students into a greater understanding of the usefulness and purpose of this ancient form of meditative movement.

—Kristy Straits-Troster, Ph.D., Clinical Psychologist, Primary Care Medicine

Dizziness is one of the more common reasons for a doctor visit, particularly in patients over the age of 50. Because the causes of dizziness can range from benign self-limiting conditions to potentially life threatening ones, a thorough medical evaluation is essential before embarking on any form of therapy. Persistent dizziness certainly has a distinct impact on the quality of life and emotional well-being of the patient. Falls, hip fractures, and lack of confidence in public often create a feeling of helplessness.

In over 20 years of experience as a clinical neurologist, I find that extensive and expensive medical evaluation including CAT scans, MRI scans, and vascular imaging studies as well as prescription medications add little to alleviating the problem. I have found vestibular rehabilitation exercises in the form of T'ai Chi classes to be a cost-effective mode of therapy. Many of my patients have opted for this nonmedication approach to treatment and have developed a sense of self-confidence through this form of exercise. In short, as a traditional medical practitioner, I frequently recommend T'ai Chi for my patients with dizziness and disequilibrium.

—Charles D. Donohoe, M.D., Neurologist

My attitude, since the first few lessons, changed, due to your effectiveness and to your ability to teach this gentle "martial art." I was suffering for symptoms related to osteoarthritis of the left coxofemoral joint, and, in addition, I was suffering from neck pain with limited motion. This symptomology disappeared with the T'ai Chi exercises. My physician's recommendation is to continue with the practice of T'ai Chi. I would pass the same recommendation to individuals with similar sedentary life styles as well as to people involved in activity, which requires exertion of the musculoskeletal system.

—Agostino Molteni, M.D., Ph.D.

"Rx: Continue T'ai Chi. — Dx: Hypertension"

—An actual physician's prescription for a patient to continue in Bill Douglas's hospital T'ai Chi and QiGong classes

Since beginning Bill's T'ai Chi program, my resting heart rate has gone from 81 to 61. It's amazing!

—Anne Bauman, Kansas

I found that the Energy Work (Sitting QiGong) and breath work, learned in Bill's T'ai Chi program, to be calming and to have that effect on those around me as well, including a returning patient who was hallucinating and having panic attacks. By walking with him and breathing deeply, the patient eventually calmed and laid down breathing evenly to await the doctor.

—Psychotherapist, Kansas City Area

After studying Tai Chi with this book's author I found an illness of the digestive system I'd had for several years has essentially disappeared. My energy levels remain high, even when I'm fighting an illness, and I get sick *much* less often.

—Tom Hansen, Lenexa, Kansas

I had surgery for a possible life-threatening infection in my head. After surgery I was recovering so fast the doctor ordered the nurses to give me more morphine. They felt I was too active and recovering too quickly. My secret—I was in bed doing Sitting QiGong [as shown in your book and videos].

—Dave Long, Washington

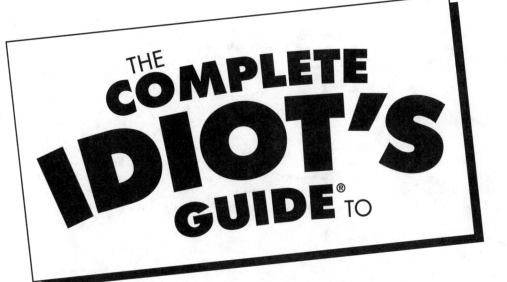

THE
COMPLETE
IDIOT'S
GUIDE® TO

T'ai Chi
and QiGong

Second Edition

by Bill Douglas

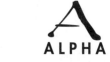

ALPHA

A Pearson Education Company

In loving memory of my father, William Edward Douglas Sr., a man who endured the horror of war and hardship like few others ... yet from that experience hungered for a world of justice and peace for all peoples of the world. Your Herculean efforts to heal your life serve as an example, enabling me to open to the profound healing T'ai Chi and QiGong offer me and the world. I hope you are up there enjoying the sight of Germans and Americans, Jews and Arabs, all playing T'ai Chi together every year. I dedicate World T'ai Chi and QiGong Day to your memory.

Publisher: *Marie Butler-Knight*
Product Manager: *Phil Kitchel*
Managing Editor: *Jennifer Chisholm*
Acquisitions Editor: *Mike Sanders*
Development Editor: *Michael Koch*
Senior Production Editor: *Christy Wagner*
Copy Editor: *Drew Patty*
Illustrator: *Chris Eliopoulos*
Cover/Book Designer: *Trina Wurst*
Indexer: *Tonya Heard*
Layout/Proofreading: *Svetlana Dominguez, Gloria Schurick*

Contents at a Glance

Contents

Appendixes

Foreword

As Bill explains in this book, although T'ai Chi and QiGong are exercises, they are integral parts of Traditional Chinese Medicine (TCM). As alternative medicine and therapies sweep the Western world, doctors now prescribe QiGong and T'ai Chi for treating stress problems, illnesses, and injuries, while many people use it as a tonic to extend their peak performance into old age. Robert Parish, one of the great NBA players, claimed T'ai Chi extended his career, making him one of the oldest *dominant* starting players in NBA history. Just as T'ai Chi protected Mr. Parish's body from the intense stress of professional basketball, it can help each of us protect ourselves from the relentless stress of a rapidly changing world.

In my 43 years of experience in Traditional Chinese Medicine, here and in the Orient, I have never heard anyone explain the premise of T'ai Chi and QiGong as succinctly as Bill does. He has the most unusual ability to explain concepts he's spent a lifetime learning in a way that is tangible and applicable to the novice student the very first day of class. You will happily realize that this book offers you, the reader, a humorous and enjoyable journey deep into the world of T'ai Chi and QiGong. After providing an extensive understanding of T'ai Chi and QiGong's profound potential, the book proceeds to very practically explain how you can dive into T'ai Chi and QiGong by clarifying such basic concepts as what to wear to class and what to call your teacher.

This book provides ways T'ai Chi can be integrated into your life on many levels through your work, social recreation, and health care, just as it has been in China for many years. Bill shares and eloquently articulates my vision that Traditional Chinese Medicine is leading a transformation in Western health care that will financially save you, the patient, untold dollars and much needless pain and suffering. This book will facilitate that transformation by making the everyday person comfortable with the commonsense approach health tools like T'ai Chi and QiGong make, and we will all be better for it.

This book, with humor and gentleness, guides you through T'ai Chi and QiGong to help you boost your immune system, sleep better, and improve everything about you effortlessly. This book is for everybody living with stress, but a must for every corporate wellness director, health care worker, and activities director. Here you can learn why T'ai Chi is the fastest-growing exercise and healing balm for modern life!

Richard Yennie, D.C., Dipl. Ac. (NCCA), Deputy Director, China Medical Assn., Research Committee, Taipei, Taiwan; President, QiGong Society of America; U.S. Representative, World Academic Society of Medical QiGong; President, Acupuncture Society of America, Inc.; Faculty Member, Waseda Acupuncture College, Tokyo, Japan; Visiting Professor at Beijing University of Chinese Medicine, Beijing, China

Introduction

Before I began T'ai Chi and QiGong classes, the stress in my life was unbearable, and depression and anxiety were almost a way of life. I actually thought at the time that that's just the way life was. It's funny what we'll settle for, when all the while there are powerful and exciting opportunities to change—just waiting for us to reach out and grab them. Back then, I returned home every night from a job I didn't like and used greasy food, overspending, too much TV, or whatever else could help me handle the stress of a life I didn't really feel too good about. I really didn't see much hope for finding any "real joy" in my life.

Then, a friend suggested a T'ai Chi class. From that day, my life began to change, to loosen, to expand and open, becoming more than I ever dreamed possible. Today I travel the world sharing the most exciting life possibilities with fascinating people all seeking to expand their lives into more than they ever imagined.

T'ai Chi enabled me to let go of my tight rigid grip on what I thought was possible in life. As it taught me to breathe deeply and allow my body's rigid muscles to let go and relax, my mind and heart began to do so as well. An open mind and open heart expanded outward into an open world. When we begin to live for what we love, the world begins to love us for it. T'ai Chi and QiGong help us loosen up, so the love within us can expand outward into all aspects of our lives. This is how we become "lovely" in the truest sense of the word. There is such beautiful potential awaiting all of us, and I am so proud and so grateful that this book has been a part of so many people's expansion—just as T'ai Chi and QiGong have been a part of mine. Enjoy!

How to Use This Book

This book is divided into six parts. Each part's information will prepare you for the next, opening your mind and imagination to concepts that will unlock your ability to expand your awareness of T'ai Chi and QiGong even more.

Part 1, "T'ai Chi: Relax into It," explains how T'ai Chi and QiGong can change every part of your life for the better. This part concludes in explaining how T'ai Chi and QiGong work by introducing you to Traditional Chinese Medicine and explaining how modern Western science is now beginning to understand how this ancient wisdom works.

Part 2, "Suiting Up and Setting Out," prepares you to dive into T'ai Chi and QiGong "big time" or "little time," depending on how much of T'ai Chi's magic you want to experience. In this part you will learn the nuts and bolts of how classes are taught, T'ai Chi etiquette, terms, wardrobe, and all the things that will enable you to choose the best class for you. You will also discover the underlying tenets of T'ai Chi and QiGong, which will dramatically enhance the benefit you get from class of video instruction beyond this book.

Part 3, "Starting Down the QiGong Path to T'ai Chi," explains how QiGong works and then leads you into an experience that is exquisite beyond words. This part ends with an introduction to Moving QiGong exercises that include the warm-ups that prepare your mind and body to dive into an ocean of T'ai Chi experience. T'ai Chi literally means "the supreme ultimate," so hold on for an incredible ride!

Part 4, "Kuang Ping T'ai Chi: Walk on Life's Lighter Side," illuminates the history of T'ai Chi and how the Kuang Ping Yang Style was brought to the West by Master Kuo Lien Ying. Then you will be led through the entire 64 postures of this powerful ancient form and instructed as to a few of the benefits of each movement. Yet, remember the benefits are endless, and since this book is only about 400 pages long, to discover them you must experience them yourself as they unfold beautifully within you every day for the rest of your life.

Part 5, "T'ai Chi's Buffet of Short, Sword, and Fan Styles," exposes you to the many incredibly beautiful forms of T'ai Chi that are available to you today. Remember that only about 30 years ago, these arts were secrets of China, so we are very lucky to have these exquisite art forms available to us now in our lifetimes. This part gives you a small, yet delicious taste of what is available. If you seek, ye shall find.

Part 6, "Life Applications," shows that T'ai Chi is much more than just a "physical exercise." T'ai Chi can help heal every aspect of our lives, our relationships, and our world. To that end, this part explains how T'ai Chi and/or QiGong can be used to help treat almost any illness or physical malady. It also explains to what extent T'ai Chi can be a powerful adjunct therapy for many mental or emotional problems, as well as a powerful tool that helps you increase your productivity and creativity in your professional life. But, even beyond healing you will see how T'ai Chi can help the world realize a much more expansive vision of possibility for our ever evolving future.

T'ai Chi Pearls

Throughout this book, I've included these five types of extra information in boxes, for your enlightenment:

> **Know Your Chinese**
> These boxes give you definitions for Chinese medical and philosophical terms related to T'ai Chi and QiGong, including pronunciation aids.

> **T'ai Sci**
> These boxes provide you modern scientific terms and insights into the world of T'ai Chi's ancient discoveries.

> **Ouch!**
> These boxes alert you to any caution you should observe in T'ai Chi practice. There won't be many of these. T'ai Chi injuries are nearly non-existent when done correctly.

> **A T'ai Chi Punch Line**
> These boxes are full of fun anecdotes and trivia about the fascinating world of T'ai Chi and QiGong, modern and old.

> **Sage Sifu Says**
> These boxes offer you tips on living the principles of T'ai Chi and maximize your understanding of T'ai Chi's subtle layers to help you get the most out of it. Sifu (pronounced *see-foo*) means "one who has mastered an art." Not only martial arts, but a master chef, or artist, might be a sifu.

Acknowledgments

A great thanks to the many dedicated Chinese creators of T'ai Chi who've spent lifetimes developing this wonderful art and health science the world now has access to. T'ai Chi and QiGong are great gifts the Chinese culture has provided for the world, and I offer them a deep and heartfelt thank you. Their efforts leave me convinced that every culture on this planet has treasures to offer the rest, and I hope we all can open our hearts and minds to truth and value no matter where it comes from.

A profound thanks to my teacher, Master Jennifer Booth, her teacher Gil Messenger, their teacher Russell Schofield, and our grand master Kuo Lien Ying, who made the daunting journey from China to San Francisco. His courage in migrating to this strange land made it possible for millions of Americans to have access to the beauty and power of Kuang Ping Yang T'ai Chi Chuan.

I would like to thank my brilliant sister Diane Douglas, her associates Jay and Sandra, my brother Ed, and sisters Barbara and Peggy, without whose insights and support, none of this would have been possible. My wife Angela and her mother Shun Oi Wong were an integral part of my T'ai Chi journey, and my father-in-law, Bonwyn Wong, embodied the humility and infinite wisdom Chinese people are famous for. My children Isaac, Andrea, and Michael led me to the doorway of change through their innocent examples of wisdom, and my parents, Evelyn and William Douglas, showed me that even the harshest tests can produce pearls in us beautiful creatures, known as human beings.

Thanks to Mulan Quan instructors Angela Wong-Douglas and Andrea Mei-Wah Douglas for their wonderful exhibitions and insights into the elegant art form of Mulan Quan basic, fan, and sword style. Thanks to Mike Sanders, Michael Koch, Christy Wagner, and Drew Patty for both their patience and profound editing expertise, and for Susan Norman's sage advice on holistic living.

With the modern stress plague ravaging the world, I want to thank the visionary educators beginning to incorporate T'ai Chi and QiGong into education systems worldwide. When every graduating senior is a T'ai Chi master, how much less drug and alcohol abuse, and how much less violence and children in prisons will there be? Thank you all for your courage, vision, and open-heartedness, to see the profound value of these tools even though they come from another culture. Thanks to all the innovative T'ai Chi teachers who are discovering new ways to teach these ancient arts, to make them fun and contemporary so that modern children (and adults) in all societies can learn to love them.

Last, but not least, I'd like to thank illustrator Jenny Hahn Neely (shikuns@mindspring.com), for her work on the more than 200 instructional sketches and her dedication to this project. Ms. Neely is an extraordinary artist with an ability to capture complex, and *even internal* T'ai Chi concepts in her illustrations. Her work has set a *new standard* for T'ai Chi book instruction. Also, thanks to Jessica Kincaid for her computer graphics (www.filigree.com), master photographer David Larson for his brilliant photos (davidlarson@ sprintmail. com), and Jeff Chappell for the cover photo (jeffreychappell@hotmail.com).

Special Thanks to the Technical Reviewer

The Complete Idiot's Guide to T'ai Chi and QiGong, Second Edition, was reviewed by an expert who double-checked the accuracy of what you'll learn here, to help us ensure that this book gives you everything you need to know about T'ai Chi and QiGong. Special thanks are extended to Master Jennifer Booth.

Trademarks

All terms mentioned in this book that are known to be or are suspected of being trademarks or service marks have been appropriately capitalized. Alpha Books and Pearson Education, Inc., cannot attest to the accuracy of this information. Use of a term in this book should not be regarded as affecting the validity of any trademark or service mark.

Part 1

T'ai Chi: Relax into It

This part explains why a simple, easy-to-do, 2,000-year-old Chinese martial art is the most popular exercise in the world today and is practiced in corporations, hospitals, living rooms, and backyards (just like yours) around the world.

If you want to find a calm center in the middle of life's storm of change, while also toning your muscles and healing your mind and body, T'ai Chi and QiGong are just what the doctor ordered—literally, *ask your doctor!*

T'ai Chi is a unique exercise that simultaneously heals the physical, mental, emotional, and spiritual body. With T'ai Chi, you can boost your energy levels, dramatically improve your health, *slow your aging process*, become more creative, and significantly lower your stress levels even in our increasingly stressful world. And this is only scratching the surface of T'ai Chi's benefits.

This part shows you that all the power you ever needed is found right in the center of where you are anytime and all the time. Providing access to the unlimited personal power that we each possess makes T'ai Chi perhaps the most powerful personal growth tool in the world. So whether you seek a simple, easy-to-do exercise, a stress-management tool, or a profoundly healthy philosophy of life, T'ai Chi may just be what you've been looking for.

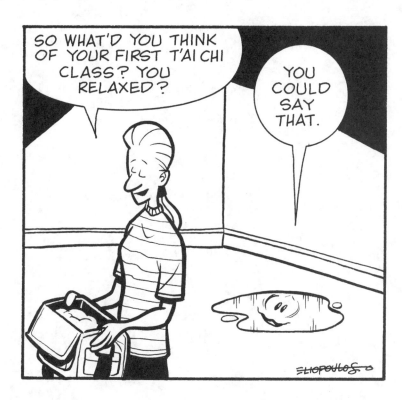

Why Practice T'ai Chi?

In This Chapter

- The reasons behind T'ai Chi's exploding popularity
- The root of T'ai Chi
- A brief history of T'ai Chi

T'ai Chi is practiced by 20 percent of the world's population and is fast becoming the most popular exercise in the world today. Its rapid expansion is largely due to one important fact—*it feels really good*. Although T'ai Chi was originally a martial art and is increasingly offered by martial arts studios, it's now practiced in businesses, hospitals, and schools everywhere. T'ai Chi is not only a valuable tool for improving health, it is a powerful business tool as well. Companies see that T'ai Chi improves productivity by helping employees to be happy, relaxed, and creative. Hospitals see T'ai Chi as a potent, yet cost-effective, therapy for nearly any condition. T'ai Chi classes can be found nowadays almost anywhere. In this chapter, I'll give you a whirlwind tour of the reasons behind T'ai Chi's growing popularity and what T'ai Chi can do for you.

Exploring the Reasons Behind T'ai Chi's Popularity

Do you ever feel like life is getting more stressful? *It is*. The increasing stress in today's world is one reason for T'ai Chi's growing worldwide popularity. T'ai Chi was designed to help people go through change with less damage by improving the way we handle stress. Studies show change is stressful, and *even though change is often good*, if the stress that change causes isn't managed it can damage your health and outlook on life. Since about 90 percent of the discoveries made in the history of the human race have been made in our lifetime, we are all going through some serious change—*and stress*. Therefore, T'ai Chi's ability to help practitioners "let go" of this stress more easily is just what the doctor ordered, *literally*.

Imagine life is a carousel upon which we ride. When life gets spinning really fast, T'ai Chi seems to slow things down, like a hand pulling us away from the "edge," back to the center of life's carousel. Here, *in the center*, we can let life spin even faster and not feel like throwing up (hardly ever anyway). In fact, by practicing T'ai Chi as you ride life's carousel, you might even catch yourself going "wheeeeeeeeeeeeee" a lot more often.

Whether you are stressed out, continually exhausted, treating a health problem, or just wanting to get in shape and feel young again, T'ai Chi is just what you need. T'ai Chi goes right to the heart of everything we do by healing and cleansing the central nervous system. T'ai Chi helps us to let go of all the nervous tension that bogs down our mental computer system (like getting a general tune up every day). This makes every-thing inside us work better, which often makes the world around us seem better, too. So T'ai Chi is really a self-improvement tool that will make you a better "anything-you-want-to-be." Unless of course you want to be stressed out, exhausted, uninspired, and feel old and out of shape. In that case, T'ai Chi won't help.

> **Know Your Chinese**
>
> The Chinese call life energy **Qi** (pronounced *chee*). The character for Qi is also the character for air or breath. QiGong (pronounced *chee kung* and often spelled Chi-Gong) means "breath work" or "energy exercise." There are about 7,000 QiGong exercises in the Chinese Medica (the bible of Chinese Medicine). T'ai Chi is a moving form of QiGong. There are sitting and lying forms of QiGong, but all T'ai Chi is done standing and moving.

People everywhere in the world are rapidly embracing T'ai Chi as "their" exercise. Although T'ai Chi origi-nates from China, it is now seen so commonly in the West that soon it will be thought of as an American thing, a British thing, a Canadian thing, or whatever. If you ask American kids what their favorite American food is, many will reply, "Pizza!" (which is originally Italian). And someday, when asked what their favorite American pastime is, Americans will say, "T'ai Chi!"

T'ai Chi Relaxes the Mind, Body, and Our Lives

Just as we flow through the changes of life (or not), our life energy, or *Qi*, flows through us (or not, if we are stressed out). Qi is the energy of life and flows through all living things. Qi animates, heals, and nurtures life. When the stress of change makes us tense, we squeeze off the flow of life energy. Physically, this feels like tension. T'ai Chi and QiGong are easy, simple, yet sophisticated relaxation exercises that encourage the mus-cles to let go of tension, the mind to let go of worry, and the heart to let go of angst. Tension, worry, and angst all block our Qi flow.

Tension, worry, and angst are usually the result of our mind, heart, or body being unable to "let go" of some-thing. The goal of T'ai Chi is to move through a series of choreographed movements like a slow martial arts routine, but *very* slowly and in a state of absolute relaxation. In order to do this, we have to let go of our mental/physical tensions, grudges, prejudices, and anything that keeps us tied to the past. This enables us to flow more easily into the future by clearing our mind and body of old stress so that we constantly get a "fresh" perspective on life.

T'ai Chi is simple and easy to do, yet benefits us on many deep and complex levels. T'ai Chi's slow, relaxed movements incorporate breathing and relaxation techniques that cleanse our mind, body, and emotions each time we go through the gentle movements. T'ai Chi is designed to uncover and release every single place we hold tension or blocked energy. When our mind or heart holds onto issues (fears, obsessions, angers, and so on) our body literally squeezes itself with tension. Going slowly through the movements is like doing an internal scan of the entire body to clear and release any place the body is gripping onto tension. There is no exercise on earth that can help you go through this wild ride toward the future quite like T'ai Chi can—which is why T'ai Chi is truly the exercise of the future.

T'ai Chi Promotes Internal Strength for Young and Old

T'ai Chi looks very much like slow-motion kung fu. David Carradine performed T'ai Chi as Kwai Chang Cane on the television series *Kung Fu*. And although T'ai Chi shares some similarities with kung fu, don't let that scare you away. T'ai Chi can be practiced by anyone at any age and in any condition.

In martial arts circles, it is known as an internal martial art. T'ai Chi promotes internal strength physically, mentally, and emotionally, which is why it can be powerful training tool for martial artists. But you don't have to be a martial artist to benefit from T'ai Chi because it can also be practiced even by those in wheelchairs, with great results.

Unlike karate, T'ai Chi has no belt or ranking system because the benefits of T'ai Chi can only be *felt* and not seen. You practice T'ai Chi to live better, more calmly, clearly, healthfully, and productively. T'ai Chi is a tonic for life. You will see your progress reflected by how you feel, how spry you look in the mirror, how much you love life, and how healthy you are. Isn't this much better than owning a black belt? However, if you do karate, T'ai Chi can help you get that black belt by improving your internal function and grace.

Also, T'ai Chi differs from most martial arts in that people of all ages can practice it. Many people with disabilities and ailments practice T'ai Chi as therapy. No one is restricted from practicing T'ai Chi, and yet T'ai Chi can benefit the fittest athletes, just as much as it benefits elderly arthritis sufferers. T'ai Chi clubs are sprouting up all over the world, with people from all walks of life.

Know Your Chinese

T'ai Chi Ch'uan (pronounced *tie chee chwan* or *die gee jwan*), sometimes spelled Taijiquan, means "supreme ultimate fist" or "highest martial art." T'ai means Supreme. Chi means Ultimate. Ch'uan means Fist.

Ouch!

Nearly one third of the adult U.S. population has chronic high blood pressure. Since some medications have side effects, physicians need to be made aware that T'ai Chi can sometimes lower high blood pressure as effectively as medication. Ask your doctor to look into T'ai Chi. However, never adjust medication levels without consulting your physician.

T'ai Chi: Finally an Exercise That *Feels Good!*

T'ai Chi is popular because it is easy to do and provides a gentle workout that doesn't leave you drained, *but energized!* T'ai Chi's "effortless" nature is a big stretch for most of us, however, because we associate exercise with *force*, *pain*, and *tension*. In fact, some exercise actually contributes to stress. When I played junior high football in west Texas many years ago, the coaches determined that we were through running when one of us started throwing up. That's right, upchucking. It was the only time in my life I ever hoped to see someone throw up.

T'ai Chi is helping the world get a healthy, enjoyable view of exercise. As a nation, we have adopted a mutant notion of exercise, exemplified by the mantra "no pain, no gain." This has traumatized many Americans, including myself, leaving an indelible mark on how we view exercise. In T'ai Chi we have a mantra, too, "If your exercise causes pain, you'll get so sick of the thought of it that you'll never want to do it again." Ours isn't as neatly poetic as "no pain, no gain," but ours makes infinitely more sense. T'ai Chi should always, always, *always*, feel good. And since it does feel good, you will look forward to it. Each morning you will find yourself grateful that you're alive and able to practice this cool exercise called T'ai Chi.

You Are Perfect, and Perfect for T'ai Chi

T'ai Chi doesn't begin with the premise that there is "something wrong" that needs to be "fixed, sculpted, lost, or burned off." It is a very accepting exercise, and helps us remember we are already *perfect* … but our ability to get better is *limitless*. Everyone is *qualified* to do T'ai Chi. You don't have to look good in tights or Spandex to do T'ai Chi, although if you do T'ai Chi enough, you'll look pretty good in whatever you like to wear.

> **CAUTION**
>
> ### Ouch!
>
> Beginning T'ai Chi is a *big step* for many of us, and it is easy to psych yourself out of taking it. Just like the first day we went to kindergarten, we thought of all the "big bad" stuff that would probably happen. But, for most of us, none of that materialized, and in fact we actually had a lot of fun. Take a chance. Dive into life by entering the waters of T'ai Chi and QiGong.

T'ai Chi and QiGong are for anybody who is dealing with stress. In other words—*everybody*. Anybody can do T'ai Chi. If you've picked up a book on T'ai Chi, you've probably experienced the *acute stress* of imagining yourself in some of those incredible (seemingly impossible) positions the T'ai Chi models pose in for the photos. Relax. Those people are models. Most people do T'ai Chi just the way you will do it. Easily and effortlessly. Although T'ai Chi was one of the original martial arts, it is now practiced all over the world as a relaxation technique by people of all ages in the same shape you are in, and sometimes *in even worse shape*.

When you begin an exercise class, you may have the illusion that everybody other than you "belongs" there, and that they are all "good" at it. You will find that everybody goes through the same trials and tribulations. As you lighten up on yourself, you'll see struggling, growing, and healing are everywhere. Breathe and enjoy; you are among friends.

When you first begin practicing T'ai Chi out in the backyard or in your local park, people may stare. Before long, your unique practice of T'ai Chi becomes part of the rich texture of the neighborhood, and if you move away, they will miss you. Just as T'ai Chi adds to your personal internal charm, your practice adds to the charm of your community.

T'ai Chi Goes to the Root of Problems

Life is very complicated, and T'ai Chi cannot solve all your problems. However, T'ai Chi can help you simplify your life in a big and relaxing way.

Imagine that you're a tree. While your mind and body are the trunk of that tree, all your "life stuff" is like the many leaves on that tree. Your job, relationships, hobbies, hopes, and problems are all dangling out there on the tips of your life. When your health is bad or you can't sleep well, this affects the whole tree. You may have problems with your job that may strain your relationships, which in turn will drain the energy you need to pursue your hobbies, making you too tired to have hopeful dreams, *and causing your problems to get seemingly bigger and bigger*. When you are already beat, trying to figure out how to heal all these sick, shriveled leaves is too much to even think about.

A T'ai Chi Punch Line

One old Chinese master lecturing his new students said, "QiGong is said to build character in its practitioners. I don't know about that, but it will definitely make you into a character."

However, what if you could pour some magic water on the roots of your tree? Magic that would heal all the sick leaves and cause them to grow larger, to catch more breezes and more sunlight, *and more fun!* This is what T'ai Chi does. By nurturing the very core of your mind and body, T'ai Chi makes you better at *everything you do*. You don't practice T'ai Chi to be better at T'ai Chi (although that happens). Each time you practice T'ai Chi, you pour healing water on the roots of everything you are. This healing water, or energy, is carried out to the leaves of everything you do, making you the freshest, greenest tree you could ever want to be.

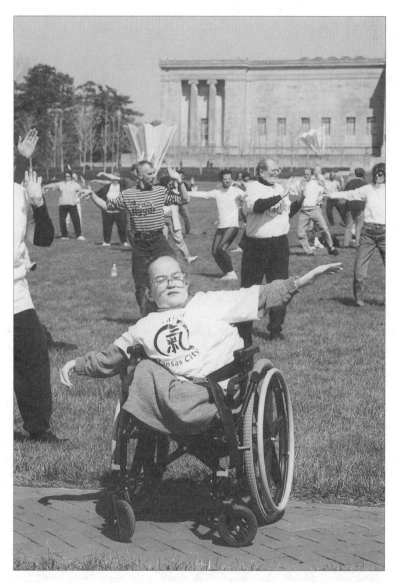

T'ai Chi is increasingly popular!

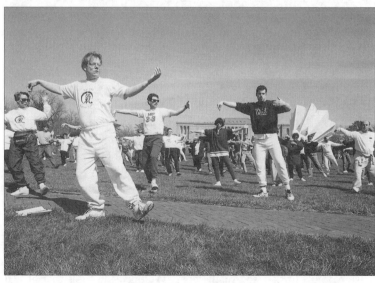

Bill Douglas (yes, the author of this book) leads the Kansas City T'ai Chi Club in the largest gathering of T'ai Chi practitioners outside China.

Getting to the Root of T'ai Chi

One name does not adequately express everything T'ai Chi is because T'ai Chi nurtures so many aspects of our lives at the root. Although originally a martial art known as T'ai Chi Chuan ("supreme ultimate fist"), the shortened name of T'ai Chi reflects how it is now viewed, as one of the most effective mind/body exercises in the world. So T'ai Chi now refers to "supreme ultimate health exercise," "supreme ultimate relaxation therapy," "supreme ultimate balance conditioner, muscle toner, beauty treatment."

T'ai Chi is the supreme ultimate because it goes right to the root of most health problems by relaxing the muscles and mind, aligning the spinal posture, and balancing the energy systems that run through the body, providing them with life energy. It is one of the most soothing, easy, and powerful things you can do for yourself. It is a profound self-improvement tool, a great toning exercise, and an incredible healing art. Whether you want to improve external beauty, mental outlook, or physical health and longevity, T'ai Chi heals the roots of your being.

All-Purpose Medicine

T'ai Chi is a highly effective therapy for many injuries or chronic conditions, whether mental, emotional, or physical. The following chapters will discuss different maladies and how T'ai Chi treats them. T'ai Chi bolsters the immune system, as well, and can actually eliminate problems long before they become an actual physical illness.

An Ultimate Beauty Treatment

Forget about covering up problems with makeup or surgery. Beautify from the inside out instead! Many cells are replaced daily, and almost the entire body is completely replaced every five to seven years. You are literally born anew on some level each and every day of your life. How those cells are reproduced is determined by how the life energy, or Qi, flows through your body. Therefore, you can have a terrific impact on how you age, look, and feel by promoting your Qi flow.

T'ai Chi's Cleansing of the Nervous System *Releases Power*

Have you ever sat back and noticed how small children never run down? Like the Energizer rabbit, on fast forward, they leap and spring, dance and chat, and chat and chat. Have you ever thought to yourself, "God, I wish *I* had that energy"? Well, you *do* have access to that energy (and without doing espresso shooters).

> **CAUTION**
>
> **Ouch!**
>
> T'ai Chi can boost your energy levels tremendously. However, it is important also to get the proper amount of sleep. Do not try to use T'ai Chi's energy boost to replace proper sleep and diet. T'ai Chi will promote an all-around healthful lifestyle as you become more subtly attuned to your body's needs. One aspect of T'ai Chi's quiet mindful movement is that it quiets you down enough to sense the mind and body's needs, whether it's more rest, water, and so on.

As human beings, we begin to block our access to that energy as we "mature" by holding onto past grudges, by shouldering responsibilities that are unrealistic, or just because of silly worries. Then we don't know how to let them go, and we get used to having less and less energy. We can think on a mental level that we want to "stop worrying" or "let go of tension," but that doesn't really work. We need life tools that help us let go of these blocks on deep levels in our mind, heart, and body, so that we can open to your flow of life energy.

T'ai Chi and QiGong will give you access to simple exercises, which feel good and can open a valve to that limitless energy you thought you had lost forever. The Chinese discovered long ago that these blocks, or our stress, are simply the mind and nervous system squeezing onto grudges, worries, or even desires. Just as our muscles can tighten when tense, our mind and heart can grip tension too, and we have to be taught how to let go of their squeezing grip on life issues. So the goal of these ancient exercises is to wash our nervous system clean, so our mind can be fresh and vibrant like a newborn baby's, while still remembering the important stuff, like stopping at red lights and dressing before going to work.

Seriously, as we let go of most of the meaningless, irritating debris bouncing around in our mind, we have more space and energy for really important ideas to surface. Important memories like the bill we forgot to pay, or realizations like we forgot to tell someone how much you care about them. T'ai Chi's slow, soothing movements provide that calm open space, even in the very center of the rat race.

A Fountain of Youth

America is not into the "aging" thing. What Americans spend on cosmetic surgery attests to that. T'ai Chi will help you get over that prejudice, while also slowing the aging process in many ways. The Chinese believe as we practice T'ai Chi it returns us to a state of "child-likeness" (but not childishness), where we see the world with fresh eyes. This allows us the freedom to reinvent ourselves easily and constantly, *just as children do*, enabling us to flow with the changes of life. We can once again be flexible and exuberant, while still benefiting from the wisdom of experience (like being able to hit our mouth with the spoon, well, most of the time). So T'ai Chi has the ability to renew us, and through that renewal enhance our strength, health, and creativity.

T'ai Chi is based on the principle that the world doesn't need to be held up by our worrying mind and tense body. In fact, we are much more helpful to the world (and far more enjoyable to be around) if we can let go of as much stress as possible. Realizing this principle is the first big step to letting T'ai Chi reopen you to your own personal rejuvenating "fountain of energy"!

> **Sage Sifu Says**
>
> I used to hold the world on my shoulders
> 'til my tense muscles felt like very heavy boulders.
> Then one day Sifu said, "This world needs no holders,
> so breathe and relax your bony little shoulders."
> … so I did!
> —T'ai Chi poem

Explaining T'ai Chi: History and Premise

T'ai Chi is unique. Although it is in a way 2,000 years old, it is at the cutting edge of modern Western medical research. T'ai Chi is ancient yet modern, Eastern yet increasingly Western. Using T'ai Chi is a way to get the most benefit out of all worlds, old and new, East and West. In fact, Western science is embracing T'ai Chi very rapidly. Almost every month a new study seems to find yet another thing T'ai Chi can treat, cure, or improve. A researcher at the University of Massachusetts-Lowell said T'ai Chi is about to explode (in popularity) as medical practitioners discover the time-tested technique.

In fact each new T'ai Chi player educates more people on T'ai Chi, and sometimes in *odd ways*. One of my students was practicing T'ai Chi in the park in a suburb of Kansas City one morning when a police officer approached him to ask if he was all right. The officer said someone had called and reported somebody was having a "problem" in the park. So it may behoove you to know a bit more about T'ai Chi in case you need to do some fast-talking. The following will help.

Historical T'ai Chi

For an exercise that is so made to order for modern life, it is amazing to realize that T'ai Chi is thought to be about 1,200 years old. Furthermore, T'ai Chi is an expanded version of a more ancient exercise called QiGong, which may be at least 2,000 years old. T'ai Chi's moving exercises are done very slowly, like slow motion kung fu. In days of old, T'ai Chi (or T'ai Chi Ch'uan) was primarily a martial art. It is believed that Buddhist and Taoist monks began practicing T'ai Chi forms in monasteries (yes, like the Shao Lin Temple) for two reasons: One, to promote health because they were out of shape from sitting around meditating all the time; and two, because they were so out of shape, they couldn't defend themselves, and bandits would come and beat them up before taking their valuables. (And you thought you had stress!)

Modern T'ai Chi

When most people first join a T'ai Chi or QiGong class, they are not quite sure what they are getting themselves into. Most have a mother, a doctor, a friend, a daughter, or son telling them, "This T'ai Chi stuff is the greatest thing since sliced bread and you have gotta try it!" However, these enthusiasts can't quite explain why you've gotta try it. So the following is for you, or whoever's been trying to explain it to you.

In modern terms, T'ai Chi and QiGong are ancient systems of *biofeedback* and classical conditioning. Traditional Chinese doctors of long ago noted that our natural tendency is to hold onto stress, which bogs down the brain. They therefore created exercises that would train the mind and the body not only to continually dump stress, but also to actually change the way the body handles future stress (not the way your kids change the way you handle stress, but *in a good way*).

> **T'ai Sci**
>
> Biofeedback uses a computer program to train people how to relax when under stress. The computer shows them when their blood pressure goes up and their heart beats faster so that they can then practice relaxing and slowing things down. Dr. Gary Green, a leading biofeedback specialist, refers to T'ai Chi as "biofeedback without the computer."

As T'ai Chi players move through their slow motion movements, their mind becomes calm, their breathing deepens and slows, and their muscles relax. All this happens while the muscles are toning, making it a very efficient exercise. But, forget about efficiency, T'ai Chi should be done as though you were going to do it forever. If you try to "hurry up and relax," it doesn't work as well.

By proceeding slowly with T'ai Chi, and *making it a game*, you will be much more likely to enjoy it and to stick with it. Chapter 2, "Let's Get Physical," explains how even in T'ai Chi's easy going way, there is great power and dramatic physical benefit awaiting you.

The Least You Need to Know

- T'ai Chi reduces stress and slows the aging process.
- Everybody can do T'ai Chi.
- T'ai Chi restores the power of youthful exuberance.
- T'ai Chi is an efficient therapy that can improve all aspects of your life.
- By clearing the mind, T'ai Chi reminds you that life is a miracle.

Chapter 2

Let's Get Physical

In This Chapter

◆ A tune-up for the whole you

◆ The benefits of an innercise vs. an outercise

◆ The ultimate performance booster

◆ The difference and similarities between T'ai Chi and yoga

T'ai Chi is perhaps the best physical exercise in the world. Unlike higher impact exercises, T'ai Chi does not harm the body. In fact, its gentle movements help the body strengthen bone mass and connective tissue, and is lower impact than even brisk walking. T'ai Chi also works on a cellular level to physically cleanse and tone the body in deep ways that you never see. However, T'ai Chi can help beautify the external physical body, too.

Depending on the type of T'ai Chi work out, you may not even break a sweat doing T'ai Chi. Therefore, T'ai Chi is a great workout you can do during a 15-minute coffee break at work, in your regular work clothes, or in your pajamas when you get up. It won't leave you out of breath and fatigued, but it will leave you feeling clear, peaceful, and at one with the universe.

According to some studies, T'ai Chi burns nearly as many calories as downhill skiing and provides many of the same health benefits as low-impact aerobic exercises. However, T'ai Chi provides balance and coordination improvements that are nearly twice as effective as the best balance training exercises in the world.

If you are an athlete, T'ai Chi could also be the best training you can do to improve your game. Golfers sometimes add a hundred yards to their drives after "playing" T'ai Chi for just a few months, while weight lifters often see results immediately. Yet even if your main physical activity is mowing the lawn and carrying groceries, the same things T'ai Chi does to benefit athletic performance will increase your physical power and dramatically reduce the likelihood of injury when working around the house.

There is no single exercise that can do what T'ai Chi does for you physically. This is why T'ai Chi is becoming the most popular exercise in the world today. This chapter tells you what you can expect from a T'ai Chi workout.

> **Sage Sifu Says**
>
> T'ai Chi provides the most benefits when it is done for fun. In fact, the Chinese refer to T'ai Chi practice as *playing* T'ai Chi. Always remember you are playing (as opposed to "working out"), and play T'ai Chi simply because playing it feels good—the benefits will come easily and naturally. To do T'ai Chi everyday and not get T'ai Chi's multitudinous benefits would be like falling down and missing the ground—you just can't do it.

T'ai Chi Acupuncture Tune-Up

T'ai Chi is a very slow exercise, performed as if you were swimming through water, or the air in T'ai Chi's case. This has many benefits. You cannot injure yourself when doing T'ai Chi correctly because the slowness allows you time to hear the body's pain signals and stop any movement that doesn't feel right. You simply adjust the T'ai Chi movements to fit your own range of mobility.

> **T'ai Sci**
>
> Acupuncture stimulates points on the body that affect the flow of Qi, or life energy. Acupressure is acupuncture without the needles. By massaging acupuncture points you are performing acupressure and getting much the same benefit.

T'ai Chi's slow standing movements also thoroughly massage the bottoms of the feet. There are acupuncture points on the feet that affect every part of the body, including every major organ. Therefore, the gentle slow massaging of the feet that your 20-minute T'ai Chi routine accomplishes treats the entire body. By the end of your T'ai Chi play time, every cell of the body will be relaxed and opened to a smoother flow of life energy. You will feel clear, bright, and renewed. The science of acupuncture is explained in greater detail in Chapter 3, "Medical T'ai Chi: The Prescription for the Future."

Innercise vs. Outercise

T'ai Chi is a mind/body exercise, or an *innercise*. That is, T'ai Chi aids the mind and body simultaneously to powerfully center us, to improve not only our physical health, but also our mental and emotional health (see Chapter 4, "Expand the Mind and Lighten the Heart"). T'ai Chi has been called an innercise because it uniquely focuses the mind on the internal condition of the body rather than on an external performance. Therefore, whereas practicing baseball makes you better at baseball and playing ping pong makes you a better ping pong player, T'ai Chi practice makes you better at everything you do.

> **Ouch!**
>
> On pain medication, T'ai Chi realizes there are no absolutes. When pain medication is needed, it is a wonderful thing to have and should be used. No one should force herself to be in agony needlessly. However, if QiGong and T'ai Chi can help reduce the need for pain medication, or help prevent injury that might result in that need, it is a very healthy option.

Advantages of Innercise

T'ai Chi improves our overall performance on a physical level because it provides us with a daily picture of how we operate. Through its slow deliberate movements we can, with a kind of inner sight, see inside ourselves to observe breath, posture, and tension levels. This allows us to correct problems before they become illnesses or injuries.

Some athletes have used medication to hide pain. T'ai Chi is the opposite of a painkiller. T'ai Chi helps us become aware of problems *before* they become acute. We do not want to hide pain because pain is the body's way of telling us that some part of us needs healing attention. However, as T'ai Chi and QiGong help the body get that gentle healing attention, they also help relieve chronic pain conditions. So T'ai Chi and QiGong help to heal injuries or illnesses that pain alerts us to, but they also help us deal with the pain as those conditions are allowed to heal. Painkillers, on the other hand, separate our mind from our body and neither heal nor grant us the awareness needed to avoid further injuries.

Having said that, if you have an existing condition causing acute pain, the pain may be so debilitating or distracting that other therapies like T'ai Chi and QiGong are impossible to attempt. This is not an either/or situation. Use medication as needed and use T'ai Chi and QiGong as needed. The two can work in concert to help you recover. As always, discuss this with your doctor.

T'ai Chi tones the muscles, increases breathing capacity, lowers stress levels, improves organ function and corrects poor posture. All these things help the body maximize its self-healing potential, which will be discussed in Chapter 3.

Problems with Outercise

We in the West suffer from the delusion that we can get our bodies fit, or even get our lives in order, without our minds being involved. For example, if you go to the health club, they will most likely have televisions above the stationary bikes or the stair climbing machines. The idea is that we can get healthy, lose stress, and get "buns of steel" while having our minds bombarded with CNN visions of world problems or the top 10 songs blasting in our ears. Of course, we can get buns of steel, but we can't get *truly* healthy that way. We've erroneously equated a hard body with health. From my personal experience, I've found that an overemphasis on the development of muscles, built up to look good to the outer world and not necessarily for health reasons, can interfere with my energy flow and natural health processes. The slow mindful exercises of T'ai Chi give me a healthy muscle tone and also seem to support my immune system function so I get sick less. This should come as a great relief to anyone who is tired of the nausea of hot, sweaty, bone-pounding exercise routines.

> **Sage Sifu Says**
>
> The Taoist philosopher, Lao Tzu, recognized that overconditioning just to look good to the outside world would not produce the desired result of health.
>
> *Stretch a bow out all the way,*
> *And you'll regret that you didn't stop in time.*
> *Sharpen a sword to its finest edge,*
> *And the edge will break very quickly.*
> *Rest when you've achieved your goal,*
> *This is the way of heaven.*
>
> In other words, if you drive yourself to pump up your muscles, you'll likely not stick with an exercise program, because its goal is in excess of your health needs. It's easier and wiser to do an exercise to make you healthy, rather than just to *look good*. This is what T'ai Chi is all about.

Overemphasizing our outer appearance is a *yang* obsession and can discount our internal, or *yin*, needs. T'ai Chi's goal is balance, and regular practice can help achieve this balance as T'ai Chi healthfully tones muscles, while attending to internal needs as well. T'ai Chi encourages us to find quiet and stillness of the mind so that our nervous system can begin to cleanse itself of accumulated thoughts and worries. This allows a deep-tissue cleansing by encouraging deep relaxation and full breath, which lets the accumulated toxins in muscles release into the body's natural cleansing systems. Our body actually holds on to anxiety in a chemical form called "lactic acids," and T'ai Chi's deep releases help cleanse that and other toxins from the body. The gentle massage of T'ai Chi movement also begins to clear the lymph glands.

T'ai Chi gives you the best of both worlds. T'ai Chi can make you more gorgeous on the outside, even as it beautifies your "terrific personality."

> **Know Your Chinese**
>
> Yin and **yang** are the Chinese concepts of universal forces. All things are an eternally flowing interaction of two opposites; the ideal is healthy balance in all things. Yin is internal; yang is external. Yin is dark; yang is light. Yin is feminine; yang is masculine. Yin is passive receptive; yang is dynamic and expressive. Even food has yin and yang qualities, so this balance determines a healthy diet.

T'ai Chi Helps You Lose Weight

T'ai Chi can be a powerful addition to the many healthy and effective weight-loss programs there are to choose from. Furthermore, T'ai Chi can help move the emphasis away from the external perception of judging negatively how you look or what you weigh, and put that emphasis on nurturing who you are (thin or heavy). By ignoring this, some fad diets only promote temporary reductions in calories rather than deep or lasting lifestyle changes. However, T'ai Chi can be a powerful ally to the many quality weight-loss programs that do attend to self-image issues, for the following reasons.

T'ai Chi works from the inside out. It promotes self-acceptance and self-nurturing. As you care more for yourself, you are drawn toward activities and foods that nurture your existence. T'ai Chi is a gradual healthy program of life change that encourages rather than demands or restricts, causing some deep internal part of yourself to draw you more effortlessly toward behavioral changes. T'ai Chi does not compete with healthy weight-loss programs, but actually may significantly expedite their benefit and improve your chances of sticking with them. QiGong research shows it can help the body metabolize fatty tissue more effectively. Plus T'ai Chi burns about 280 calories per hour, surprisingly providing, despite its slow and gentle pace, many of the immediate results gained from other exercises. To put this in perspective, realize that downhill skiing burns only 350 calories per hour, making T'ai Chi nearly as effective in calorie consumption. Moreover, T'ai Chi is very safe, low impact, takes no equipment, and can be performed in the conference room at work during break time or even in the bathroom when you sneak off for an unofficial stress break.

The great feeling that comes from doing T'ai Chi is a terrific incentive to keep you coming back to it again and again. T'ai Chi gives you that "special time" alone for yourself to just enjoy how your body feels as it lets go of stress and relaxes. This makes it a much easier routine to stick with. And the good feelings it promotes in your body help you learn to love your body more and to accept it the way it is. Surprisingly, the more we accept the way we are now, the easier it is to change to the way we want to be.

Another powerful component to T'ai Chi's effect on weight loss is how it helps us let go of stress and nervous tension. Most evening snacking is "nervous snacking." This is an attempt to repress feelings of unease by stimulating taste buds and other sensations. That's why we usually want really greasy, salty, or sweet foods to munch on at night when we are trying not to feel our stress; the strong tastes distract our mind.

> **Sage Sifu Says**
>
> Even though T'ai Chi promotes healthy weight loss, remember not to hold on tightly to a desired outcome. T'ai Chi is always most effective when we do it for the simple enjoyment of how it feels. Let everything else be an unexpected surprise.

Yet T'ai Chi does even more to promote healthy weight loss. T'ai Chi's physical, emotional, and mental centering helps us feel very pleasant. The Chinese call this state "smooth Qi," while modern psychologists call it "homeostasis." But no matter what you call it, it feels good. As T'ai Chi and QiGong get us more and more in the habit of "feeling good," we become more aware of what habits reinforce that lovely feeling. We then begin to realize that certain junk foods take us away from our feelings of smooth Qi. We also begin to understand in deep ways that proper sleep, diet, and making time to enjoy life all contribute to our smooth Qi. The more we feel that way, the more we want to feel that way. This helps our body to find a healthy weight effortlessly as we learn to love things that promote this feeling, such as light healthy foods and our T'ai Chi and QiGong.

T'ai Chi Tones Muscles, Too

Not only does T'ai Chi tone muscles but it does so while promoting a more elegant elongated form. Many exercises are designed to "buff us up," giving us a shorter, stockier appearance. T'ai Chi, on the other hand, may actually lengthen the body over time, making us more lithe. As we age, it is our tension that shortens our bodies more than gravity. By practicing T'ai Chi's relaxed movements every day, we allow the muscles to release tension as they seemingly let go of one another and release their grip on the bones and connective tissue. We can actually lengthen each time we do T'ai Chi.

T'ai Chi's attention to posture really improves your grace, whether you want to move like Grace Kelly or Gene Kelly. Plus, as T'ai Chi smoothes your moves, it also heals your body.

T'ai Chi recognizes that the body always wants to be in the best, most healthful posture. However, our tension sometimes wrenches the bones or vertebrae out of place. This causes pain and eventually physical damage, not only to the back, but also to associated organs because all parts of the body are affected by spinal alignment.

By practicing T'ai Chi and QiGong each day, the muscles seem to begin releasing their tight grip on the bones, which can relieve pressure on the vertebrae caused by muscle tension. This allows the spine to realign, along with other bones and joints. You will be more graceful, more spry and energetic, and more charming because you will have less and less chronic pain.

T'ai Chi Oils the Joints

As we age, we often lose mobility, feeling like the rusty Tin Man in *The Wizard of Oz*. In fact, this "rusting" can start at about any age; we need only to stop using our bodies fully. There are two reasons we lose mobility. The first is because calcium deposits that normal usage would wear off build up in our joints. The second is because our liquid systems function less well when we are sedentary. Therefore, our joints get more brittle and stiff.

T'ai Chi can solve both problems better than any other exercise. T'ai Chi movements require the body to rotate about 95 percent of the ways it can be rotated, thereby working out the potential calcium deposits wherever they may be lurking. No other Western exercise comes close to this. Swimming, for example, only rotates about 65 percent of the body's potential movement. Second, T'ai Chi stimulates the liquid systems of the body to keep joints and other tissue more supple, even into advanced old age.

Ouch!

Never force joints to be more mobile than feels good. T'ai Chi is more about being quiet enough to "hear" what the body tells you than about moving in any certain way. When doing T'ai Chi or anything else, be aware of your current limits. Then play at easing up against that limit day after day after day. You are limitless. Enjoy the ride!

T'ai Chi's Like a Day at the Spa, but Without the Bill

Like a day at the spa, T'ai Chi leaves you with a healthful glow caused by increased circulation, energy flow, and the resulting nourishment of each cell of the body, including skin. The beauty salons of the future will provide access to these exercises (some already do). T'ai Chi can help you feel as though you spent everyday at the spa, except your credit card won't feel the pain.

Yet, ultimately T'ai Chi allows us to achieve the only real beauty. The beauty of being a real and caring human being.

Discover Dan Tien—Your Physical Center

T'ai Chi provides us with much more overall energy during the day and much more power for specific tasks. It does this by getting us to quiet our minds enough to become aware of the way we move and of our postural alignment while we are moving.

T'ai Chi movements are done by focusing our awareness on two things. Our *dan tien*, or center of gravity, is located about $1^1/_2$ to 3 inches below the navel near the center of the body—our vertical axis, or our line of posture. In the hard martial arts like karate, they know of the power of the dan tien. The ability to exert extreme force for breaking boards and bricks comes from awareness of moving from the center of our body, which is the dan tien. But again, that same power can help us lift our laundry basket or turn over our mattress with much less chance of hurting our back or pulling a muscle. For those who have some physical problem, awareness of dan tien may make you more capable of simply functioning more normally again.

Express Yourself with Dan Tien

No matter what form our physical expression takes, the internal self-awareness of moving from and breathing into the dan tien will add power. Whether you are making a board room presentation, ironing the clothes, or running a marathon, your performance will be simultaneously more effortless and much more powerful.

All great coaches know that real power comes from the dan tien. Even if they have never heard of the term, they all know that dan tien is the source of expressive power. Singing or acting coaches talk of "speaking from the diaphragm," golf coaches speak of "swinging with the belly button," and baseball coaches teach batters to "squash the bug," which is another way of saying to swing with the pelvis by pivoting the back foot as if squishing a bug. But, no matter how they describe it, they all are saying that any great athletic performance or physical expression is powered by centering the movement from the dan tien.

Move Effortlessly from the Dan Tien

Becoming aware of the dan tien means moving from the core of your physical being. Remember playing with spinning tops as a child? If you put your hands on the outside edge of the top and tried to spin it, it was a lot of work, and it didn't spin very much. However, once you learned to place your thumb and forefinger around the center spindle of the top, you found that just a little flick of the thumb and finger sent the top spinning like mad. This is what moving from the dan tien is all about. This is why moving from dan tien makes a boxer's punch harder, a golfer's swing more powerful, and a lawn mower's job easier, and easier on the back.

As T'ai Chi teaches us to move from the dan tien, it also helps us realize that we can let most of our muscles relax while the dan tien moves us around our harried lives. At first this concept of effortless movement sounds odd, but with practice, as you get better and better at it, it makes sense. The more we allow the body to relax, the more the raw power of the dan tien's movement comes through in our golfing, housework, or verbal and physical communication.

Know Your Chinese

Dan tien is an energy center located slightly below the navel inside the body. In T'ai Chi, it is known to be the center of gravity, and all T'ai Chi movement is directed by this point, while the torso and limbs are extensions of this central point.

Ouch!

The old adage "lift with your legs, not your back" is a modern version of T'ai Chi's admonition to "move from the dan tien." T'ai Chi makes you very safety conscious. Yet, this awareness of how to move, push, and lift in ways that don't hurt you will become almost instinct as you practice T'ai Chi over the years.

Know Your Chinese

Soong Yi-Dien (pronounced *shoong yee-dee-en*) is often heard in Hong Kong's famous garment district. It means "the suit is too tight, loosen it up, loosen it up!" Our bodies are our mind's suits, and we are all wearing our suits way too tight. Chinese T'ai Chi masters will therefore say, "Soong Yi-Dien" as well.

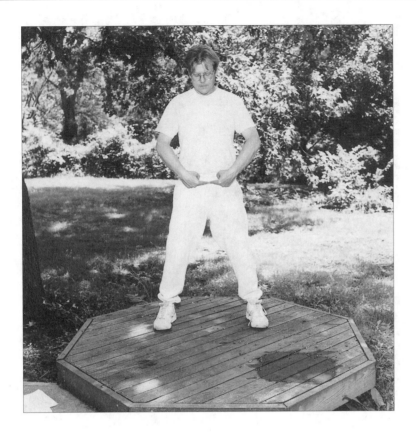

The dan tien is located about 1½ to 3 inches below the navel, near the center of the body, although slightly toward the front.

When our bodies are tight, the power of the dan tien is watered down. Even if a baseball batter squashes the bug well and swings with his pelvis or dan tien, if his arms and shoulders are tight, the dan tien's power can't flow through them. So to maximize the power of dan tien, we must also teach the body to relax enough to allow that power to pour up through the arms or down through the legs.

Knowing that relaxing our body increases our power does not automatically translate into increased power. In fact, trying to memorize too many of T'ai Chi's benefits will tighten you up. Let this information wash over you effortlessly. Chapter 11, "Sitting QiGong (Jing Gong)," will give you an exercise that will teach your body how to be effortless. In Part 3, "Starting Down the QiGong Path to T'ai Chi," you will learn how QiGong will relax your mind, which will in turn relax your body. This maximizes the expression of whatever magic we are here in this world to express by allowing dan tien's power to flow through us unimpeded by tension. T'ai Chi's practice of moving from the dan tien makes T'ai Chi a great athletic trainer. Therefore, QiGong's ability to help us release the tension inhibiting dan tien's power makes QiGong perhaps the world's greatest self-improvement program. Come back and reread this chapter after practicing the Sitting QiGong exercise in Part 3. This will help you see how T'ai Chi incorporates powerful health and performance tools into not only your way of moving, but also your way of thinking and living.

Ouch!

Whenever you catch yourself trying too hard or notice your head and shoulder muscles tightening—just stop. Take a few breaths, and on each sighing exhale, let the world roll off your shoulders. It is amazing how well the world holds itself up each time your bony little shoulders take a break. Take more breaks from holding the world up.

This photo illustrates how a loose frame sends the full force of the dan tien's motion up through the body, out the bat, and into the ball. Note that the batter's back foot "squashing the bug" sends the dan tien into motion toward the ball.

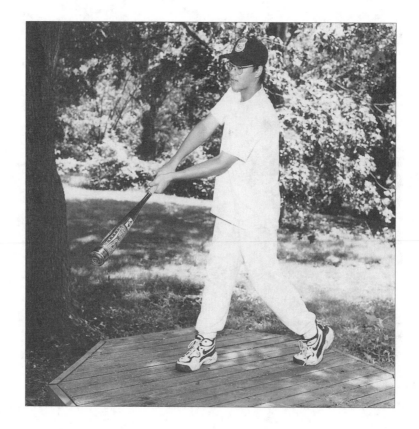

Stay Loose, Bruiser!

The goal of T'ai Chi is to move through life as effortlessly as possible. This doesn't mean we run from challenge and adventure. T'ai Chi teaches us to breathe easily and relax, no matter how much adventure we are going through. However, as we practice T'ai Chi, we may find that some of the negative drama in our lives is self-created; as we let go of unnecessary stress, we will likely find more calm. This will save our energy for adventures that are really fun.

So T'ai Chi teaches us to let the body let go of itself. Using only the muscles that are absolutely necessary for each movement, thereby conserving energy for when we really need it.

The most beautiful way to express this concept is found in a French fencing (sword fighting) term. The French fencing masters speak of how you should hold the foil, or sword: Hold it lightly like a dove, so not to crush it in your grip, and yet firmly so it does not fly away. This is the lesson for life that T'ai Chi brings to mind and body again and again, and powerfully affects how we view our world. If we hold onto possessions or loved ones too tightly, it will reflect in our muscles, health, and relationships. We will squeeze all the magic out of life, just like we can squeeze all the power out of our sports performance. This is why great sports heroes never hold onto the idea of a championship; they just relax into the moment.

> **Sage Sifu Says**
>
> The facts and figures on the benefits of T'ai Chi are valuable only if they encourage you to stick with it. The benefits of T'ai Chi and QiGong come pleasantly and effortlessly by breathing, relaxing, and celebrating the miracle of your physical body.

Dan Tien Awareness Improves All Activities

In T'ai Chi we move and think from the dan tien, the center of physical gravity. This also centers our awareness and maximizes the power of any physical effort. As T'ai Chi teaches us to loosen, breathe, and enjoy, everything we do improves.

T'ai Chi's and QiGong's mental centering of our awareness in the dan tien area is coupled with a feeling of flowing energy (see Part 3). This cleanses our nervous system of all cloudiness and distortion, clearing communication between mind and body. By focusing our awareness within and letting go of the stress of the day, we become more focused on what we are doing right here and right now. So if we are hitting a golf ball right here and right now, or cooking dinner, or making a speech at the PTA meeting, we will be more likely to make a record drive, a spectacular meal, or an inspired speech.

T'ai Chi vs. Yoga

Students always ask what the difference between yoga and T'ai Chi is. When Jay Leno's character on *The Tonight Show*, "Iron Jay," was asked that question he said, "T'ai Chi, dat's a little spicier den yoga, *ain't it?*"

Without tackling which is spicier, let's begin by looking at what makes them similar. Both T'ai Chi and yoga are excellent mind/body fitness tools that are being practiced by more and more people around the world. Both help us let go of stress and cultivate a sense of well-being in our lives. Both can be very gentle and used by almost anyone.

Now, some differences. T'ai Chi is more easily practiced by those in wheel chairs because T'ai Chi is done upright, whereas many yoga positions require lying down. T'ai Chi's standing motion continually challenges your balance, which explains why T'ai Chi is the best balance conditioner in the world. And since it is done standing up, T'ai Chi can be performed about anywhere outdoors. Furthermore, T'ai Chi can be practiced in any type of clothing, making it much more convenient for corporate settings. While yoga postures are often static poses, T'ai Chi's postures flow one into the other, just as life's changes flow one into the other, making T'ai Chi's effortless changes a model for life.

While yoga is practiced to prepare the body to experience a blissful meditative state, with T'ai Chi, the QiGong meditative state is often practiced *before* movements. This is because T'ai Chi's goal is to bring the blissful state of enlightened awareness into our physical lives. Yoga goes to a place of peace, T'ai Chi brings that place of peace into our daily activities. Both are wonderful habits and can each enhance the effectiveness of the other. I recommend yoga highly.

T'ai Chi and yoga are complementary disciplines, and your T'ai Chi practice may prepare you to dip your toe into yoga, or vice versa. There are strengths that both offer uniquely, and although I advocate making T'ai Chi a part of your daily life, I encourage you to try yoga as well. Life is a great experiment.

The Least You Need to Know

- ◆ T'ai Chi tones, beautifies, and empowers you and everything you do.
- ◆ T'ai Chi done wisely does no damage to your body and can help keep it working for as long as you need it.
- ◆ By teaching self-acceptance, T'ai Chi makes you more adventurous in life.
- ◆ T'ai Chi can enhance athletic training, no matter what your game.

Medical T'ai Chi: The Prescription for the Future

In This Chapter

◆ Discover the health benefits of T'ai Chi

◆ Unlock your healing mind using the T'ai *Key*

◆ Explore the links between acupuncture and T'ai Chi

◆ Find out what Western medicine knows about T'ai Chi and QiGong

◆ Find how T'ai Chi and QiGong are rapidly integrating with medicine

The doctor of the future will prescribe no medicine, but will interest his patients in the care of the human frame …

—Thomas Alva Edison

T'ai Chi and QiGong's medical benefits have been studied for nearly 2,000 years in China and for only about 20 years in the West. However, Western medical research is rapidly discovering what Chinese medicine has long realized, that T'ai Chi provides more medical benefits than any other single exercise. That's why this ancient Chinese exercise is at the cutting edge of modern medical research.

This chapter gives you both an understanding of how Chinese medicine views our health and also the emerging Western scientific research that validates these ancient views. The bottom line is we are very lucky to live at a time when these wonderful tools are available to us in the West. We are also lucky to be able to see scientific proof that they work because as practitioners of Traditional Chinese Medicine understood centuries ago, our faith is the greatest healer. So if we know in our minds that T'ai Chi works, our bodies will allow it to do its magic, and we will be the big winner.

The Health Benefits of T'ai Chi

We live in a stressful world; only recently has Western medical research come to recognize that stress is at the root of most health problems. Therefore, the health crisis that stress is causing in the West has actually created a great opportunity for us because it is opening us up to the wonders of Traditional Chinese Medicine and tools like T'ai Chi and QiGong. In fact, the following list of T'ai Chi's measurable health benefits indicates how this opening to T'ai Chi may save us from our health care crisis. T'ai Chi can …

- Boost the immune system.
- Slow the aging process.
- Reduce anxiety, depression, and overall mood disturbance.
- Lower high blood pressure.
- Alleviate stress responses.
- Enhance the body's natural healing powers such as recovering from injury.
- Increase breathing capacity.
- Reduce asthma and allergy reactions.
- Improve balance and coordination *twice* as well as the best balance conditioning exercises in the world.
- Help to ensure full range mobility far into old age.
- Provide the lowest impact weight-bearing exercise known.

The Chinese character for "crisis" is a combination of two other characters—one for "danger" and the other for "opportunity."

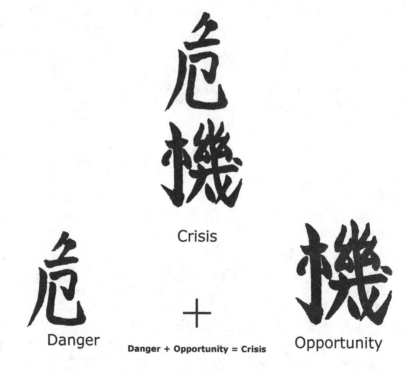

Crisis

Danger

Danger + Opportunity = Crisis

Opportunity

However, before adding T'ai Chi to your physical therapy program, consult your physician to see if T'ai Chi might affect your medication levels. For example, many with high blood pressure find their blood pressure lowers. Your physician should know if T'ai Chi can alter your current therapy for such conditions and then can lower your medication safely.

Mind over Matter

T'ai Chi's artful beauty can make us forget that it is actually one of the most highly evolved health technologies on Earth. The Chinese realized that our mind or consciousness is the root of who we are. Our health and our lives are merely reflections of our state of mind. Therefore, T'ai Chi's mindful quality incorporates the mind and body into a powerful healing force.

Interestingly, Western science now sees that Traditional Chinese Medicine's ancient insights were right on the money. A new science called *psychoneuroimmunology* has found that our mind constantly communicates to every cell of our body.

Emotional chemicals, known as neuropeptides, flow throughout our bodies, communicating every feeling to the entire body. So when hitting every red light on the street aggravates us or we become anxious in every line we stand in, we walk around in a state of perpetual panic (or as Bruce Springsteen sang, "Yer life is one long emergency"). This negatively affects our heart, brain, and entire circulatory system. In fact, those effects in turn affect other organs, which can cause a breakdown of the entire system over time, causing, for example, kidney failure, heart enlargement, and hardening of the arteries.

But don't fret, T'ai Chi helps us do just the opposite. We can decide to let issues slide right off us, literally breathing fears out with every sigh and yawn. As we sit in QiGong meditation or move in T'ai Chi's soothing postures, we let a nourishing healing flow of Qi, or life energy, fill every cell of our body.

Don't try too hard to memorize any of these details on Traditional Chinese or Western medicine. Rather, let the concepts wash over your relaxed mind. The important stuff will stick, and you can always go back to look up details later.

> **T'ai Sci**
>
> Psychoneuroimmunology is a modern science studying how the mind's attitudes and beliefs affect our physical health. *Psycho* means "mind," *neuro* means "nervous system," and *immunology* means "system of health defenses."

Sage Sifu Says

Traditional Chinese Medicine (TCM) differs from the Western approach in that its focus is holistic. *Holistic* means it views the body as an integrated whole. A TCM doctor does not treat only symptoms, but rather tries to discover the root of health problems.

For example, if we have allergy problems, Western pharmaceuticals might send chemical missiles in to dry out the sinuses. This does stop the runny nose, but some medications may result in irritating the surrounding tissue by drying it out or other undesirable side effects. Acupuncture, on the other hand, or T'ai Chi in the long run, will enable the body's natural balancing to occur, reducing the incidence of sinus problems in a way that nurtures the tissue. This is done by re-establishing the blocked flow of Qi that is at the root of the problem.

To fully appreciate T'ai Chi's medical benefits, it may be helpful to understand how Traditional Chinese Medicine views the body. Traditional Chinese Medicine has known for centuries what Western science is only now discovering—that our mind and body are two inseparable things. In Traditional Chinese Medicine, there is a joke that "the only place the mind, body, emotions, and spirit are separate is in textbooks." In real life and T'ai Chi, it just isn't so. T'ai Chi's slow mindful movements are the epitome of this union of mind and body.

So when your body's muscles are rigid, your thinking will likely be more rigid, too. Likewise, if your thinking is harsh and rigid, this will in time be reflected in stiffness in your muscular frame. This stiffness impedes the

Know Your Chinese

The energy meridians are known as **jing luo**. *Jing* literally means "to move through," and *luo* means "a net." So energy meridians are a network of channels.

A T'ai Chi Punch Line

There are also acupuncture maps for animals. In fact, some racing horses have their own personal acupuncturists. Many veterinarians are beginning to use acupuncture as part of their practice.

flow of Qi, which diminishes our health. Therefore, your mind and your thoughts have as much, or maybe more, to do with your health than the food you eat or the exercise you get.

Energy meridians, or *jing luo*, link all the organs and the entire physical body to the mind and emotional systems. This explains how T'ai Chi and QiGong's mind/body exercises integrate all aspects of the self into a powerful self-healing system.

What are these energy meridians that T'ai Chi helps to unblock? By now you know that Qi flows through and powers every cell in your body, the way electricity powers your house. Without Qi, the cell would be dead, for Qi is the life force. The meridians are how Qi gets to the cells. You can't see these meridians; you can only detect the energy that moves through them, just as you cannot see an ocean current in the water, but you can detect its motion.

There are ancient maps of these meridians, made thousands of years ago by Traditional Chinese doctors. These acupuncture meridian maps show 14 main energy meridians that carry Qi throughout the body internally and externally. The names follow, listed first by the modern acupuncture abbreviation, then by the English name, and a few followed by the Chinese name in italics.

- CV = Conception Vessel or *Ren Mai*
- CX = Pericardium Channel
- GB = Gallbladder Channel
- GV = Governing Vessel or *Du Mai*
- HE = Heart Channel
- KI = Kidney Channel
- LI = Large Intestine Channel
- LU = Lung Channel
- LV = Liver Channel
- SI = Small Intestine Channel
- SP = Spleen-Pancreas Channel
- ST = Stomach Channel
- TW = Triple Warmer or *San Jiao* Channel
- UB = Urinary Bladder Channel

Acupuncture and T'ai Chi

There are three aspects of Traditional Chinese Medicine: acupuncture, herbal medicine, and T'ai Chi/QiGong. All three share a common premise that Qi pours through the body, and our health is diminished when the energy flow gets blocked.

So whether an acupuncturist is treating you with needles, an herbalist is prescribing herbs, or you are practicing T'ai Chi, you are trying to balance the imbalances, or unblock the energy that flows throughout your body. Millions of Americans are now using alternative therapies like acupuncture and herbs. If you practice T'ai Chi daily, your relaxed state will help herbs or acupuncture work even more effectively.

The energy meridians, which flow throughout the interior of the body, have 361 points that surface at the skin, and these are the most common treatment points acupuncturists use. But the whole body and even the mind can be treated with acupuncture because these meridians that surface at the skin also flow inside the body, through the brain and other organs.

T'ai Chi and QiGong affect the same energy flow that acupuncture does, although acupuncture can be better for acute problems, whereas T'ai Chi is a daily tune-up. Therefore, acupuncturists often recommend T'ai Chi to their patients, and T'ai Chi teachers recommend acupuncture to students with chronic or acute conditions, as a supplement to the students' standard medical treatments. T'ai Chi and acupuncture are very complementary, and each makes the other more effective.

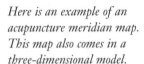

T'ai Sci

Modern acupuncturists often call the Qi meridians bioenergetic circuits.

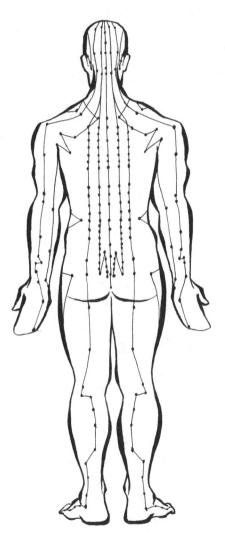

Here is an example of an acupuncture meridian map. This map also comes in a three-dimensional model.

Say, "OOOOHHHHHMMMMMM"—OHMMeter, That Is

It is mind-boggling when you consider that many modern acupuncturists find acupuncture points with electronic equipment, not unlike an Ohmmeter. What's amazing is that acupuncture maps were made long before electronics was developed, some believe over 2,000 years ago.

How did they know where those points were back then? They might have felt them. As you practice T'ai Chi and QiGong, you will eventually begin to feel the Qi flowing from your hands or in your body.

Get an Acupuncture Tune-Up

Acupuncture sees the body holistically, meaning that each small part of the body contains connections to the whole body. Therefore, an acupuncturist can treat any problem in the whole body through, for example, the ears. Likewise, any part of the body, or even the mind, can be treated through the hands or the feet.

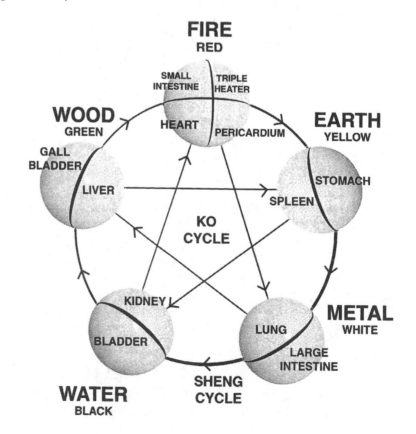

Know Your Chinese

Zang Fu literally translated means "solid-hollow." Organs within the body considered to be hollow, like the stomach or large intestines, are Fu organs, while the solid organs, such as liver and lungs, are Zang organs.

One of the powerful health benefits T'ai Chi provides is a daily acupuncture tune-up. Because T'ai Chi is so slow and the weight shifts so deliberate, with the body very relaxed, the feet are massaged by the earth during a T'ai Chi exercise. The bottoms of the feet have acupuncture points that affect the entire body, and the mind, too. Acupressure is acupuncture without the needles. So the foot massage is a 20-minute T'ai Chi session that stimulates all the acupuncture points on the foot through acupressure, thereby treating the whole body. No other exercise provides this type of slow, relaxed motion, making T'ai Chi unique in providing you an acupuncture tune-up each time you do your daily exercise.

Don't Be Zang Fu-lish

Another profound benefit T'ai Chi provides is a gentle massaging of the internal organs. Because T'ai Chi moves the body in about 95 percent of the possible motions it can go through, it not only clears the joints of calcium deposits, but it also gently massages the internal organs.

In Traditional Chinese Medicine (TCM), this is a powerful therapy for optimum health. TCM recognizes that the body is an integrated whole whereby all the parts are connected by the flow of Qi. In fact, the Chinese system of medicine is built upon a Zang Fu graph, which shows how organs interact with and depend on one another for good healthy function.

The Zang Fu system uses a memory model, applying each organ to one of the five elements of the earth. The Chinese see the world as made of Earth, Metal, Water, Wood, and Fire. The energy flow affects different organs through the Sheng Cycle and the Ko cycle. This figure shows how organs are interactive and interdependent on one another for healthful function.

Therefore, because T'ai Chi massages all the organs through its gentle full rotations, it helps to balance all the integrating activities of the Zang Fu systems.

Be Kind to Your Emotions

Acupuncture, herbal medicine, and T'ai Chi/QiGong use the Zang Fu system to understand how the body, mind, and emotions integrate. A problem with a particular organ may have emotional symptoms. Likewise, a chronic emotional state may have a physical impact on the organs. The following list explains the Zang Fu connection between organs and emotions commonly related to imbalances with those organs or their energy channels:

> **Sage Sifu Says**
>
> If you go to a Traditional Chinese Physician, she may likely ask you about your emotions as well as your physical symptoms because emotional states may help lead her to understand which organ's energy is deficient or in excess.

- ◆ Liver = Depression, anger
- ◆ Heart = Excess joy (such as manic behavior), excess mental function
- ◆ Spleen = Obsession
- ◆ Lung = Anguish, grief, melancholy
- ◆ Kidney = Fear, fright

So T'ai Chi benefits the mental and emotional states, not only by encouraging us to let go of the day's problems by focusing on breath and movement, but in other ways as well. T'ai Chi stimulates the organs with gentle massage, while stimulating the acupressure points on the feet and throughout the body, with its gentle relaxed postures. The breathing in T'ai Chi is full, yet effortless, encouraging internal releases of mental and emotional blocks that also help the internal Zang Fu systems become less restricted, more free flowing, and healthful on mental, emotional, and physical levels. Chapter 4, "Expand the Mind and Lighten the Heart," will explain how T'ai Chi and QiGong can provide mental and emotional healing.

Increase Flexibility

T'ai Chi not only increases flexibility by regularly stretching the muscles very gently, but through the Zang Fu system as well. As we age, especially but not exclusively men, we often find a depletion in our kidney energy. The kidney energy is responsible for the function of the liquid systems of the body. Therefore, the decrease in kidney energy that accompanies aging causes our connective tissue, such as tendons, to become brittle. We are then much more likely to tear, or otherwise injure, our bones or joints when we stumble or fall.

So the tremendous balance improvements T'ai Chi offers are only part of why T'ai Chi practitioners are much less likely than other people to suffer falling injuries. The improved performance of all organ functions enhances the entire physical body's health. In fact, in this way, sitting QiGong may also increase flexibility, even though it is a nonphysical exercise.

Western Medicine's Research on T'ai Chi and QiGong

After reading this section you should be satisfied beyond a doubt that *T'ai Chi works*. So when you get to the QiGong and T'ai Chi exercises in Parts 3, 4, and 5, you won't have to think about their benefits. The mind is the greatest healer. Therefore, if you believe in the value of your therapy, it will be much more effective for you.

Stress Is the Symptom

By now you know that stress is the chief cause of illness in the modern world. As Western medicine discovers that T'ai Chi and QiGong are effective stress-reducing exercises, these powerful mind/body health tools are being used in more and more hospitals and are prescribed by more and more doctors.

Studies show that reaction to stress can damage the entire body. It causes chronic hypertension (high blood pressure), which can cause the arteries to harden, kidney damage, and enlargement of the heart. Stress also has been shown to impair our ability to think and actually shrinks the hypothalamus and the hippocampus parts of the brain. Yikes!

A T'ai Chi Punch Line

Traditional Chinese Medicine sees the body and mind intertwined. So a rigid body can cause us to think rigidly as well. Or perhaps more accurately, a rigid mind can cause us to have a rigid body.

Who Ya Gonna Call?

T'ai Chi is a stress buster. An article in *Occupational Therapy Week* explains that T'ai Chi's emphasis on posture and diaphragmatic breathing (breathing from your diaphragm) accounts for a practitioner's reduction in muscular tension and the stress it causes. Patients using T'ai Chi report a greater ability to cope with fear and anxiety, as that physical relaxation is reflected in their mental attitude.

Bellevue Psychiatric Hospital in New York City provided T'ai Chi to both staff and patients. Their Activity Therapy Supervisor said, "T'ai Chi is a natural and safe vehicle to *neutralize* rather than resist the stress in our personal lives, an ability which we greatly need to nurture in our modern fast-paced society."

T'ai Chi Is Your Heart's Best Friend

Harvard Medical School's *Women's Health Watch Journal* reported that, "T'ai Chi has *salubrious* effects," and that "practicing T'ai Chi regularly may delay the decline of cardiopulmonary function in older adults ... T'ai Chi was found to be as effective as meditation in reducing stress hormones."

A Duke University study recently announced that managing stress controls heart disease even more effectively than exercise. Since T'ai Chi provides both powerful stress management and gentle exercise, T'ai Chi is your heart's very best friend. Now, go out and play nice with your new friend.

Sage Sifu Says

With all these T'ai Chi and QiGong facts swimming through your mind, now is a good time to practice QiGong's mind-clearing tools. Take a deep breath from your abdomen to your chest, and on the sighing exhale, let your shoulders relax away from your neck as they sink towards the floor. Repeat this several times, and as you release the breath, imagine that every cell in your body is relaxing as you release each breath. Now as you let go of the breath, let all your cranial muscles release their grip on your skull, and as you let go, allow your mind to release all the facts and figures it is trying to remember.

Ironically, you will find that the more your mind lets go of trying to hold onto facts, the more easily it can absorb information.

T'ai Chi Reduces Mental Stress

A study cited in the *Journal of Psychosomatic Research* claimed T'ai Chi study subjects reported less tension, depression, anger, fatigue, confusion, and anxiety; they felt more vigorous and, in general, had less total mood disturbance.

The *Journal of Black Psychology* states that many African-Americans suffer from chronic high blood pressure. The article explains that hypertension is a physical result of psychological stress. The article proposes T'ai Chi as a holistic way for treating psychosomatic illnesses, or those illnesses caused by stress.

T'ai Chi may also help us think better. Research has shown that stress can limit the development of the hippocampus, the part of the brain that deals with learning and memory. So T'ai Chi's ability to reduce stress responses may actually enhance our ability to learn and remember.

Know Your Chinese

T'ai Chi and QiGong have long been known to boost the immune system. Ancient Chinese medicine understood the concept of the immune system, which the Chinese called **bu qi, bu xue,** meaning "tonify the Qi and blood." When Qi and blood are strengthened, we are better able to fight off infection and disease.

T'ai Chi Lowers Body Stress

Working Woman magazine's article on T'ai Chi said, "increasingly mind/body workouts are replacing high-impact aerobics, and other body punishing exercises of the 1980s. These mind/body workouts are kinder to the joints and muscles and can reduce the tension that often contributes to the development of disease, which makes them especially appropriate for high-powered, stressed-out baby boomers."

A Boost to Your Immune System

Prevention magazine reported a study on T'ai Chi's effects on the immune system. They found that regular practice of T'ai Chi may increase the body's production of T-cells. These T-cells are T-lymphocytes. "Lympho-whats?" you might ask. It doesn't matter. What matters is that these little T-cells help the immune system destroy bacteria and possibly even tumor cells. If T'ai Chi can make more of these little buggers, what are we waiting for. Let's T'ai Chi one on!

In China, QiGong is commonly prescribed as an adjunct to chemotherapy and radiation. Studies indicate that when QiGong is combined with standard cancer treatments, favorable results are obtained, treating virtually all forms and stages of cancer. Part of the reason for this success is that QiGong helps patients feel less helpless. Studies show that feelings of self-empowerment can have powerful healing benefits on the course of almost any disease, including cancer.

A T'ai Chi Punch Line

I was once studying T'ai Chi and QiGong in Hong Kong. Because of the time difference, I was waking up at 3 A.M. With nothing else to do, I became a particularly diligent student and practiced Gathering Qi or Standing Post for nearly an hour and a half each morning. After about a week of this, I began to visually see the Qi flowing around people, especially their heads. I noticed that those who seemed to be enjoying the day had large pluming expanses of energy around them, while those appearing driven and stressed had tiny restricted energy emanating from them.

How Does T'ai Chi Fight for the Immune System?

American QiGong master Ken Cohen has dubbed a hormone called DHEA the Health Hormone. In his book, *Qigong: The Art and Science of Chinese Energy Healing*, Mr. Cohen explains that this hormone is believed to be linked to Qi.

DHEA is short for dehydroepiandrosterone. Yeah, I know, *forget about it*. But don't forget that DHEA is related to youthfulness, less disease, and a more functional immune system.

According to Mr. Cohen, low DHEA levels have been directly linked to cancer, diabetes, obesity, hypertension, allergies, heart disease, and most autoimmune diseases.

When we are under a lot of stress, our body exhausts itself of this important hormone. Therefore, by practicing T'ai Chi, we can increase DHEA levels, thereby increasing our immune systems ability to fight whatever steps in the ring with it. Let's rumble!

T'ai Chi does two wonderful things to help us age healthfully:

◆ It maximizes the body's full potential to regenerate healthy cells, which actually slows the aging process.

◆ It promotes a deep self-acceptance and self-awareness, so that as our body goes through the challenges of aging, we are much better able to handle and adjust to those changes, both physically and emotionally.

DHEA and T'ai Chi, Back Together Again

DHEA is also involved in the aging process. This hormone's levels tend to decline with age, but the decline is much worse when under chronic stress. Add natural aging and chronic stress, and you have an express train to an old body. However, our old friend T'ai Chi once again comes to the rescue. T'ai Chi's gentle movements and breathing techniques promote the serenity that can keep DHEA from being depleted.

Of course, the increased circulation of blood and Qi also fully oxygenate the skin, which provides nourishment to your outer beauty. The Zang Fu system's being balanced by T'ai Chi's stimulation of acupressure points and massage of the internal organs also moves the liquids and oils of the body to the tissue that needs them, further adding to your external beauty and internal health.

> **T'ai Sci**
>
> Free radicals are atoms with an extra electron that bounce around wreaking havoc throughout the body. We see this with our eyes as aging. The calming effects of T'ai Chi and QiGong not only affect the mind, but can also reduce the damage done by free radicals, thereby slowing the aging process.

> **Know Your Chinese**
>
> **Fan lao huan tong** means "reverse old age and return to youthfulness." This is what the Chinese believe T'ai Chi and QiGong offer, and, of course, Western scientific methods are beginning to tell us how and why that happens. East meets West.

Aging's Radical, Dude! (Free Radicals, That Is)

There is a pesky little *free radical* atom in your body called "super oxide" that causes the body to age. Not only does it cause wrinkles and age spots, but it can also weaken cartilage and joints. In fact, this super oxide may even induce cancer or other immune system disorders. *Obnoxious little thing, isn't it?*

However, regular T'ai Chi and QiGong practice can protect your body from these pesky free radicals by activating an enzyme called *superoxide dismutase* (or *SOD*). SOD is our cellular superman and defends our cells from the ornery super oxides that break down our health systems.

A study of those who practiced QiGong for a half-hour a day for one year showed that their levels of SOD increased dramatically compared to people not doing QiGong. Another study showed a large increase in SOD after only two months of QiGong practice.

Make No Bones About It, T'ai Chi Does Your Body Good

The National Institute of Mental Health released a study showing that women under chronic stress with depression had weaker bones than those in normal emotional states. In fact, the stressed/depressed women had the bones of 70-year-old women, even though they were only 40 years old.

T'ai Chi lessens the incidence of depression and the body's stress responses, and is a gentle weight-bearing exercise. These abilities may make T'ai Chi the best thing you can do to keep your bones healthy, even into old age.

T'ai Chi Does an Incredible Balancing Act!

For aging Americans, the simple act of stumbling and falling can often be fatal. The sixth largest cause of death for older Americans is complications from falling injuries. This costs our country about $10 billion a year and causes tremendous suffering for older people. We are all paying for our nation's poor balance in human suffering and in higher healthcare and health insurance costs.

T'ai Chi was part of a balance study by Harvard, Yale, the Center for Disease Control, Washington University School of Medicine, and Emory University. T'ai Chi practitioners fell and injured themselves only half as much as those practicing other balance training. This is an amazing finding that can change the lives of older Americans.

Although many of us are not in the age group that is likely to suffer serious injury from falling, we can all benefit greatly by having better balance. Better balance puts much less stress on the body throughout the workday, and you will find that you have much more energy as T'ai Chi practice improves your balance.

> **T'ai Sci**
>
> In a university study on balance, researchers were testing a rather expensive computer model designed to improve people's balance. The researchers were stunned to find that a simple inexpensive exercise called T'ai Chi was in some ways nearly twice as effective as the expensive computer model.

T'ai Chi's Dirt Cheap and Can Be Done on Grass, Too

Compared to the best balance training in the world, T'ai Chi is about twice as effective. Some of the other balance exercises studied in the Ivy League study on balance were very expensive computer models that required participants to go into a lab and practice. The simple exercises of T'ai Chi are therefore not only much more effective than the other exercises, but they are very cheap.

You don't have to get a gym membership or an expensive physical trainer, or any fancy clothes or equipment. All you need are these terrific toys called your mind and your body. Now, *go play!*

T'ai Chi's Gentle to Arthritis and Your Joints

T'ai Chi is an exercise few doctors will ever tell patients to stop practicing. It provides perhaps the lowest impact weight-bearing exercise there is. We all need weight-bearing exercise to help build bone mass and connective tissue, but for those with rheumatoid arthritis or some other conditions, weight-bearing exercise is a problem. For these people, weight-bearing exercise can aggravate joints, causing tenderness or swelling.

However, a study cited in the *American Journal of Physical Medicine and Rehabilitation* wanted to see if T'ai Chi would harm rheumatoid arthritis patients. To their pleasant surprise, T'ai Chi did no damage whatsoever and provided them with the safe weight-bearing exercise they seriously needed. The forms were modified for these patients, and everyone with arthritis or knee problems should be sure they only do forms that feel good to them. But this T'ai Chi discovery is good news for all of us because it gives us all a weight-bearing exercise that is safe even into old age.

T'ai Chi: The Healthcare of the Future

Most Chinese hospitals have long integrated Western crisis medicine with Traditional Chinese Medicine. This is now rapidly happening in the United States as well. The American Medical Association recently recognized acupuncture as a valid treatment, which is causing Western doctors to look at T'ai Chi and QiGong even more intently.

Growing numbers of neurologists, cardiologists, general practitioners, physical therapists, hypertension specialists, and psychologists are already prescribing T'ai Chi and/or QiGong as treatment, or as supplemental treatment, for many conditions. In Part 6, "Life Applications," you will find T'ai Chi prescribed for specific conditions.

As more Western scientific research is completed on the benefits of T'ai Chi and QiGong, this trend will expand, and we all will benefit greatly by lower healthcare costs.

T'ai Chi and QiGong's Healing Powers

When you first hear of the benefits of T'ai Chi and QiGong, it may sound like snake oil. This is because it is effective for helping to treat all things on all levels. "How can it do that?" you may ask. It does this by connecting us to the most powerful healing tool there is—the healing power of the mind. It is the power of the mind that is at the heart of our healing.

> **A T'ai Chi Punch Line**
>
> Studies have shown that if patients "believe" that something can cure them, the possibility that it will is much higher. Cynicism is found to be one of the single most hazardous behaviors for our health. I always tell students, "If I have a choice between being smart enough to realize I'm incurable, or stupid enough to fool myself into curing myself—I'll be the fool any day."

It is estimated that placebos can positively treat about 60 percent of our health problems. Placebos are sugar pills (or fake treatments) doctors sometimes give to fool patients into curing themselves. This gets the mind/body to trigger its own internal healing processes, by the mind simply telling itself it's okay for the body to heal. This indicates that the body has a tremendous potential to *self* heal, *if we believe in the cure*.

T'ai Chi and QiGong are not placebos. They are powerful health tools that can give us access to the tremendous natural healing power of the body, the power behind the placebo. Many of these healing benefits are documented, and new research is emerging all the time. It's important for you to understand just how powerful these tools are so that your mind will allow them to do their magic.

The Least You Need to Know

- T'ai Chi facilitates the flow of Qi and health to your cells.
- Narrow thinking squeezes off life energy.
- T'ai Chi integrates the mind, body, and emotions.
- By toning our Qi, we tone all our healing systems.
- Only T'ai Chi provides an acupressure treatment and organ massage, while promoting circulation and centeredness.
- You don't have to memorize how it works, just relax and do it.

Chapter 4

Expand the Mind and Lighten the Heart

In This Chapter

◆ Discover the power of calm and peace

◆ Know that you can be as powerful as you want to be

◆ Accept that you are perfect

◆ Flex your imagination muscle

The problem with the rat race is, even if you win the race, you're still a rat.

—Lily Tomlin

Our mental and emotional well-being is ravaged by the demands of the day-to-day rat race. T'ai Chi is not only a great physical workout and health tool, but can heal us mentally and emotionally by changing the way we look at life. T'ai Chi shows us that life does not have to be that hard.

The simple ways T'ai Chi and QiGong look at movement and life can be powerful self-improvement tools, as well as a soothing balm to our frazzled nerves.

T'ai Chi Calms the Rat Race

Chinese masters constantly repeat, "*Soong Yi-Dien*" (loosen up). This instruction is not just to encourage a physical loosening, but a mental, emotional, and social loosening as well. The goal of T'ai Chi is to weave silken threads of calm into our lives, soothing us as we face the daily rat race. The calmer we are, the calmer our workplace and our home are.

However, at first, rather than bringing T'ai Chi's calm to the rat race, students often unconsciously bring the rat race into the T'ai Chi class or into their T'ai Chi practice at home. They do this because they want to "efficiently" learn T'ai Chi. Our work, lives, and technology are all geared toward making things happen faster and faster. So we naturally want to "hurry up and

Ouch! _____

Many Western students feel hopeless upon learning that T'ai Chi is a lifelong process. We in the West are conditioned to expect immediate, short-term results. Don't be discouraged. T'ai Chi is the lifelong process that gives immediate results. Even if you just took one T'ai Chi class and practiced what you learned, you would get great benefit. It just gets better and better for the rest of your life.

relax." This can't happen. We have to let go of urgency and efficiency in order to truly and deeply experience what T'ai Chi offers. However, much to the surprise of many T'ai Chi students (including me), we soon realize that as T'ai Chi helps us become less urgent, we actually become more efficient. If this sounds impossible, read on.

Frantic Action vs. Efficiency

T'ai Chi's ability to calm, energize, heal, strengthen, and tone the mind and body in a short half-hour workout is unequaled. However, if you try to do T'ai Chi efficiently, it doesn't work as well. It's when you relax and don't try that T'ai Chi works its magic.

The idea that we can get something very worthwhile done without being in high anxiety to hurry up and do it is a new concept for most of us.

T'ai Chi Is Smelling the Roses

Our heart and mind seem to be in a constant state of turmoil. With the tidal wave of information the information age has swept into our lives, we always feel two steps behind the pack. We struggle to understand the latest technology, knowing full well that a newer version will be out before we learn the one that just came out. We forget to breathe and enjoy the *learning* in life, which is pretty much all there is to life when you get down to it. We are not and never will be done learning. So we might as well smell the roses on the way.

Learning to "love the learning" of T'ai Chi is one of the most important lessons T'ai Chi offers our frantic lives. In T'ai Chi classes students sometimes come in gung-ho to learn one set of forms and move on. The concept that T'ai Chi is a lifelong process comes as a big shock. Students think they can hurry in, get fixed, get calmed, get healthy, and then get going. They want to hurry up and *finish*, so they can hurry up to finish the next thing they want to hurry up and do. But by living this way, our lives just become a lot of hurrying. There is no finish in T'ai Chi or in life.

T'ai Chi's calming effects can be felt immediately the very first day of practice, but not if you hurry up to feel them. You have to let go of outcome and let the nice feelings be a pleasant surprise, rather than an urgent demand.

T'ai Chi's movements flow one into the other, just as life's events do. By learning how to breathe and relax the body, while moving through these events, we become an island of soothing calm even when in the center of the rat race. Our habit of letting the frantic demands of the day fill our mind becomes easier and easier to let go of as we practice T'ai Chi.

" " **Sage Sifu Says** _____

Go ahead—take a deep breath right now! Don't wait until you are in a quiet retreat or on the top of a mountain to use your T'ai Chi tools. Begin to weave the ideas of effortless breathing release into everything you do. If you remember to breathe, everything else will most likely take care of itself.

Remember to Breathe—Everything Else Takes Care of Itself

The very first thing students do in T'ai Chi class is to close their eyes and breathe. Take deep breaths all the way into the bottom of the lungs and then let go of the breath, the muscles, and the day. Let go of everything you've done before getting there and everything you plan to do later. Just be here and now, breathing.

As your mind fills with remembering to breathe through your T'ai Chi movements and gravity forces you to focus on your balance, you must let go of the worries of the day. You cannot do T'ai Chi without letting go of thoughts about what to defrost for dinner or the laundry that needs to be done.

T'ai Chi does not advocate starvation or wearing dirty clothes. It does, however, advocate being 100 percent in the moment, whether it's doing T'ai Chi or washing clothes. This is what is called mindfulness, or being here and now. You'll find that the more you can let go of the dinner and the laundry to feel your breath, your muscles releasing, and the silken flow of your T'ai Chi movements, the more you'll enjoy doing the laundry or cooking dinner when you do get to it. The T'ai Chi practice of being here and now will seep into your daily life by reminding you to breathe as you move. As you do the laundry, you'll slow down and breathe, you'll feel the pleasure of the warmth of the clothes coming out of the dryer, and really enjoy the sweet scent of clean clothes. While making dinner, you'll relax and breathe, enabling you to truly smell the fragrance of dinner.

We don't have to race if we are always where we like being. Then we never have to fear looking in the mirror and seeing a racing rat.

> ### Sage Sifu Says
> As T'ai Chi helps us "feel good" on a regular basis, we want more of that feeling. You may find yourself spending more time with people who nurture you and less time with those who put you down. This is a powerfully healthful transformative part of doing T'ai Chi. As the movements in T'ai Chi teach you to ease around areas of discomfort in the body so as to expand mobility without injury, this echoes out into our lives. You begin to find nurturing ways to move and live socially.

The Power of Effortlessness

In our fast-paced dog-eat-dog world, it is hard to believe that we can be more powerful when we are not straining. However, that is exactly when we are most powerful, not only mentally and emotionally, *but also physically*. Because we are so conditioned to be mentally and emotionally straining all the time, many students feel "guilty" taking quiet still time to heal their minds and emotions from the strains of the day. Those students need a real physical example of how we function more effectively when relaxed. If you are a victim of this guilt, the following exercise will help you let your mind and emotions get the most out of T'ai Chi's effortless ways.

The Unbendable Arm

The unbendable arm is a terrific physical example of the concept of "effortless action" and how powerful that kind of action is. In the West we tend to think of big straining muscles and bursting head veins whenever we think of power.

T'ai Chi can rescue us from that sweaty, head-pounding delusion. In T'ai Chi, our goal is to move and stand with as little effort as possible. Ancient *Taoist* poets tried to explain in words the seemingly limitless power found in living lives of effortlessness with calm minds and quiet hearts. However, the concept of effortless power is so strange to Westerners that the following demonstration of the Unbendable Arm is worth a thousand words. (Note: If you have any arm or shoulder injuries, you may not want to do the Unbendable Arm exercise. Also, if you have difficulty performing it, you may want to practice the Sitting QiGong exercise in Part 3, "Starting Down the QiGong Path to T'ai Chi," and then try again.)

> ### Know Your Chinese
> The focus of **Taoist** (pronounced *dowist*) philosophy is the invisible force of nature's laws. When we are calm and still in our hearts, minds, and bodies, we can "feel" or "sense" the subtle direction of Tao. Living the Tao is the most effortless, meaningful way to live. In the West we may call the sense of the Tao a hunch or an intuition, or what feels right.

Notice that the person is able to bend my arm even as I use all my muscular strength to resist.

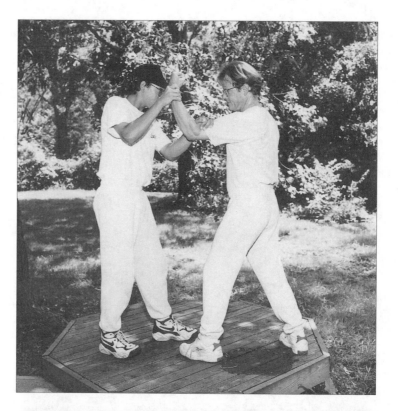

However, notice here that my arm is relaxed, yet the other person cannot bend it.

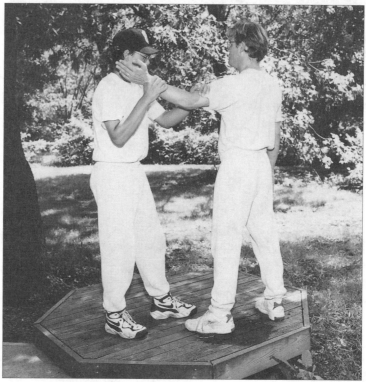

The Unbendable Arm is a powerful physical example of this principle of effortless power. In my class demonstrations I will ask the largest, most powerful-looking student to try to bend my arm. Resisting with all my muscular strength, they nevertheless eventually bend my arm. However, when I completely relax my mind and body, thinking of an empty flow, or of airy relaxation pouring through my head, shoulder, arm, and on out my fingers through the walls of the building, they can't bend it. The students strain to bend my relaxed arm, yet find they cannot.

Our Flexibility Is Our Strength

This Taoist principle of effortless power is even more meaningful in our mental and emotional lives.

I use the Unbendable Arm not to demonstrate the physical power of effortless motion (although it does demonstrate that), but to dispel the myth that our straining is equivalent to productivity. The Chinese say the most powerful T'ai Chi is like a supple bamboo, flexible and bendable, because obviously a rigid stick can be easily broken. Just as we relax our arms to make them strong, we can relax our minds to become more effective in life. We can relax our hearts and experience more profound and meaningful feelings. When we breathe and relax while typing at the keyboard or answering the phone, we are so much more effective and real. We have time for the people in our lives, instead of always rushing past them to get to the next urgent task.

> **T'ai Sci**
>
> Taoist philosophy is a model used by many Western psychotherapists as they encourage patients to let go of obsessing on outcome and rather enjoying the "process" of life. In fact, T'ai Chi exercises are recommended as an active model to achieve these healing ends.

Patterns vs. Chaos

T'ai Chi helps our bodies be more effective by relaxing the muscles. This allows a more ordered pattern of muscle use, so that muscles aren't fighting other muscles. Well, T'ai Chi has the same effect on the mind. By quieting the mind of all the daily "noise," our mind can open to more orderly patterns of thought.

Coaching the Mind Team

Similar to the way that the body fights itself physically with muscle tension, the mind also keeps itself in needless chaos with noisy thoughts spinning around in it. T'ai Chi and QiGong can end this internal battle and enhance the power of the mind and imagination. Just as the slow deliberate motions of T'ai Chi calm the body and get the muscles to work together more powerfully (as demonstrated by the Unbendable Arm), that same calmness gets the mind to organize.

 A T'ai Chi Punch Line _____

When studying T'ai Chi in Hong Kong as a young man, I was intrigued by the construction workers there. At the time I was in great shape, being a karate enthusiast who trained very hard. However, I was humbled by the much smaller thinner Chinese construction workers hauling enormously heavy bags of cement up bamboo scaffolds on their thin shoulders. They showed barely any exertion. Whether the workers practiced T'ai Chi or not, they had obviously absorbed some of its principles.

Imagine that life is like a football game, and we keep getting batted around by really big linemen that we call problems. The noise in our heads is deafening, as every time we get up from being knocked down, another big problem bangs into us. It's hard to even think about solutions when big problems bang into us one after another.

Now, imagine that we could somehow be lifted up above the chaos to look down on what's happening from a higher, clearer angle, like a coach in the upper deck of the stadium. We would see patterns, or plays, forming. We would see how waves of linemen or problems flow. We could make adjustments before problems are right in our face, enabling us to choose the path of least resistance, not only making it easier, but getting much more yardage, or success, with each play. T'ai Chi practice continually lifts our mind to that higher clearer perception.

> **Sage Sifu Says**
>
> The Taoist philosophers took a holistic approach to the world, meaning that they saw each little thing as kind of a model for bigger structures. For example, each cell in our body makes up the whole body, as individuals we make up our family, our family makes the neighborhood, which makes the city, state, and society. Therefore, the most powerful contribution we can make to the world is to be the healthiest we can be, physically, mentally and emotionally. If our health heals the world around us, then a healthier world around us also heals us. This is the kind of cycle that needs to spin out of control.

Innercise Integrates Outer Relationships

Phil Jackson, former head coach of the World Champion Chicago Bulls, is a Zen practitioner, and he introduced the entire Chicago Bulls basketball team to Zen exercises. T'ai Chi and QiGong exercises are from the same roots as Zen exercises and are often indistinguishable from them.

> **A T'ai Chi Punch Line**
>
> The Chinese Character for Qi, or life energy, and the Latin root *spir*, as in spirit, mean "the air we breathe." Both ancient cultures obviously saw how our breath connects us to the life force. When considering that each of us has breathed an atom of oxygen that was breathed by Jesus, Buddha, and Mohammed, the Taoist claim that we are all connected becomes a very real concept.

The year that the Bulls were introduced to Zen practices, was the year that they became the winningest team in the history of the NBA. This is no coincidence. The choreography displayed by the Bulls that year was mind-boggling; the team often resembled one living entity, rather than five separate players. As Zen exercise allows the mind to clear itself of its daily chatter or rubble, it also clarifies the communication between people. So, just as the Bulls players began to quiet and clarify their own internal function by relaxing muscles and quieting thoughts they didn't need, they simultaneously clarified their player-to-player communication. This clarity is what we saw in the incredible plays the Bulls made that year.

This same clarity we cultivate through our daily T'ai Chi or QiGong exercises can help us clarify our relationships with others at work or home. Most social breakdowns are rooted in a lack of clarity, for if we aren't clear on what we want and need, we can never expect others to support our efforts. Whether its our love life, our family, our work, or social relationships, T'ai Chi's soothing way of moving through life will make relationships more healing and effortless.

People around us become easier to deal with when we are easier to deal with. T'ai Chi shows us how much of the external world reflects what goes on in our own heart and mind. *Dressage*, the national magazine for the Olympic horseback riding style, promotes T'ai Chi as perhaps the most effective exercise a rider can perform to enhance riding skills. What's fascinating is why.

The article said that horses pick up on the riders mental and emotional stress levels. Therefore, if the rider does T'ai Chi before mounting his horse, the horse gives a smoother and quicker ride.

Imagine how much your unconscious mental and emotional turmoil affects those around you at home or work. Then think of how much your life would change if you did T'ai Chi before riding in.

T'ai Chi-Hut-Hut-BREAK from Old Patterns

This is what T'ai Chi and QiGong can do. T'ai Chi's physical model of moving with the muscles relaxing off of the bones is a model for letting go of mental and emotional obsessions. T'ai Chi allows us to let go of the chaos of life and lets our mind lift and observe, unattached to outcomes, grudges, or obsessive desires. It allows us to see more clearly the patterns that cause us to bump our head into the same old walls again and again.

Letting go of attachments or stepping out of the game from time to time gives us a fresh perspective. Fresh perspective is what allows us to exercise our "imagination muscle." It's the most effortless thing you can do. However, it's not always easy because it requires you to let go of all your thoughts, plans, and regrets. Creating space or breathing room in our busy days with T'ai Chi and QiGong helps our mind let go of old patterns. This allows our mind to open to the pure inspiration that wants to bubble up inside it.

> **Sage Sifu Says**
>
> The life force is clarity and simplicity and holds no need to compete. By letting go of desires, utmost calm is realized, and all the world arrives at effortless peace.

T'ai Chi Dispels the Idea of Wrongness

The most mentally and emotionally healing concept T'ai Chi has to offer our hypercritical world may be that T'ai Chi dispels the idea of "wrongness." When you practice T'ai Chi, you never ever do it "wrong." You just do it. Each time you do it, you relax a little more, you breathe a little easier, and your T'ai Chi gets a little better.

T'ai Chi Is a Model for Life

The effortless sustenance T'ai Chi offers our lives is the understanding that we are always "perfect," that our lives are ever-evolving perfection. When we learn things about T'ai Chi that we can improve, it is much easier to adopt the new ways if the old ways don't have to be "wrong." This is one of the ways T'ai Chi makes a terrific model for life in general.

Our culture's concepts of wrongness constipate the ability to let go of old ways and move into new ways more easily. If something must be wrong before it can be discarded, we judge ourselves as wrong for having done it that way. If we see things in an ever-evolving state of improvement, then nothing is wrong, and there are always better ways. Then we can see that we were right for having done it the old way, but can be even "righter" for doing it a new way.

The only wrong thing you can do in T'ai Chi is to tell yourself you're wrong.

> **Ouch!**
>
> If you study with a T'ai Chi instructor who is hypercritical, you may want to find another one who has more fun with T'ai Chi. However, be aware that if you are hypercritical of yourself by nature, you may unconsciously project that onto the instructor. Relax and enjoy yourself when in T'ai Chi class and when practicing at home. This will help your instructor relax, too.

T'ai Chi Breaks Limits

T'ai Chi's way of seeing exercise (and life) as a process leaves us always content with where we are, while always taking us past our old limits. When we obsess over getting things "right," whether we know it or not, we limit ourselves by thinking we are "done" when we get it "right." By giving up that myth, we begin to feel a limitlessness to life. T'ai Chi helps us feel bigger, dream bigger, and love bigger.

Each time you do T'ai Chi, you relax a little more deeply and become a little more self-aware, enabling you to continually improve your T'ai Chi.

Know Your Chinese

The character for **Qi** (pronounced *chee*) represents steam rising from rice, meaning "the air of life," a symbol for effortless sustenance.

Sage Sifu Says

"When problems arise, use your energy to fix the problem, rather than wasting energy fixing the blame. Fix the problem, not the blame." This concept goes right to the heart of what T'ai Chi offers our harried lives.

Notice that the Qi character is a combination of steam or air (the top half) and rice (the lower half).

When we stick with T'ai Chi long enough, we realize that our T'ai Chi improves each time we do it. More important it helps us see that we never did T'ai Chi "wrong," for T'ai Chi is not a destination where a fixed level of perfection exists. Like our lives, T'ai Chi is an unfolding rose of improvement that blooms endlessly, more perfectly, and more beautifully each new day that we practice it. An 80-year-old T'ai Chi teacher was being interviewed about his 60 years of T'ai Chi practice. The interviewer asked him, "At what point did you feel you mastered T'ai Chi?" The old teacher replied, "I'll let you know as soon as I do."

T'ai Chi Enhances Life

Does T'ai Chi make life perfect? No, not more perfect than it already is. And it is always perfect, although sometimes it may seem perfectly miserable. T'ai Chi encourages you to let go of outcomes, and simply pour your energy into whatever nourishes life, your life and all life. The flow of Qi through the body is like water through the roots of a plant. It doesn't fix anything in particular, it just enhances life. As the Taoist philosopher Lao Tzu put it, "The best people are like water. Water nurtures all things and never is in competition with them."

Qi

Steam rising off rice is the Air of Life, *or Qi*

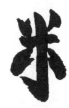

Steam rising off rice

Rice

T'ai Chi and QiGong Strengthen the Imagination Muscle

Sitting QiGong is a motionless exercise. So if the slowness of T'ai Chi makes it seem ineffective to many Westerners, the stillness of QiGong may seem like a colossal waste of time. However, this could not be further from the truth.

These slow mindful exercises bring the brain into a very calm state known by scientists as the alpha state. This is a highly creative state of mind. In fact, three of the great discoverers of our time had their greatest insights while in alpha states. Albert Einstein, Thomas Edison, and Nikolai Tesla all claimed to get their greatest discoveries while in a state of mind that Einstein called "wakeful rest."

Why is the alpha state such a creative state of mind? There are two reasons. One is that when our mind is filled with normal daily worries, plans, and television/radio noise, there is no room for creative thought. Two, there may be a deeper knowledge within our minds that we can't access when our minds are busy with daily problem solving. The psychologist Carl Jung said there is a "collective unconscious" that holds great knowl-edge, and that we all have access to it. But when our mind is busy with balancing the checkbook or worrying about our next raise, we can't open up to that great knowledge. This collective uncon-scious is the ocean of information our minds get ideas from. It is like all the information on the Internet, and our minds are like a computer that can download that information.

When we are tense, our minds are tight and closed to new ideas. This resembles the problem with the Internet. The Internet has loads of great information, but most computers seem to take for-ever to access it. This is because information bottlenecks when it passes through the system's modems because these modems have a limited bandwidth. If your brain is like your computer, and ideas are like the Internet, then QiGong and T'ai Chi are a way to increase that bandwidth to allow much more access to informa-tion.

We've all experienced this whether you know it or not. Have you ever faced a really tough problem that you couldn't solve. No mat-ter how hard you tried, you couldn't see the solution. Then when you gave up, and went for a walk, or sat on the back porch, or went for a drive, the answer came to you. You saw a pattern you missed when your mind was too busy trying to put pieces together. Then when you gave up, your mind put the pieces together very eas-ily and very effectively.

This is what T'ai Chi and QiGong help us learn to do more often and more easily. They open our mental bandwidth by allowing the mind to let go of its clutter. Things get clearer. So Einstein, now you can see that T'ai Chi and QiGong are far from a waste of time.

> **Know Your Chinese**
>
> The **alpha state** is a fre-quency of brain waves that occurs during a state of relaxed concentration. It is one of four brain wave frequencies: delta is the slowest, prevalent during infancy or in adults during sleep; theta is present in drowsy barely conscious states; alpha, during QiGong relaxation exercises; and beta is common when the mind is busy or restless.

> **A T'ai Chi Punch Line**
>
> Bet ya your brain's in beta! The stress we feel in our busy lives is partly because our mind spends too much time in beta brain waves, or "busy brain waves." QiGong can help you drop into a calm state even when you're in line at the supermarket.

The Least You Need to Know

- ◆ T'ai Chi heals your mind and heart.
- ◆ Real power comes from peace of mind.
- ◆ T'ai Chi teaches that life is limitless.
- ◆ Stress closes the mind, but QiGong opens it.

Chapter 5

Find Your Center

In This Chapter

- Being here and now
- Letting go of the fight or flight response
- Understanding what constitutes T'ai Chi mastery
- Discovering the master in you
- Using T'ai Chi to change your world

Usually we don't think about being in or out of "center" until life is completely out of hand. Then we know we are out of it, but we're still not sure what *it* is that we're out of. We often think we are just out of our minds.

This chapter can make you an expert on what the center is. Then all you need to do is practice the QiGong exercises in Part 3, "Starting Down the QiGong Path to T'ai Chi," and the T'ai Chi in Part 4, "Kuang Ping T'ai Chi: Walk on Life's Lighter Side," to feel how good the center feels when you're in it. Being in center reduces the melodrama in your life, so you can focus more attention on the big stuff.

Standing in the center means aligning our physical, emotional, mental, and spiritual selves so that we function at our very best, using everything we've got in everything we do. This centering capability of T'ai Chi may seem spiritual, but it is really a kind of science that understands that our mind, body, emotions, and spirit are all intertwined, and that if we integrate them through T'ai Chi practice, we become more powerful. If our body and mind work together to nurture our emotional and spiritual well-being rather than against each other as they sometimes do, life may be less dramatic but much more fulfilling.

T'ai Chi-ing Zen and Now

A wonderful American interpretation of Zen philosophy is, "No matter where ya go, there ya are." All the toys, trips, and movies in the world cannot take you away from yourself. T'ai Chi is about being right in the center of where you are right now, rather than running from it.

T'ai Chi helps us stand right in the center of our lives by focusing the mind and body to release stress that blocks awareness of our spiritual nature and needs.

> **Know Your Chinese** _____
>
> The word **Zen** is a Japanese translation of the Chinese word *ch'an*. Both are translations of the original Sanskrit word *dhyana* (pronounced *jyana*). They describe an art often called "just sitting," or *za-zen*. While one sits in Zen meditation, the mind does not calculate or figure, but is still and calm within, like a glass of muddy water slowly becoming clear as it sits still.

Often, it seems like life is a merry-go-round, and we're hanging on by our last fingernail as the demands of life pull at us with everything they've got. This is what being "out of center" refers to. When we are out there on the edge just trying to survive, we are not very creative. In fact, we often complicate our lives even more with various coping behaviors. Some people cope by overcharging their credit cards on compulsive spending. Others smoke compulsively or turn to alcohol or drugs. Still others become adrenaline junkies who can't slow down and have to be doing something all the time. All these behaviors have one thing in common: They all distract us from the turmoil going on inside our own minds and hearts. T'ai Chi is like a Zen exercise. Zen is an art of *being still*, not running from problems, but being here and now.

> **A T'ai Chi Punch Line** _____
>
> Lao Tzu (pronounced *low* [as in "OW!"] *dzoo*) wrote, "In doing nothing, all things are done." He wasn't advocating laziness. He meant that by breathing, relaxing, and enjoying whatever it is that we do, all things get done, yet seem so effortless that we feel like we did nothing.

T'ai Chi slows us down inside and out. As our body begins to move more slowly, our breathing slows down. As we hear our breathing slow, our mind begins to ride on the rhythm of that relaxed breath, letting go bit by bit of the storming thoughts of the day. As the mind calms it has a resonant effect on the heartbeat, the blood pressure, and the healing systems of the body. On some level we begin to realize we are not in a state of mortal danger after all, which is a state that our ancient "fight or flight" response produces in us. It is this response more than the world around us that makes life seem like it is spinning way out of control.

Fight or Flight—or T'ai Chi

Feeling panicked by life is something we all experience much more often than we want to think about. This feeling is a product of the reflex response called the *fight or flight response*. This reflex response is like an old memory held in the cells of our body, a cellular memory from our caveman (or cavewoman) days, when we were the grade A prime rib for saber-toothed tigers. We automatically respond to stress by breathing shallowly and tightening every muscle in our bodies so as not to be heard and to be ready to run like heck or bash the head of our would-be diner.

> **Sage Sifu Says** _____
>
> The natural breathing that T'ai Chi and QiGong promote is a powerful antidote to the fight or flight response. Just remembering to breathe when crisis hits can significantly affect your ability to better handle it.

T'ai Chi Bring Caveman to Modern World, Ugh!

Our modern problem is this. Our cells still think they live in a prehistoric world where mortal danger is everywhere. Our outdated response to stress often leaves us in a minor (or not so minor) panic at every red light, supermarket line, or computer glitch we encounter.

This response worked well back then because we really didn't have many options. It does not, however, serve us very well today. Although sometimes the thought of either attacking the source of our anxiety or running away from it seems mighty appealing, it doesn't bode well for our next job performance review.

Room for improvement: Bill should attempt to attack fewer co-workers this quarter, and an emphasis on not fleeing from customers is highly recommended.

T'ai Chi Stops the Fight and Slows the Flight

On a cellular level the fight or flight response is just as inappropriate. When we go into that mode, our heart pounds, our blood pressure elevates, oxygen consumption increases, and blood lactate levels (anxiety levels) increase. If it happens often enough, it can actually cause our brain to shrink.

When we enter this state, the energy flowing through our body becomes very erratic, like a stormy sea. When we practice our T'ai Chi and things begin to calm and center, our energy begins to flow more smoothly and evenly. The Chinese call this "smooth Qi." Smooth Qi is a healthful state produced by doing T'ai Chi. It soothes our body and begins to sooth our mind as well. Some would say T'ai Chi actually starts calming the mind, and then the body becomes calm. Either way it is a pretty helpful thing to be able to do.

Withdrawal from Adrenaline

Many of us have actually become addicted to the feeling of anxiety, just like a cigarette smoker gets addicted to the energy level nicotine doses provide. So at first T'ai Chi or QiGong may cause you to feel drained.

T'ai Sci
Studies show that about 80 percent of illness is due to stress, and that the six leading causes of death are stress related. Most stress-related damage is caused by adrenaline addiction. According to these studies, most of our illnesses are self-inflicted, which means that we are creating our own healthcare crisis. T'ai Chi could help us to break our adrenaline addiction, while also helping to dramatically lower healthcare and insurance costs in the long run.

If this happens, hang in there. You are going through an adrenaline withdrawal. As you continue to practice your T'ai Chi and QiGong, you will eventually break through that wall of drowsiness and boredom. You will discover that you can have the best of both worlds. You will experience the relaxed energy that T'ai Chi creates in you as you find your center.

As the flow of Qi opens up throughout your mind and body, you will have limitless energy, but without the edge. You will run with plenty of juice, but be attuned to when it's time to rest, and you will be able to rest when it's time. You'll feel less and less need to be endlessly busy all the time, but you'll have limitless energy for the truly important things in your life. Furthermore, the calmness that T'ai Chi fosters will grant you the wisdom to know which activities are important and which are not.

Today is a good day to get off adrenaline and get to the real juice. Breathe, breathe some more, and do T'ai Chi.

A T'ai Chi Master: What's That?

T'ai Chi and martial arts abound with myths of superhuman feats performed by masters who defy physical reality. These feats may be true. Some masters have been known to break bricks with their heads. Although, having never been attacked by a brick, I'm not sure what the point is. I'm usually only attacked by stress, fear, and anxiety.

Actually, these performances are compelling demonstrations of the power of internal effortlessness and focus. Often, however, these bizarre demonstrations are a distraction from the real point of these wonderful tools. What T'ai Chi and QiGong offer us is much more miraculous than the ability to break bricks; they help us understand ourselves and how we fit into the world. They make us masters of our own destiny instead of victims of circumstance. Of course, real masters understand that we are never in control, but merely co-pilots of our destiny. However, a copilot is preferable to and more powerful than being an unwitting passenger on this first class ride we call life.

Manifest (Physical) vs. Unmanifest (Energy)

Does it seem like life is one surprise after another? Look again. Our physical bodies are the manifest part of who we are. Our thoughts are the unmanifest part of us that creates our body. So our bodies are like reflections of our mind. Our thoughts are energy that triggers feelings or emotions and that actually changes our physical body. These emotions turn the energy of thoughts into physical responses, just as chronic worry can create ulcers.

Consider this: Remember when Old Yeller died at the end of the story? It broke your heart and made you cry, didn't it? *Come on, you know it did*. Well, the thought about Old Yeller dying at the end of the movie caused a deep emotional swell; our eyes water, and it actually feels like our heart is about to break. So thoughts change our bodies through the communication of emotions. Put simply, our mind in some ways creates our body.

One of the fascinating things QiGong shows us is that the thoughts we are aware of are actually just reflections of what goes on inside us on even deeper levels. Most of our consciousness is subconscious, or below the surface of our awareness. Our thoughts and emotions, and lastly our physical bodies, are results or reflections of an even deeper part of us. That deeper part is the unmanifest part of ourselves. QiGong and T'ai Chi's ability to connect us to that deeper, unmanifest part of ourselves is a potent self-improvement tool.

> **T'ai Sci**
>
> Centuries ago, Chinese Taoist philosophers wrote that all things are formed from the same field of potential energy. As modern physics explains it, all atomic particles emerge from the same energy field, meaning that all things in the universe are made of the same essential energy. We are all, therefore, connected to everything else, to each other, and to the universe.

> **Know Your Chinese**
>
> **Taoism** (pronounced *dowism*) is an ancient Chinese philosophy of life. Its premise is that life flows through all living things the way ocean currents flow through the ocean. The Tao nurtures life and cannot be defined because it applies to all things. Taoists believe we should flow with the Tao, the way a surfer rides the waves, while adding our own flair and best intentions to its currents.

Imagine that our lives are like a big fountain drink of 7Up in a clear glass. If you stand up and look down into it, you only see the bubbles bursting up into the air from the surface. This represents the manifest, or obvious, part of life. From this angle you don't see the deep liquid below that formed these bubbles.

As we experience events in our lives, we are only seeing the bubbles popping up from the surface and not what formed them. These emerging bubbles may take the form of successes, or recurring problems. Perhaps we go from one bad relationship to another or constantly fight with our kids.

However, T'ai Chi meditation, and especially QiGong meditation, let us sit down and look at the "7Up glass of life" from the side, allowing us to see the source of the bubbles. Here we can see that those bubbles, or events of our lives, actually form way down below the surface. This is the unmanifest, or unconscious, part of life.

So our quiet meditations place us sitting on the side observing the true depth of life. Here we see experiences are really end results rather than big surprises. Events in our lives are actually results of patterns or habits we have below the level of what we usually see and feel. We set ourselves up for success or failure by how we think of ourselves every day. If we think of ourselves as valuable human beings, capable of success, then we're much more likely to form bubbles that pop on the surface of our lives in the form of success stories.

Likewise, if we continually think of ourselves as bad or worthless, we will probably form bubbles to reflect that worthlessness in the form of relationship problems. Because if we believe that we are worthless, then we will attract people into our lives who will reinforce that reality. "Pop, pop, pop." Seeing only the pops makes us feel like victims of life.

Masters Are No Longer Victims

Being a T'ai Chi or QiGong master means we are no longer content to remain ignorant of the unmanifest part of life.

However, it's not enough just to know that our responses and actions in life have deeper roots. We have to find ways to change the patterns that form those bubbles way down below the surface of our lives. T'ai Chi and QiGong can help us do this. By quieting our mind and body, they can allow us to feel inside where we hurt or hate. By feeling the source inside, we can begin to let it go. For example, if we have a grudge or unresolved hatred in our heart, we may walk around with a chip on our shoulder. The world will quickly give us confirmation for our grudge or hatred because people we meet will seem cold to us as we greet everyone with the chip on our shoulder, which makes us seem cold to them.

Another example: Sometimes I get angry with my kids, but what I'm actually responding to are things I hold inside. When I realize this, my responses change. I find that practicing my quiet T'ai Chi or QiGong meditation when I get home allows me to be clearer with my kids. I clear out stuff inside, so that if I do have a problem with their blasting stereo or whatever, I am responding to that and not to something I brought home from the office (or from my childhood). By being more aware of the dynamics of our lives, we feel less like victims. We can begin to affect our world more clearly.

As our lives become less cluttered with bubbles of discord, there is more room for a limitless, flowing geyser of life energy or Qi to course through us. We become a geyser watering and nurturing everyone and everything lucky enough to be around us.

T'ai Chi and QiGong's daily pattern of reminding ourselves that we can *change* with ease, and feel safe in the world without constant muscle-tensing apprehension, is a powerful tool. Sometimes it seems as though the body literally squeezes past burdens within each and every cell. T'ai Chi's ability to allow the body to release those burdens held from the past so each cell can fill with and be nurtured by life energy is a powerful way to affirm that we are worthy of success and love. On levels deeper than we can ever understand, T'ai Chi's easy and pleasant tools help create bubbles in the deepest part of our hearts and minds that burst outward and upward in lives that reflect our very best potential. Cheers, Master! Yeah, that's you.

> **Ouch!**
>
> Modern psychology says that we are bombarded on many levels by information and stress that we never consciously perceive. Therefore, trying to attach mental reasons to feelings of being out of control, frightened, or stressed is often a futile exercise. T'ai Chi helps us let go of stress on deep levels that we will never even notice.

> **Know Your Chinese**
>
> The *I Ching* (pronounced *ee-ching*), also known as *The Book of Changes,* is an ancient Chinese book of divination. This book is used to tell fortunes or to advise people on life decisions.

> **Sage Sifu Says**
>
> The Kuang Ping Yang Style of T'ai Chi is a series of 64 integrated postures, one always changing into the other. The 64 postures symbolize the 64 possibilities of change represented in the *I Ching.* The essence of the *I Ching* is that life is a constant flow of changing circumstances. Its lesson is that we cannot find security by holding onto any one thing or way of being, but by learning to change easily and smoothly as life dictates.

Master Your Own Self

As discussed earlier, the six leading causes of death are stress related. Since stress is something that we *can* control by practicing T'ai Chi and QiGong, using these tools means that we can powerfully affect our future in a positive way.

Luck of the Draw

We all are born with natural tendencies to height or weight, or for some, diabetes or heart disease. Our genes give us those tendencies. However, we can play a big role in how those genes play out. If we drink or smoke heavily and ignore a healthy diet, we can help increase the possibility of the onset of diabetes and heart disease, while likely stunting our growth in length and expanding our growth in width.

On the other hand, we have been lucky enough to live in an age when T'ai Chi is as available as Coca-Cola. We have the ability to put an eternal ace up our sleeve, which heavily stacks the odds in our favor to live long, healthy, productive lives.

Gut Feelings: Tuning Your T'ai Chi Antennae

My T'ai Chi classes for children always began with one simple question, "Can you feel the inside of your bodies?" With little hands pressing into tiny rib cages, their puzzled faces would usually answer no. My next question was, "Have you ever felt a stomach ache or a headache?" Obviously, they all had.

T'ai Chi and QiGong are about moving the body, but it is also about feeling the body from the inside. We can feel pain inside, so we can also feel pleasure, and awareness of these feelings enables us to detect normal or abnormal function at a very early stage. By becoming attuned to our internal function, by quieting down, moving slowly, and listening to the signals inside our body, we tune our T'ai Chi antennae. We become conscious of our heart beat and our respiration rate.

What amazes most people is that we can affect our heart rate and respiration rate by using some simple QiGong methods to becoming aware of them. This is only the beginning. In my children's T'ai Chi classes, I asked children how it felt when they got nervous in school or were in trouble. They described feelings of "tight shoulders," "tight hearts," "tight chests," "hard to breathe," and so on. I asked them to make themselves feel that way, having them clench their shoulders and tighten their chests. Then I asked them to take in a deep breath and to let their chest and shoulders relax like a cloud floating in the sky on the exhale. I asked them to close their eyes and repeat this until they could feel their shoulders and chest relaxing and expanding from the inside.

Try it. Pull your shoulders way up by your ears until your shoulders are very tight, and you can feel that tension. Tighten up all your head muscles as well, and feel that tension. Now, take a deep breath, close your eyes, and let go of everything as you release the breath; feel every cell of your body releasing that breath—absolute effortlessness, absolute letting go on a cellular level. Feel how good that release feels in the muscles in your shoulders and back, and how with every breath you let out, they relax a little more. Enjoy the tingling as blood and Qi flow back into those areas.

Our body is a playground of sensation. T'ai Chi exercises and QiGong methods are games we can play in that playground. It's fun, and it makes us healthy. What a deal!

> **CAUTION**
> **Ouch!**
>
> Dr. Andrew Weil, the Harvard-educated medical doctor who now promotes Traditional Chinese Medical tools as part of his medical practice, claims shallow breathing is the main threat to our health. By becoming more conscious of our breath and breathing more fully, we may avoid the health problems many of our shallow breathing peers seem condemned to.

T'ai Chi Can Affect the World Around Us

As you practice T'ai Chi daily, you begin to find that it has an effect on the world around you, not just the world inside your body. Shao Lin folklore spoke of T'ai Chi masters being invisible. What that may have referred to is the way their nonabrasive personalities allowed them to blend in unnoticed. For example, if two men walk into the same bar, one pushy and ill-tempered and the other very unassuming, the bar will be more dangerous for the ill-tempered man.

What You See Is What You Get

In many ways we create the world we see by our expectations. If we push ourselves relentlessly, not taking time to enjoy life, we will likely see a hard-driven merciless world around us. If we are cantankerous and mean, we will likely draw out those aspects of the people we meet. If we are filled with endless desires for things that we do not have, we will see a world of scarcity and desperation. Conversely, we are generally content with what we have, we will see a world of plenty. T'ai Chi is a celebration of our existence. It slows us down each day, long enough to remember how wonderful it is just to be able to move and breathe, live and feel. It nourishes our contentment. This makes us a healing force in our world, and a healthier world makes us a healthier person.

T'ai Chi and QiGong Are Inner-Space Suits

T'ai Chi and QiGong can help us focus our view of the world.

Look out your window. Do you see a tree, the sky, traffic, smog? Move your chair until all you see is the most pleasing aspect of what your window offers you. Each time you take a break from your work, resume this position and enjoy the view.

Our lives are our minds looking through a window at the world. At any given time we can see the best our world can be or the worst it can be. In fact, the state of our world has as much or perhaps even more to do with where *we are* as it does with where the world *is*. Two people can look at the same situation and see two entirely different things. For example, one person could look at a family and see a miracle they were blessed to be a part of, while another might look at the same situation and view it as a burden on his life, a prison he is sentenced to. In fact, the same person may see his life as either of those things on any given day.

After seeing our world from space, astronauts have experienced a dramatic change in the way they viewed life. They spoke of how precious life on Earth seemed from out there; even the things we think of as annoying, the arguments, and traffic, seemed so precious from outer space.

By helping us to let go of our attachments to life's annoyances and allowing our minds to travel to "inner space," T'ai Chi and QiGong give us a view adjustment. We begin to notice that the things our children or co-workers do that are irritating are irritating because of the way we look at them. With T'ai Chi and QiGong, we get to pull back and remember how precious each moment is. What could be more helpful?

The Least You Need to Know

- ◆ T'ai Chi puts you in the center, right here and right now.
- ◆ T'ai Chi helps you cope with modern life without stress.
- ◆ T'ai Chi helps you think creatively.
- ◆ T'ai Chi changes the world, by changing your view of it.

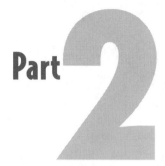

Suiting Up and Setting Out

This part prepares you for your first T'ai Chi class, fashionwise and otherwise. However, for those with T'ai Chi experience, it may also provide valuable insights on how to make your on-going T'ai Chi experience even more meaningful, both internally and externally.

Knowing when and where to do T'ai Chi can enrich your T'ai Chi experience and can even help treat certain health conditions. You will also learn the ins and outs of T'ai Chi etiquette and how to get the most out of T'ai Chi by becoming aware of the different ways it is taught.

Even advanced T'ai Chi students can benefit from this part's explanation of some of the mental and emotional challenges T'ai Chi practitioners encounter. If you're an advanced student, this part will validate your own experiences. If you're a beginner, these insights will prepare you for those same challenges so that you can ride them out and hang in there for the long beautiful haul with T'ai Chi.

This part concludes by providing you with interesting and helpful T'ai Chi and martial arts terms, so that when you enter class you'll know what's being said. More important, Part 2 will enlighten you as to the deep and long-term goals of T'ai Chi exercises, enabling you to enjoy T'ai Chi's benefits right from the beginning.

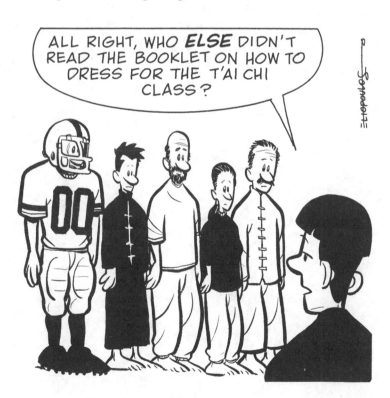

Chapter 6

Know What You Want: Finding the Right Class

In This Chapter

- ◆ Finding a place to learn
- ◆ Choosing a class
- ◆ Choosing an instructor and style that's right for you

There are many ways to learn T'ai Chi. T'ai Chi's main lesson is to find the most "effortless" way to live. Therefore, you do not want to force yourself into a square hole, being the round peg that you are. You want to find the class that best suits you. Since everyone is different, T'ai Chi is perfect because T'ai Chi can be learned in many different ways.

This chapter helps you decide what class is right for you, informing you of what's available and providing you with some questions to ask yourself. The more clear you are on what you want from T'ai Chi, the easier it will be for an instructor to fulfill those needs or to point you to another class that can.

Locating a T'ai Chi Venue

Just as T'ai Chi is good for so many different things, it is also offered in many different venues. What benefits you seek from T'ai Chi may help determine where you want to study T'ai Chi. Your options include the following:

- ◆ **Businesses.** Many company Wellness Programs are beginning to offer T'ai Chi classes for employees. Ask your employer. Of course, you may want to study T'ai Chi outside of work or in addition to the company class. Don't limit yourself to taking only the classes at work (however, many company classes are subsidized, so this can be an incentive to do it at work). If you take a work class and enjoy the instructor but would feel more comfortable with a class outside of work, ask the instructor about other classes he or she offers.

◆ **Martial arts studios.** Many of the "hard" martial arts studios specializing in karate, kung fu, or kenpo are beginning to offer T'ai Chi classes as well. In fact, a few have offered them for many years. Be aware, however, that martial arts studio classes will often focus on the martial applications of T'ai Chi. Usually, these classes will be more comfortable to someone who is interested in a more athletically demanding form of T'ai Chi. These classes may involve a gentle sparring technique known as Push Hands, although Push Hands has many mental and emotional purposes as well.

Even if you are not interested in T'ai Chi's more athletic or martial applications, you should not rule out a martial arts studio until you speak with the instructor. Instructors have their own style, and where they teach may not necessarily indicate how they teach or what their focus is.

◆ **Senior centers.** Many community centers or senior centers offer T'ai Chi classes geared toward seniors. If you have a chronic condition that limits your mobility or are rehabilitating from an injury, you may find these classes very helpful. These classes generally progress at a slower, gentler rate than T'ai Chi for the general population.

Being a senior, however, doesn't mean that these are the classes you need. Many seniors want to learn more quickly and are up to more physical challenges. As a senior, you may enjoy a general community class or even a martial arts studio class. You can't judge a T'ai Chi-er by his cover. In fact, the more you do T'ai Chi, the younger your "cover" is going to look.

◆ **Community center and hospital classes.** Many cities' parks and recreation departments now offer T'ai Chi classes, as do many hospitals. These classes are usually for the general population and will include students of all ages. Generally, these classes will progress through learning movements at a little faster pace than the senior program classes do. However, even the briskest pace is usually quite manageable if you spend a little time each day practicing between your weekly or semi-weekly classes.

◆ **Church classes.** Many houses of worship now offer T'ai Chi classes. Understanding T'ai Chi is to know that it is a health science and not a religion. Yet, T'ai Chi's promotion of quiet mindfulness is beneficial to anyone's spirituality. Therefore, if your church offers T'ai Chi classes, you may enjoy the spiritual focus of the instructor.

◆ **Colleges and universities.** Usually T'ai Chi is part of the adult continuing education departments of colleges and universities, although many schools now offer accredited T'ai Chi programs. In the continuing education departments, these classes are often introductory courses that give you a sample of what T'ai Chi offers. This tendency occurs because colleges require minimum enrollments to continue classes. Since advanced classes are often too small to sustain through colleges, many quality instructors will offer these intro programs so that students can meet them and then continue advanced study through private studio programs.

◆ **Support groups.** Many support groups for Parkinson's disease, multiple sclerosis, fibromyalgia, or AIDS (to name a few) may facilitate ongoing T'ai Chi classes for their members. In the Kansas City area, for example, I am working with the local Veterans Hospital to provide T'ai Chi classes specifically geared toward wheelchair practitioners. I am also encouraging hospitals to design rooms with hooks in the ceiling for "climbing harnesses," thereby enabling people with balance disorders to practice T'ai Chi without worrying about falling injuries.

If you are a wheelchair practitioner, you can participate in regular T'ai Chi classes by simply modifying the movements to suit your needs. Interview instructors to find one who can fit your needs. You will need to make your own innovations of the movements if the instructor has no experience with wheelchair students. Also, you may want to take the beginning class more than once since you will have more to cover than your standing peers will.

If you have special needs or conditions, you should contact your local hospitals to request T'ai Chi classes geared to your needs. If you have a support group, organize them to encourage the hospital to innovate. T'ai Chi is about forming lives that fit our needs, and creating your T'ai Chi class can be a great T'ai Chi exercise. Have fun and be creative!

Sage Sifu Says

Try not to use only your head when choosing a T'ai Chi class. Just because the school looks nice, or the credentials sound great, or the instructor has studied for a gazillion years doesn't mean that it is the right school for you. When you talk with the instructor, ask yourself, "How do I feel about this person?" That is the most important question.

Also, do not compare yourself to other students in your T'ai Chi class. Some will be more flexible, some will be less flexible, and none of that matters at all. Lao Tzu said that he who does not contend is beyond reproach. You are always perfect, now and after years of practice.

Choosing a Class

Again, choosing your class depends on your needs. What can you afford? What do you seek to accomplish? Once you decide on the questions to ask, call around and speak to many different instructors. If they are available, take workshops or sample classes through community education programs. This will give you an opportunity to meet the instructors face to face and experience their instruction before enrolling in a long-term class (although most T'ai Chi classes run for only 6 to 10 weeks at a time).

What Is the Cost?

It's helpful to look at T'ai Chi as if it were health insurance. If you pay now with a little money for the class and some time each day to practice, you will reap the benefits for the rest of your life. You will also likely be more productive and make more money in the future. You'll be more relaxed and do less "impulsive" buying, which will save you money, too. T'ai Chi is a very inexpensive investment with a very high return.

T'ai Sci
Research shows that stress costs businesses $7,500 per employee per year, driving up our health care costs. To fight stress-related health costs, some insurance companies and health care providers now pay for or subsidize the cost of T'ai Chi and/or QiGong classes for their clients. Call your insurance carrier to ask if your T'ai Chi class tuition can be rebated or credited on your premiums. Get a receipt from your instructor.

The cost of T'ai Chi classes is often determined by the location and by the quality of the instruction. For example, many martial arts studios have longer contracts, which, of course, requires a larger up-front investment. Each studio is different, though, so call and inquire.

No matter what your income level, you will likely be able to find T'ai Chi you can afford. There are many T'ai Chi hobbyists that offer very low-cost classes through YMCAs or other community centers. Although these instructors may not be as highly trained as those teaching in the more expensive locations, you can still benefit from attending these classes. Also, higher cost does not guarantee higher-quality instruction. If an instructor has studied for many years, he will likely be better than one who has studied for only a year or two, no matter the location.

However, to maximize your T'ai Chi experience, you will likely have to pay a bit more. Still, even the highest-quality instruction is usually no more than $10 or $15 per class or $80 to $120 per 8-week session (cities vary in cost). In most cities, this is about the cost of a movie, popcorn, and a soda. Not a bad investment for something that can change your life. Also, if you are a member of a senior center or support group, your organization may be eligible for a grant. Available grants may enable you to get very high quality T'ai Chi instruction at little or no cost to participants.

How Often Should I Go?

Different locations will offer different programs, but one T'ai Chi class per week is the most common arrangement. Each class usually runs between an hour to an hour and a half. Some studios may offer two or more classes per week.

> **Ouch!**
>
> Most people don't practice enough, but don't go berserk and burn yourself out either. Once or twice a day is good for a full session. However, if you're having a tough day at work and want to sneak off for a quick T'ai Chi session in the bathroom or empty boardroom, go for it.

There is nothing wrong with going to several classes a week if you can afford it, as long as you don't do it to the point of burn out. However, one class per week is more than enough, as long as you practice at home during the week. In the beginning you may only practice at home for about 10 minutes a day, but over time your practice will get longer as you learn more movements. Eventually you won't have to think about practicing because you'll look forward to it. Whenever you're having a rough day or maybe when you want to celebrate having a good day, you may find yourself slipping out to "play" T'ai Chi. You'll also want to do T'ai Chi when you get home so that you'll be in a better mood to fully enjoy your evening.

Evaluating an Instructor

There are many things to consider as you look for your T'ai Chi instructor. The degrees or awards your potential instructor holds matters very little. More important is whether your instructor's temperament feels good to you. Another consideration is the style of T'ai Chi you want to learn.

> **Sage Sifu Says**
>
> Because it's new and slow, you may at first find T'ai Chi a little frustrating. This is not uncommon. Remember to breathe and let go of frustrations you feel as you release your breath. Also, you may catch yourself displacing your frustration on the instructor. Be aware that this can happen so don't give up on a good instructor for the wrong reasons. The more you can lighten up on yourself, the more the people around you can lighten up as well, including your instructor.

Instructor Personality

One good question to ask a prospective instructor is, "Do you still study with other T'ai Chi teachers?" If a T'ai Chi teacher still studies, it tells you that she understands the great depth and endless width of the art and science of T'ai Chi. T'ai Chi expands for a lifetime, just as we expand as living beings, always growing and learning.

> **Ouch!**
>
> If doing a particular movement doesn't feel right, discuss it with your instructor. Make adjustments on your own as well; everybody does T'ai Chi his own way. Of course there is a proper form, but it takes time for the body to adjust, and for some with injuries or physical conditions that limit movement, although your range of motion will increase, you may never do it just the way your instructor does, and that is perfectly okay. The way you do it is perfect for you.

Secondly, what is your focus? Are you interested in treating an illness, growing spiritually, or the martial applications of T'ai Chi? The answer to this question will help you know what to ask your prospective instructor. For example, if you have a high-stress corporate career, you may feel comfortable with a T'ai Chi instructor who has experienced that lifestyle and can offer you ways to use the tools he teaches in ways meaningful to your life. Or if your desire is spiritual growth, you may seek an instructor who focuses more on that aspect of T'ai Chi. If you have a particular health problem, you may connect well with a teacher who has the same problem. T'ai Chi is, however, multidimensional in approaches and benefits, so any instructor from any walk of life will be good for you if you feel comfortable and accepted in their presence.

What I needed personally as a T'ai Chi student was patience. I needed an instructor who didn't scold and patiently allowed me to grow at my own pace. Of course the art of patience is at the core of T'ai Chi, so if your teacher isn't patient on a regular basis, they probably aren't living their T'ai Chi.

You will want a teacher who actually uses the tools they teach and has benefited from them in their lives. You don't want a teacher who's simply teaching because the health club or hospital they work for told them to learn it so they could teach it. If a T'ai Chi teacher is actively using the tools, they are getting better at using them, and they are growing and expanding as a human being, which makes them better at everything they do, including teaching T'ai Chi.

T'ai Chi instruction is not like a regular job. The instructor should be someone who uses the tools and is immersed in the art of personal growth. This doesn't mean that they are some kind of saint. Don't fall into the trap of thinking the T'ai Chi instructor is "above" the trials and tribulations of normal life. A good teacher is someone who lives all that stuff and is lucky enough to have learned the wonderful tools T'ai Chi offers to make the absolute most out of what life offers. A good teacher is therefore not above fear, stress, and worry, but they are learning how to use T'ai Chi to grow as best they can and can communicate to you how they've coped, and how T'ai Chi might help you cope as well.

A T'ai Chi teacher doesn't tell you what's right or how to grow. They explain how the growth tools that T'ai Chi offers has helped them grow. Whatever truth resonates to you is what you take. A T'ai Chi teacher's life, or health, or balance, may not even be as good as yours, but it is much better than it would be if they didn't practice T'ai Chi. Therefore, a T'ai Chi instructor can teach a prize fighter how to punch harder and a basketball star how to shoot better, even though the athlete could soundly defeat the T'ai Chi teacher in their sport. A T'ai Chi teacher teaches the tools of growth, but we all grow in our own ways and at our own pace.

T'ai Chi Styles

The teacher is more important than the style; however, if all teachers are equal, you may decide on a T'ai Chi class by which style you are attracted to. There are several different major T'ai Chi styles. They all have most of the common benefits, and which you choose depends on what looks good to you. The major styles are listed the following list. Most style names reflect the family name of their original creators.

There are many styles of T'ai Chi and every style can be done by everybody. If 30 different people are in a room doing the same style, you'll see 30 different ways to do it because we all move differently. A good instructor will realize this and may correct a way you are doing it, but will accept it when you say, "My body doesn't do it that way, yet, but I'm working on it." So while always striving for perfection being continually contented with where you are, grounded in the reality *that you are always evolving perfection*.

The following list of styles is not comprehensive. It only lists some of the more popular styles. Your local bookstore or the Internet are good resources for finding information on a wider selection of T'ai Chi forms.

- The extent **Yang Style,** founded by Yang Lu-chan who studied under Chen Style creator Chen Chang-hsing, is widely practiced in the United States and China. Yang Lu-chan was eventually invited to teach T'ai Chi to the Imperial Court, and became known as "Yang the Unsurpassed."

◆ The **Kuang Ping Yang Style** of T'ai Chi exhibited in this book, was brought to the United States by Kuo Lien-ying in the 1960s. Kuo trained under Wan Ch'un (a student of Yang Pan-hou, the son of Yang Founder Yang Lu-chan).

◆ The **Chen Style** founder, Chen Chang-hsing, is only four generations removed from T'ai Chi's originator, Cheng San-feng, making the Chen Style closest to the original creator of T'ai Chi. The Chen family split into two forms referred to as the "New Frame" and the "Old Frame." The more extent New Frame is based on the same original 13 postures the Yang, Wu, and Kuang Ping Yang Styles are.

◆ The **Wu Style** was founded by Wu Quan-yu, a student of the originator of the Yang Style, Yang Lu-chan, and his son, Yang Pan-hou. Wu Quan-yu was Manchurian by race and worked as a bodyguard in the Imperial Court in Beijing. Because of his skill in T'ai Chi and his renown, he did much to help spread knowledge of T'ai Chi Chuan. Some say that the smaller and more restricted movements of the Wu style were due to Master Wu's training in the restrictive clothing of the Imperial Court, and would therefore be an ideal self-defense training for use in modern street clothes.

◆ **Mulan Quan** is a modern form, founded by Sifu Mei Fing Ying. Mulan is named after the legendary young woman Fa Mulan (who's name translates to "wooden orchid"). Besides its basic hand form, Mulan Quan offers a Sword Style, as do some other forms, and also a somewhat unique Fan Style. Although derived from the nearly extinct form, Hua Chia Chan, its founder simplified its forms and added more *wushu* (martial arts). The form was approved by martial arts masters and named Mulan Quan in 1988.

Each style varies a bit depending on the instructor. T'ai Chi is a living art, and it changes and grows as it is passed down through the generations. The Chinese masters said, "Learn T'ai Chi exactly as you are taught, your personality will polish it effortlessly." So, for example, even if you study Yang style T'ai Chi, your forms will likely be a bit different from other schools of the same style. No one is wrong or right, just different. Just as each rose has its own *unique* beauty, but each is beautiful. It would be comical for a rose to strut around the garden proclaiming that its beauty was superior.

However, there are certain tenets that all T'ai Chi adheres to and must be observed by all students. Some concepts include the dan tien, vertical axis, effortless flexibility, and mindfulness, which will be discussed in detail later in Chapter 9, "Saddle Up: Horse Stance and Other Terms."

Some styles have modified "fast" versions. In fact, all T'ai Chi can be done at varying speeds, and it is fun to experiment with different rhythms and speeds. However, in class your instructor will probably move quite slowly. Some styles also offer advanced students variations that use swords or fans.

> **CAUTION**
> **Ouch!**
>
> If you have arthritis or a balance disorder, be cautious of the "fast" forms. It doesn't mean they are bad for you, but you have to be your own best advisor as to what you want to do. Listen to your body; do what feels right.

The Least You Need to Know

◆ T'ai Chi classes can be found almost anywhere.

◆ No matter your needs, a class can be found to fill them.

◆ No matter what your budget is, T'ai Chi is affordable.

◆ Ask your insurance carrier if they pay for T'ai Chi.

◆ Attend class weekly and practice daily.

◆ The best instructor for you is one you like.

◆ The best style is the one that looks fun to you.

Chapter 7

Plan Ahead: Where and When to Practice T'ai Chi

In This Chapter

♦ Finding the best place and time to do T'ai Chi

♦ Getting the most for your T'ai Chi bucks

♦ Ways to make time for T'ai Chi

This chapter explains where and when to do T'ai Chi, as well as what to wear. You will discover that these questions are not only a matter of etiquette or convenience, but can also affect the health benefits you get from T'ai Chi.

You will discover the advantages of a large class vs. private instruction, video/book instruction vs. live classes, and also tips on how to make time for whatever T'ai Chi program you choose.

Home Practice vs. Class Study

Although practicing at home by yourself on a regular basis is how T'ai Chi's benefits are realized, studying with a qualified instructor is an essential part of the success of your home practice. No matter how many years you study T'ai Chi, you can still benefit from studying in classes. T'ai Chi, like life, is an endless growth process.

Most of us in the modern world want fast answers. We like to take classes or workshops and move on. And sometimes our educational motivation has more to do with getting our hands on a piece of paper that says we know something, than with personally being changed by the knowledge.

Therefore, most people rush through a T'ai Chi course to learn a few moves and then think they are done. Of course, you do get some benefit from any exposure to T'ai Chi. You can learn things on the first day that can benefit the rest of your life. But why stop there? T'ai Chi can offer you a deep ocean of experience. After 20 years of T'ai Chi practice, I still study with my instructor, and even though the very first class was beneficial and wonderful, I still find benefit that carries into my home practice in each and every class.

T'ai Chi provides life-long benefits and should be practiced for the rest of our lives. However, this isn't a marriage contract. Don't feel smothered by this. Drop in and out of T'ai Chi as often as you like. T'ai Chi will always be patiently waiting for you when you come back, like a touchstone or a port in a storm. Eventually you will do T'ai Chi simply because you feel pretty spectacular when you do. Besides finding classes personally enjoyable, you will discover that T'ai Chi attracts interesting people, and the social aspect will draw you as well.

Bookworm T'ai Chi

T'ai Chi books are great for helping you understand the philosophy, art, and science of T'ai Chi, and as supplements to classes. However, a book cannot replace a live instructor or the other benefits of a class.

It is difficult in books to explain how the body moves through movements because books are dependent on still photographs. The ability to see an instructor move and to ask for clarification or hear the questions of other students is invaluable. Also, it is easier in person for instructors to explain things in stages while you relax, whereas when using a book, facts must be remembered because the instructor isn't there to remind you.

Video T'ai Chi

If you do not have access to T'ai Chi classes, a video is the next best way to learn. Also, you can use books to supplement your understanding of what videos teach. Using books and videos together can help maximize the benefit of your T'ai Chi practice. As the videos teach visually and audibly enabling your mind to relax, the books round out your intellectual understanding of the movements and exercises.

Consider that the average 8-week introductory T'ai Chi class entails at least 12 hours of instruction. The average T'ai Chi video is one hour. You can see that it is difficult for an instructor to explain a 2,000-year-old art and science that is so rich in benefits in a 1-hour video. Some videos are done in multivolume, several-hour sets, which is the best way to go if you do not have access to live T'ai Chi classes. Your author, Bill Douglas, offers multivolume T'ai Chi video courses for individuals and corporate wellness programs in the back of this book. These are great if you have no access to live classes, but again go for the live class if you can.

Videos can be great supplements to your ongoing T'ai Chi class, especially if your instructor has produced one or approves one for the class. Be aware however that even if a video covers the same style you are studying, the style may look different. If you are in a class, check with your instructor before purchasing a video. Bookstores, magazine ads, and martial arts stores are usually good places to find an assortment of T'ai Chi videos.

The Horary Clock

Acupuncture, Chinese herbal medicine, and T'ai Chi understand that the body has natural rhythms that align with certain organs and functions. You can actually use this "horary" (hourly) clock to treat problems. Each organ has certain hours called peak hours. These peak hours are generally the best for treating these organs and are listed in the chart below:

- 11 A.M. to 1 P.M.: Heart
- 1 P.M. to 3 P.M.: Small intestine
- 3 P.M. to 5 P.M.: Bladder
- 5 P.M. to 7 P.M.: Kidney
- 7 P.M. to 9 P.M.: Pericardium

- 9 P.M. to 11 P.M.: Triple burner
- 11 P.M. to 1 A.M.: Gallbladder
- 1 A.M. to 3 A.M.: Liver
- 3 A.M. to 5 A.M.: Lung
- 5 A.M. to 7 A.M.: Large Intestine
- 7 A.M. to 9 A.M.: Stomach
- 9 A.M. to 11 A.M.: Spleen

> **Know Your Chinese**
>
> In Traditional Chinese Medicine, the word **tonify** means to strengthen, energize, and imbue with health. Therefore, it can be applied to Qi, blood, tissue, organs, or processes in the body or mind.

In Part 3, "Starting Down the QiGong Path to T'ai Chi," I will introduce some QiGong exercises for specific organs. However, T'ai Chi can generally tonify all the aspects of the body and every organ. Therefore, T'ai Chi practice at a peak hour could provide a good therapy. Yet, if your peak hour is in the middle of the night, you may prefer a sitting or lying QiGong exercise to focus Qi into the desired organ. The sitting QiGong exercise in Part 3 will give you a great technique to use in peak hours.

Outdoor vs. Indoor

The single most important thing about practicing T'ai Chi is that you actually do practice it. Where you practice is secondary. The following recommendation to do T'ai Chi outdoors should not be construed to mean that you should not practice inside. If you can do T'ai Chi outdoors, do so. However, if you don't feel comfortable doing it outside because of where you live or the weather, then by all means do it inside.

Practicing Outdoors

The purpose of T'ai Chi and other QiGong exercises is to promote the flow of Qi. Qi's life energy flows through us and all living things. Therefore, the Chinese have always advocated performing T'ai Chi outdoors where you can enjoy and benefit from the Qi of other living things. In fact, Traditional Chinese Medicine teaches that when we do T'ai Chi, our relaxed body and mind benefit from nature's healing energy even more.

We all know that just being in nature has a soothing quality, so if T'ai Chi can magnify this benefit, all the better. The word "mesmerize" is derived from the name of the famous Dr. Mesma. Dr. Mesma worked with patients suffering from psychotic episodes. Reportedly, Dr. Mesma would instruct his patients to sit with their backs up against a tree whenever they felt an episode coming on, and his patients were said to benefit greatly from this "nature therapy."

As you practice T'ai Chi in your backyard, the park, or even around the plants in your house, you may experience the benefits of this therapy for yourself.

Choosing a Surface

T'ai Chi should be practiced on a level, predictable surface, especially when you are beginning. As you play over the years, you may experiment with more uneven and challenging surfaces.

T'ai Chi can be performed on grass, sand, dirt, or pavement. It is good to practice on varying types of surfaces because this gives your mind/body communication even more information for improving your balance.

> **Sage Sifu Says**
>
> Your balance fluctuates from day to day, yet like a bullish stock market it is always improving. So on days when your balance is at its worst, don't think you are not benefiting from T'ai Chi. Rather, let go of constantly measuring your progress. Enjoy your loss of balance even as much as you enjoy the T'ai Chi on days when your balance is great.

Try to choose a flat area, out of direct sunlight. Soft morning sunlight or evening light is all right, but do not practice in direct sunlight during the hot part of the day. You will discover that practicing T'ai Chi in different light is challenging as well. Doing T'ai Chi in the dimming light of sunset challenges you to use more internal and less external balance references.

Practicing Indoors

The benefits of doing T'ai Chi indoors are pretty obvious if it's freezing, smoldering hot, or the mosquito population is in full production. Though outdoors is optimum, T'ai Chi benefits can be had anywhere and anytime.

> **CAUTION Ouch!**
>
> When you run out of room doing T'ai Chi, you adjust by moving back two steps and then resume. Most people live in cities, and this "apartment T'ai Chi" is how most T'ai Chi must be done. Don't psych yourself into thinking you cannot practice T'ai Chi because your house isn't big enough. These are not limitations but opportunities to learn flexibility in mind as well as body.

Again, when you are having a tough day at the office, it's great to slip off to the restroom or the supply room to drift into a T'ai Chi getaway. If you practice T'ai Chi at home before work or in the evening, it is often just more convenient to practice inside.

One problem students encounter indoors is space. As you move through your T'ai Chi repertoire, you often will cover more ground than your living room provides. If the next step takes you through a wall, just remember where you are at, move back a couple steps, and pick up where you left off. Eventually, you won't even think about it. T'ai Chi pours into your living room, just like it easily and naturally flows into your life. Just as T'ai Chi encourages an almost liquid relaxation of mind and body, its use and benefits can seem to pour into every nook and cranny of our lives with much benefit.

Last, but not least, when doing T'ai Chi indoors, you should minimize noise by turning off the TV and stereo; don't let noises beyond your control be an issue. Noise is in the ear of the beholder.

Large Class vs. Private Class

Surprisingly, learning in a large class has several advantages over more expensive private lessons, although both have their own strengths, depending on your needs.

The Pros and Cons of Large Classes

If an instructor is in great demand, their classes will inevitably be larger. Therefore, you will get less personal attention but will benefit from their quality of instruction. On the other hand you may find instructors in less demand with smaller classes that can provide you with more personal instruction. Decide what your priorities are and then choose a class size that meets your needs.

You can learn very effectively in a large class setting. In fact, there are distinct advantages to being in a large class. As fellow classmates ask questions for clarification, you can benefit by their inquiries. Also, you will discover that there is a group energy to T'ai Chi classes. Just as plants emit life energy, so do other people, and as your classmates practice T'ai Chi, you can bask in the glow of their presence.

Usually, an accomplished T'ai Chi instructor will have numerous advanced students who will help as assistants. In a larger class, you can benefit from the expertise these students have to offer. Note that advanced students probably are less than perfect, but so is the instructor. You will learn T'ai Chi in layers, and the advanced students can give you a layer of instruction that the instructor can add to or polish over the months and years.

T'ai Chi classes will benefit you even if you take them for a short time, providing you with tools you can use for the rest of your life. However, it is best to take classes for a lifetime. It is fun, beneficial, and a great way to meet interesting people, so why not? By doing so, you have no deadline or rush to progress at a certain speed. If you practice everyday for a few minutes you will likely learn the forms quite easily. However, if you need to repeat the beginning class again, and again, that is no problem.

If you are in a large class, you may have to move around a bit to see what the instructor is doing. Move to wherever you need to be to see. T'ai Chi is very informal. Usually, in a very large class there will be advanced students positioned in various locations so that you can follow them if you cannot see the instructor clearly. If you aren't sure what is being taught, raise your hand and ask for clarification. Don't be shy about this. The best T'ai Chi classes are ones where students interact and ask questions. The least productive classes are those where the teacher does all the talking.

> **Ouch!**
>
> Do not assume the instructor is aware of a problem you have with a movement or the class program. Ask questions during class to clarify instruction. However, if you have concerns about the program, discuss it with the instructor after class. Before you stop attending a T'ai Chi class in frustration, discuss concerns with the instructor. Most instructors want to help you get it—that's why they're there.

The Pros and Cons of Private Lesson

Very few people get private lessons. Part of the reason is that they can be very expensive. A good T'ai Chi instructor usually will begin at about $75 per hour and can go up significantly from there.

However, some people, such as emergency room physicians, have erratic, demanding schedules and are forced to take private lessons. This is a highly effective way to learn the T'ai Chi forms in a very short period of time because the instructor's entire focus is on your learning.

Private lessons can also be beneficial to those learning to be instructors, thereby enabling them to learn minute details and background on movements and their purpose.

> **T'ai Sci**
>
> Any malady should be discussed with a physician. However, in addition to your medical doctor, you may want to discuss your condition with a certified doctor of Traditional Chinese Medicine. Using QiGong on your own can be a powerful adjunct therapy for a condition you may be treating; however, if used under the direction of a Traditional Chinese Medical practitioner, it may be even more effective.

Time Out for Class and Practice

To maximize your benefit of T'ai Chi practice, it's best to spend about 20 minutes in the morning doing T'ai Chi or a sitting QiGong meditation exercise. Spend another 20 minutes in the evening doing whichever one you didn't do in the morning. Usually the first response to this suggestion is, "I don't have an extra 40 minutes a day!"

If that is your response, ask yourself the following questions:

- ◆ Do you spend 40 minutes a day watching television?
- ◆ Do you spend your morning and afternoon breaks drinking soda or coffee and chatting?
- ◆ Do you ever spend time eagerly waiting to access the Internet, or waiting for the computer to print, or dinner to bake?

For most of us, the answer to at least one of these questions is yes. This shows you that you probably do have an extra 40 minutes a day. So the main difficulty in doing T'ai Chi isn't really having the time, but deciding to do it. When we decide to do it, we find that we will make time. Beginning new life habits is one of the single most difficult things people attempt. But T'ai Chi is worth it.

Life Habits Are Hard to Change

T'ai Chi is new for you. You will find that it will take time to get used to doing it every day. Don't punish or scold yourself when you forget. Just enjoy it when you do it. The following example will help you see just how difficult it is to change life habits, so you can go easy on yourself as you begin to adapt to a new life with T'ai Chi.

A study of cardiac recovery patients shows just how difficult it is to change. Patients were given a choice of two therapies to follow after their heart attacks. The first was only to take medication and be released within days. Unfortunately, that first choice carried a prognosis of another possible major heart attack within a few months. The second choice involved staying in the hospital for a much longer period to learn stress-management techniques and new dietary changes and offered a much rosier forecast of the patients likely going several years before another coronary. Amazingly, nearly all the patients opted to leave immediately, even though it increased the likelihood of a premature death.

What is ironic about T'ai Chi is that even though it may be difficult to incorporate into your life at first, it will make all other healthy life changes much easier. Again, T'ai Chi is a technology designed to help us change with less effort and stress. Therefore, the longer we practice T'ai Chi, the easier it is for us to change. So if you decide to go on a healthier diet, stop smoking, or start getting out in nature more, the effort you make to learn T'ai Chi will make all these other efforts to change more "effortless."

T'ai Chi Is Positively Effortless

Studies show that when we change for positive reasons, we are much more likely to change our habits. Therefore, rather than do T'ai Chi because your blood pressure is high or your stress levels are unbearable, do T'ai Chi because it feels good. Don't rush through your T'ai Chi, but make it a little oasis in your busy day. Slow down enough to feel the pleasure of the movement and the stretches. Enjoy how good it feels to breathe deeply and let the whole body relax. This will condition you day by day to love the feeling T'ai Chi gives you, causing you to look forward to it and miss it when you don't do it.

Make a Calendar

Create a T'ai Chi calendar and place it on your refrigerator door. Every time you do your T'ai Chi or QiGong, mark a big X on that day's square. As you begin to get a few days in a row, you will want to keep that string going. You will also begin to notice that the more Xs you have on the calendar, the better you feel. Your awareness becomes more subtle and pleasant, which will help you make the transition from doing T'ai Chi for the calendar accomplishment to doing it for how it makes you feel.

Social T'ai Chi

T'ai Chi clubs are increasingly popular in the United States, as they have been in China for centuries. This is because even though T'ai Chi is a terrific personal exercise and is thoroughly enjoyable alone, it can also be a terrific social event. There is a group energy that T'ai Chi clubs offer that can heighten the pleasure T'ai Chi provides.

T'ai Chi clubs also are very supportive and encourage T'ai Chi players to practice on their own. When we have a class or a club to get together with, we are much more likely to practice on your own at home. We want to improve our T'ai Chi so that we can play more complex T'ai Chi games using mirror image forms and other games involving several players. Therefore, continuing with a T'ai Chi class or club for the rest of your life is a great way to stick with T'ai Chi for the long haul. Social T'ai Chi is also terrific since T'ai Chi practice can extend your life substantially; if you outlive all your peers you won't be lonely because you'll still have your T'ai Chi club to hang out with.

The Least You Need to Know

- ◆ If you don't have access to live classes, videos and books can be used.
- ◆ Although outdoor T'ai Chi is optimum, indoor T'ai Chi is great, too.
- ◆ Treat certain organs by using the "horary" clock.
- ◆ Large classes can be great if you ask questions.
- ◆ Use a calendar to get used to practicing, until T'ai Chi becomes an integral part of your life.

Chapter 8

Be Prepared: Your First Day of Class

In This Chapter

- ◆ Picking your T'ai Chi wardrobe
- ◆ Preparing mentally and physically for class
- ◆ Knowing what is expected of you
- ◆ Learning the terms

In this chapter, you will learn what to wear to do T'ai Chi. Yet beyond fashion concerns, this chapter also prepares you mentally, emotionally, and physically for your first day of class. Even those currently involved in T'ai Chi will find these mental and emotional insights into T'ai Chi challenges helpful.

This chapter will provide you with many ways to get the most out of T'ai Chi training by explaining class structure, what is expected of you, and clarifying terms you may encounter in class.

Choosing Your T'ai Chi Wardrobe

Ultimately you can do T'ai Chi in any kind of clothing, but certain clothing *is* suggested for class. Typically, T'ai Chi students wear anything they want. It is helpful to wear something loose and stretchy and to leave jewelry at home; however, the rest is often up to you. The most common T'ai Chi suit is a T-shirt and sweat pants. Spandex or body suits, although not prohibited, are not typically worn in T'ai Chi. Also, longer dresses can make it more difficult for an instructor to see posture or leg placement, but if your class is in an office environment, don't worry about it.

If you practice T'ai Chi at the office, everyone will likely be wearing office clothes, but they will kick off their heels. If you go from the office to a studio or community class or if your company holds classes in an exercise area, bring some sweats and tennis shoes to change into.

Some studios, especially martial arts studios, may require more formal attire. If they do, they will direct you to a martial arts supply store that sells the appropriate garb, or the studio may provide them.

> CAUTION
>
> **Ouch!**
>
> Some Chinese masters caution against practicing T'ai Chi barefoot because it opens the feet up to "pernicious influences." This sounds sinister, but it may only mean that you could chill if the ground is cold or pick up an infection if the ground is dirty. Conversely, others say it is good to practice barefoot because it connects you to the earth, whereas your rubber shoes electrically isolate you from it.

Footwear depends on the location. For most T'ai Chi classes, tennis shoes are fine. However, some studios that offer T'ai Chi, such as martial arts or yoga studios, will require bare feet. It is not advisable to wear only socks in these studios because socks can be slippery. If you need arch support and attend a class in these locations, you may be able to wear tennis shoes that have never been used on the street or Chinese kung fu shoes. These nonstreet shoes will not damage the floor, but check with the instructor before purchasing them.

The only hard and fast rule that all instructors follow on footwear is that you cannot wear heeled shoes. This is hard on your back, makes balance difficult, and changes the way the whole body moves. If doing T'ai Chi at the office, just kick off your heels, or bring tennis shoes if they feel more comfortable.

Considering External and Internal Hygiene

T'ai Chi has very few external hygiene rules, but internally, it is good to prepare yourself mentally and emotionally by letting go of some myths about yourself and exercise.

External Hygiene

Unlike most other martial arts, T'ai Chi usually requires no contact between participants. Therefore, hygiene rules are pretty much like daily life. You will be in fairly close proximity to others, so if your job leaves you a little ripe, you may want to shower prior to T'ai Chi class. However, if you come to class from the office, there shouldn't be a problem. The only concern might be if you attend class at a studio that requires you to go barefoot. If you go straight from the office to one of these classes, you might just buy some handy-wipe wet towelettes and clean your feet off prior to going into class.

Don't wear heavy cologne or perfume into class because the deep breathing in T'ai Chi may make it overwhelming to others. Again, jewelry should be left at home, especially jangly jewelry.

Internal Hygiene

The clutter in our mind, heart, and body is the most important thing to cleanse prior to attending your first—or one hundredth—T'ai Chi class.

In the long run T'ai Chi will help relieve allergy problems, but if you have heavy allergies and are heavily medicated, it may be helpful to lighten up on the medications prior to T'ai Chi. That is, if your medications make your balance more difficult or make it harder to focus. However, never adjust prescription medication without your doctor's approval. If you haven't tried acupuncture for your allergies, try it. It can be a terrific nonpharmaceutical way to alleviate allergy symptoms with great results. Acupuncture treatments cannot harm, but can enhance your clarity or balance.

T'ai Chi and Massage Therapy

T'ai Chi is meant to loosen the mind and body and increase internal awareness. Tension disconnects the mind from the body. Therefore, you may find it very complementary to begin massage therapy prior to your first T'ai Chi class and to continue massage therapy for the rest of your life. Most good T'ai Chi teachers will advocate massage therapy as part of your T'ai Chi training, just as many good massage therapists will recommend T'ai Chi to their clients. You also will find that massage therapy will be helpful in relieving chronic problems such as allergies.

> **Sage Sifu Says**
>
> As T'ai Chi teaches the body to move and change more easily and effortlessly, it provides a model for the mind and heart to change more easily, too. Therefore, as you continue with T'ai Chi, you may discover you eat healthier, drink more water and less soda, get better rest, adopt habits like regular massage therapy, and spend more time with people who make you feel good about yourself.

Resistance to Change

T'ai Chi helps us change. Our mind and body get accustomed to the way we have always done things, even things that are not really that good for us. Therefore, on a subconscious level, parts of us resist good changes that T'ai Chi fosters because we don't want to let go of the way we have always been. Part of us likes to be a "couch potato" and doesn't like the way T'ai Chi is getting us more involved in an active life. Resistance to change may manifest itself in many ways.

Resistance may do the following:

- Cause you to scold yourself, to tell yourself you are too clumsy, too uncoordinated, too slow, or too tired to do T'ai Chi.
- Tell you T'ai Chi is for other people who are better, smarter, stronger, or more coordinated than you are.
- Tell you that the teacher doesn't like you or that T'ai Chi is dumb and useless.
- Tell you that it would be much more fun to watch TV and eat potato chips tonight, rather than going all the way out to your T'ai Chi class.
- If you miss a class, resistance will tell you, "You're already too far behind; don't go back there."

If you hang in there long enough, however, you will discover that after nearly every T'ai Chi class, you will feel much better than you did before going. If you become conscious of the voices of "resistance," you will be more likely to stick with T'ai Chi.

"Wrongness" Is Our Culture's "Resistance"

Your T'ai Chi progress will be held back by something that affects our entire culture. If you understand this, it will take a great deal of pressure off of you and your instructor. Most Western students are obsessed with learning the T'ai Chi movements "perfectly," and this causes them stress, which slows their ability to learn and enjoy T'ai Chi. In fact, we often convince ourselves that our attempts to learn are so "imperfect" that it is pointless to continue with our study.

T'ai Chi will show you on a very basic level that you are never "wrong." You are growing and learning how to do things better and better each and every day of your life. T'ai Chi is simple enough to use the very first day of practice, but its richness is so

> **Ouch!**
>
> Students often obsess on remembering each detail the instructor tells them; some even bring a pad and pencil to class. Don't do that. Relax. Good instructors will repeat important things over and over. Let yourself enjoy the class. Don't make T'ai Chi class another "important," "serious" thing in your life. Let it be playtime.

subtle that you can refine your T'ai Chi movements for the rest of your life. Therefore, you do not need to "perfect" the first movement before learning the second. You learn a layer of the movements, and learning that layer changes who you are and how you function. Your new and improved self can then learn the movements at yet a deeper, more subtle level, and so on for years and years. T'ai Chi leaves you in an endlessly blooming state of perfection.

Attending Your First Class

When entering your first class, you probably aren't sure what it will look like, how to treat the instructor, or what is expected of you. So let's look at these expectations one at a time.

Mainly, you will be expected to relax and enjoy yourself. You will also have a little homework, but as you'll see, this could be the best homework you ever had.

How to Address Your Instructor

The question of how to address your instructor has several possible answers. The safest way to find out what is right for the class you enroll in is to simply ask the teacher how they would like to be addressed. The formal Chinese term for T'ai Chi teacher is *Sifu* (pronounced *see-foo*), meaning "master of an art or skill." However, many T'ai Chi classes in the West are very informal. Most instructors simply go by their first name.

If a Chinese teacher asks you to call him or her Sifu, this is not because of an ego trip. Actually, this is a great compliment. This means that they consider you a worthy student, and that is an honor.

> **Sage Sifu Says** _____
>
> You can get all the benefits from T'ai Chi without straining. You don't have to memorize all the terms, or do the movements exactly like your teacher does, or read any certain books. T'ai Chi's amazing benefits will come to you by simply breathing deeply, relaxing your mind, and playing T'ai Chi in class and every day at home. Play T'ai Chi every day, and everything else will take care of itself.

Class Structure

T'ai Chi is informal, and each class is different. Some classes begin with a sitting QiGong exercise, using chairs forming a circle. For this relaxation exercise, the instructor will likely lead the group through an imagery exercise as they sit quietly with their eyes closed. Other classes will not use chairs and may begin with a standing relaxation exercise, also with the students' eyes closed. Still other instructors may begin the class by leading students in warm up exercises without practicing a QiGong or relaxation exercise.

> **CAUTION** **Ouch!** _____
>
> Your main goal in T'ai Chi class should be to relax and breathe. By not trying too hard, you learn more easily. Students who frustrate themselves by mentally repeating that they "can't get it" usually prove themselves right. If you really can't learn the movement, just follow the other students as you breathe and relax. You'll feel good after class, and you can repeat the session again, and you'll be the expert in class the second time around.

Once relaxation exercises are done, the physical class structure will probably have students staggered throughout the room facing the instructor in lines. The instructor usually faces the class, which forms lines throughout the room, giving each student enough space to swing their arms without striking one another. However, smaller, more informal classes may form a circle. An instructor may alternate facing the class or with his or her back to the class, and may move around the room as well giving students different angles to see from.

In a class formed in lines facing the instructor, find a place where you can see what the instructor is doing. Many large classes will have advanced students to help, and you can watch them if you can't see the instructor. If you can't see what's going on, ask questions or change places. Be clear of your needs. The teachers want to help you understand the movements, but in a larger class, they may not know you need further explanation. Don't be afraid to speak up—they want to help you understand.

The following list gives you an idea of the process a T'ai Chi class might go through; however, each instructor has their own format.

- Sitting or Standing Relaxation Exercise (if your class performs this).
- T'ai Chi warm-up exercises—gentle, repetitive movements that prepare you physically and mentally for T'ai Chi (many warm ups are moving QiGong exercises and are discussed in detail in Part 3, "Starting Down the QiGong Path to T'ai Chi").
- After warm-ups, the instructor may teach individual movements to practice, or if she teaches by exhibition, she will begin performing the entire T'ai Chi set and you will be expected to follow along.
- Your homework is the movements themselves, although it is highly recommended to begin using the QiGong relaxation exercises at home for your own health and pleasure.

T'ai Chi usually does not require anyone to sit or lie on the floor; however, some instructors may have warm up or cool down exercises that require it. If you are unable to do so because of an injury or physical limitation, discuss alternatives with the instructor.

How Are T'ai Chi Movements Taught?

T'ai Chi forms involve a series of choreographed martial arts poses that flow together like a slow motion dance. How these movements are taught can vary. Some classes are taught by example. Meaning, the instructor will lead the group all the way through the entire T'ai Chi form, and the students mimic until over time they remember all the movements.

However, many classes are taught for different levels, whereby the movements are broken down into one or two movements per class. If you are an average learner, these classes are preferable. It is much easier to learn one movement at a time and practice it all week than it is to try to assimilate an entire T'ai Chi form. I'll mention here that your learning will be much easier if you don't miss classes. It's easier to memorize movements in smaller bites. For each class you miss the bites get larger.

The following points lay out how T'ai Chi is taught or might be studied, in an effort to help you get the most out of your classes.

- Warm-ups and relaxation techniques are usually repeated weekly, although if you practice these everyday on your own you will be all the better for it.
- The actual T'ai Chi movement of the week must be learned and practiced on your own that week.
- Each week a new T'ai Chi movement will be added to your growing form or repertoire.
- The form will get longer and longer each week until you learn the entire form.
- Long forms of 20 minutes take between 6 and 8 months to learn.
- Short forms of 10 minutes may take 2 to 6 months to learn, depending on the instructor and the form.

- Advanced students often repeat beginning or intermediate classes for years to refine their performance of the T'ai Chi forms.

- Advanced students may serve as assistant instructors in class.

- As an advanced student, you may be asked to assist new students learning the forms for the first time. T'ai Chi, like all martial arts, is based on a mentoring system. As an assistant, you'll usually teach the first of the following three stages of T'ai Chi instruction.

- T'ai Chi's taught in these three stages.

    - First, the movements are learned.

    - Second, the breath is incorporated into the regimen by learning an inhalation or exhalation that is connected to each movement.

    - Third, a relaxation element or awareness of the flow of energy through the body is learned. Although the first step offers many benefits from the first day, the benefits get richer and deeper with each level you learn.

Sage Sifu Says

Normal T'ai Chi exercises can be easily adjusted to conform to your living room's size. Also, the more advanced sword or fan forms that some styles teach, although more challenging, can easily be done indoors, too. For example, retractable swords are available and can be left retracted when practicing indoors. The bottom line is, you can always practice T'ai Chi, no matter what style or where you are.

You Mean There's Homework!?!

T'ai Chi class exposes you to the movements, then you must practice those movements at home. There are two ways to look at this: either as another burden on your life's full plate or as a chance to take a break from the rat race and let all the weight of the world roll right off your shoulders.

The very first movement you learn on the very first day of class is a fantastic QiGong relaxation exercise that can help you begin to dump stress, if you do it in the right frame of mind. If you only do the T'ai Chi movement to prepare for the next T'ai Chi class, it won't be that relaxing. However, if you breathe deeply and let every muscle of your body relax, allowing the burdens of the week to roll off your shoulders each time you practice the movement, it'll feel great!

Ouch!

At first it will be difficult to discipline yourself to practice daily. If you fall behind in class, just play along and repeat the multiweek session again. There are no deadlines. You'll get it eventually. Don't sabotage yourself into thinking you just can't get it. Regular attendance and daily practice make T'ai Chi effortless and fruitful. If you miss class, although some instructors may help you catch up individually, you can't expect it.

To learn T'ai Chi, you will need to practice at home. But the reason we learn T'ai Chi is because it feels good, so why wouldn't we want to practice something that makes us feel good?

T'ai Chi Etiquette

Most instructors are happy to get questions during class. The rest of the class, or at least some of them, are probably facing the same uncertainties or challenges as you. A good instructor has been studying many years and may not remember all the challenges new students have, so your inquiries help him to help you and the other students. If your questions are criticisms of the format or structure, it would be best to offer them to the instructor personally after class. The instructor may not be able to fix it, but he may explain why it is done the way it is.

Knowing Your Martial Terms for T'ai Chi

Since T'ai Chi was originally a martial art, an introduction to some martial arts terms may be helpful. When you learn T'ai Chi, your instructor may use these or similar terms to describe the T'ai Chi movements. Understand that any one of these martial arts movements can be done any way that you need to do it for your own comfort. So if you have an injury or condition that limits your movement, do it in a way that feels comfortable to you. Never strain yourself to do something that doesn't feel right; just modify it a bit, kick lower, or reach less. As you play T'ai Chi in a way that feels good, over the days, months, and years, your kicks will get higher and higher.

Punches

In T'ai Chi there are punches. They are not hard grunting punches, but soft relaxing punches. There are generally three types of punches used. Both punches illustrated in the following figures begin with your fist by your hip, with the palm side of the fist turned up toward the sky. The first is a common T'ai Chi punch and begins with the fist at waist, palm turned in toward body, with no rotation of the fist as you punch. The other two are slightly more complex and therefore shown in the following figures. However, then you do a full twist as you send it out to punch in front of you, so the fist ends up with the palm facing down to the ground.

A T'ai Chi Punch Line

Many of the movements in T'ai Chi have martial arts applications and were patterned after the movements of creatures or images in nature. Therefore, T'ai Chi movements serve practical self-defense purposes and simultaneously are soothing natural motions which encourage the flow of Qi through the body just as Qi flows through all of nature.

The second punch is a Half Twist Punch. This begins with the fist near the hip with the palm turned up. When you throw the punch out, the fist rotates only a half turn, leaving the knuckles lined up in a row, top knuckle toward the sky and pinkie knuckle toward the ground.

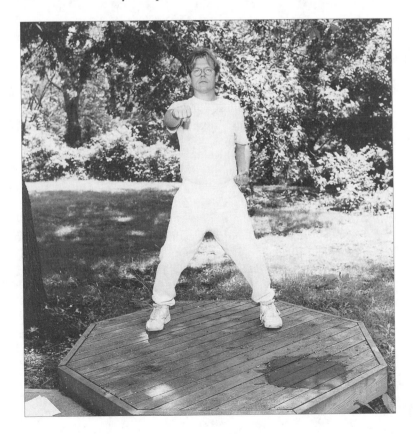

In the Full Fist Turn Punch, the fist ends up palm down.

The Half Twist Punch is more common in T'ai Chi, with knuckles ending up vertical.

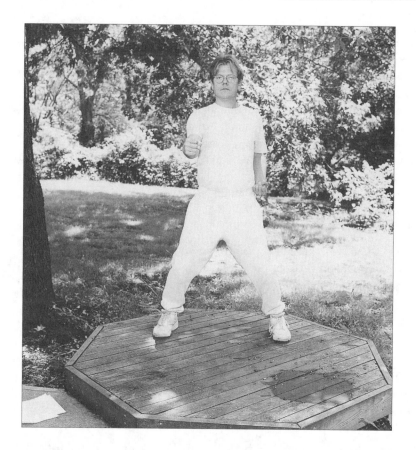

Punches are generally not thrown out in big circular haymaker punches like John Wayne threw. They come straight out from the hip like a piston, with the elbows tucked in. The elbows usually don't extend out from the sides, but stay in near the body.

Because of the many Western movies we've seen, most Westerners also try to punch with the whole upper body, actually leaning into the punch. However, in T'ai Chi and all martial arts, you do not normally lean into the punch. When the punch is complete, your head will still be posturally aligned above the dan tien.

Although there may be exceptions to how punches are thrown in various T'ai Chi forms, usually the rule of not leaning forward is always observed. However, there are times when the fist may circle around, rather than punch straight out from the hip. In Part 4, "Kuang Ping T'ai Chi: Walk on Life's Lighter Side," you will see an example of this in the Box Opponent's Ears movement.

Blocking

There are three types of blocks—In Blocks, Out Blocks, and Up Blocks. Their names explain whether the arm is blocking in toward the center of your body, out away from the center of your body, or up away from the body. One other less-used block is the Down Block, which looks like an Out Block in reverse. An example is seen in Part 4's Wind Blowing Lotus Leaves movement.

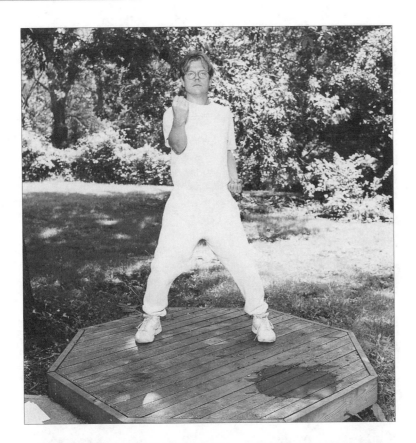

An In Block begins with the fist near your ear and then pull the arm in a circular motion across the front of your body.

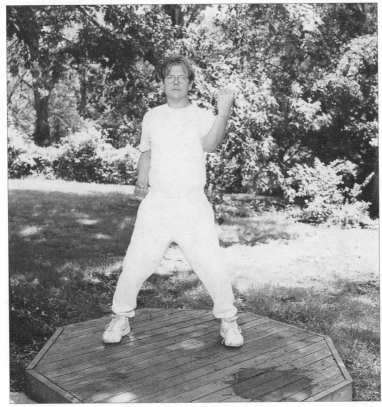

An Out Block begins with the fist near your groin, and then pull the arm in a circular sweep up across the body to block outward.

An Up Block begins with the fist palm facing your face, and then twist the palm away up to the sky, blocking up and away.

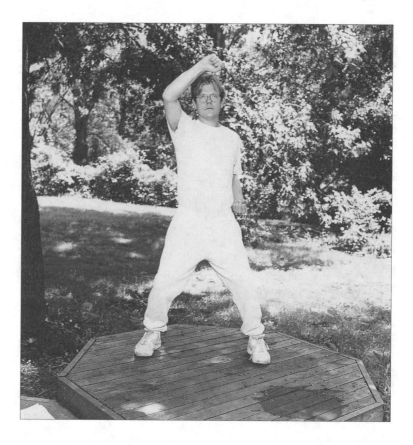

Kicks

T'ai Chi generally uses three kicks, Side or Separation Kicks, Crescent Kicks, or Front Kicks. Examples of these kicks can be viewed in Part 4, where the side kick is called "Separation of the Right Foot (and Left Foot)," the Crescent Kick is called "Wave Hand over Water Lily Kick," and the Front Kick is called "Front Kick."

The Least You Need to Know

- ◆ Ask the class instructor what to wear.
- ◆ T'ai Chi can encourage healthful lifestyle changes, such as massages or drug-free treatments for health problems.
- ◆ T'ai Chi makes life changes easier.
- ◆ Instructors will tell you what is expected of you.
- ◆ Practice because it feels good.

Chapter 9

Saddle Up: Horse Stance and Other Terms

In This Chapter

- ◆ Understand the importance of T'ai Chi posture
- ◆ Learn how T'ai Chi protects your joints
- ◆ Discover how T'ai Chi's moves teach effortless living
- ◆ Know that breath is the beginning of everything

This chapter explains the core concepts that will ensure a rich T'ai Chi experience for you whether you are beginning classes or a video instruction program. You will discover the basic concepts of T'ai Chi, how its movements are to be performed, why they are performed that way, and how to breathe when performing them. By understanding that T'ai Chi is very different from Western exertion exercises, you won't make it harder than it is, and by relaxing into it, you unlock its full effortless potential.

T'ai Chi Posture Is Power!

I introduced the dan tien in Chapter 2, "Let's Get Physical." In T'ai Chi we move from the dan tien by first sinking into the horse stance. This is how we sink our Qi, which makes us more solid, more balanced, and more down to earth physically, emotionally, and mentally.

Make a triangle with the thumbs over the navel and forefingers extending downward. The fingertips will meet at the level of the dan tien.

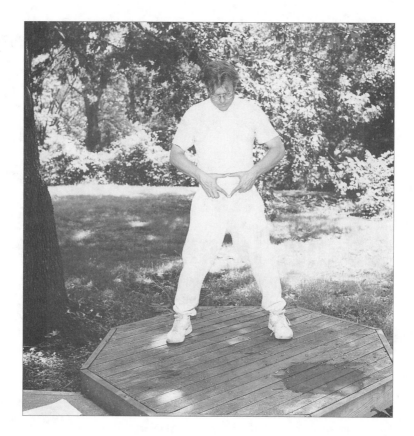

Where Is the Dan Tien?

Where the dan tien is located on the outside of the body only tells its height, for the dan tien is actually inside the body. The following describes how to find the dan tien inside:

♦ With the fingers forming a triangle as described in the previous figure, point fingers as if they could extend inside the body.

♦ Now, your fingers are pointing toward the dan tien; however, the dan tien is near the center of the body, so it can only be felt on the inside.

♦ Now tighten your sphincter muscles, as if you were pulling up your internal organs from within, and then immediately relax. Repeat this over and over, until you experience a subtle tugging sensation inside, just beyond where your fingers are pointing to your upper pelvis or lower abdomen.

♦ The place where you feel that subtle tugging feeling is where your dan tien is. That isn't your dan tien itself—that was a muscle tugging, for your dan tien is an energy center.

♦ Dan tien can only be experienced as energy, tingling, or other light sensations. This is where all powerful movement or action comes from, and cultivated awareness of the dan tien with T'ai Chi makes any action you take more powerful, with less likelihood of injury.

The Horse Stance and Dan Tien Ride Together Again

The dan tien is the basis of the Horse Stance. The Horse Stance is the basic stance for all martial arts, including T'ai Chi. It aligns the three dan tien points, *upper*, *middle*, and *lower*, to give you the best posture and most effortless movement.

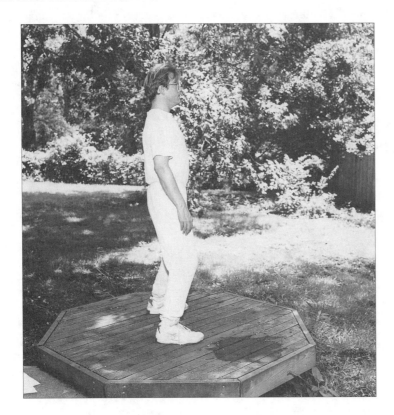

Note that the head is drawn upward toward the sky, as if a string were pulling from the center of the head. The chin is slightly pulled in, and the tailbone or sacrum is dropped down. This has the effect of lengthening the spine.

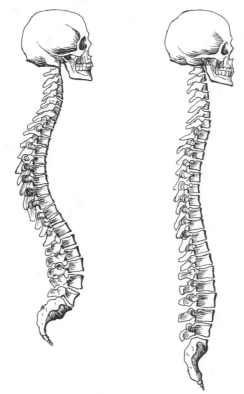

This figure illustrates how the spine is lengthened as you drop into the Horse Stance, although this is an exaggeration.

The Vertical Axis and You

Many lower back injuries are caused by poor performance posture. T'ai Chi will encourage you to maintain good posture and will remind you when you get sloppy. Proper posture is found in aligning the three dan tien points over the soles of the feet, with the weight slightly more to the heels than the front. As you practice T'ai Chi's slow gentle forms, your back will experience discomfort whenever you forget posture and let your butt creep out too much. However, the slow, low-impact nature of T'ai Chi will alert you to correct posture long before real damage occurs. This is what sets T'ai Chi apart from other training. If done correctly, slowly, and gently, T'ai Chi enables you to become aware of any poor physical habits long before physical damage is done. In fact, you often don't become aware of problems in high-impact sports until the doctor is telling you not to play that sport *ever again*.

Everything and the Sinking Qi

T'ai Chi is about sinking. This isn't like heaviness as in a ship sinking, but more of a weightless release of muscles, allowing the skeleton to effortlessly hold the weight of the body. Let your relaxed shoulders sink away from your neck as you sink into your movements. It's as if you were swimming through an atmosphere of effortlessness as you move through your forms.

Sinking Your Weight

Each T'ai Chi movement is associated with an inhale and/or an exhale. When you move and exhale, you allow the body to sink into a feeling of effortlessness. This is how it's done: As you transfer your weight from one leg to the other, relax the entire weight of the body down into the weight-bearing leg. The Chinese call this "sinking your Qi." By practicing this in T'ai Chi you will move more effortlessly, and your balance will improve. This also promotes blood and energy circulation through the body and encourages less joint damage by removing chronic tension from your daily movements. Tight muscles make tighter joints.

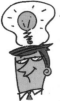

A T'ai Chi Punch Line

An advanced T'ai Chi student went to study with a grand master in China. The grand master told him to stand on one leg and said, "Keep standing, I'll be back." The grand master returned 15 minutes later and reached down to squeeze the student's calf muscle on the leg he was standing on. The master scoffed, "Too tight! Why is your leg so tight? Keep standing, I'll come back and check later."

Ouch!

There are some T'ai Chi styles that do require pivoting a weight-bearing foot. To accomplish this with no damage to the knee, you lift the dan tien at the same time so as to relieve pressure on the knee. If you have knee problems, I recommend not performing these types of pivots. But you can modify the form to be safe for you.

Don't Tear the Rice Paper!

In the TV series *Kung Fu*, you may have seen Kwai Chang Cane walk across the rice paper for his graduation ceremony at the Shao Lin Temple. This looked very mystical, but it was actually a very practical test.

The purpose of the test was to discover if he was pivoting the foot that was carrying his weight. In most T'ai Chi, you do not pivot the weight-bearing foot because this can destabilize your balance. More important, doing this can also cause knee damage. Styles that do pivot on weight-bearing legs do so rarely and take certain precautions to prevent injury. These pivots are not recommended for arthritis sufferers.

T'ai Chi movement is a process of "filling" and "emptying" each leg of Qi, or weight. The position of the dan tien over a leg determines that it is full, and the other leg is empty. You "fill" the opposite foot by shifting your dan tien over that opposite foot. Then your "empty" foot has no weight on it and can be pivoted with zero damage to the knee.

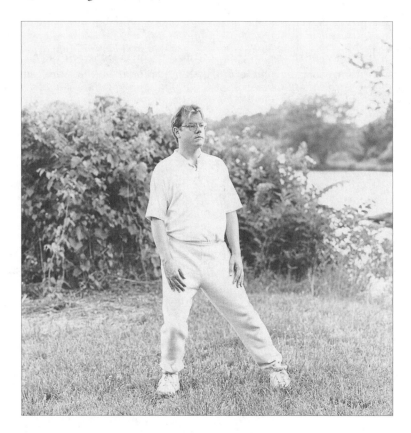

The vertical axis of the head and heart dan tien points lines up over the lower dan tien. This axis moving over a leg is filling that leg with Qi, or weight. As you let your breath out and relax your body weight onto a leg, you sink your Qi into that leg.

Active Bones Under Soft Muscle

T'ai Chi is unlike any exercise you have ever done because it is done best when done easily. T'ai Chi's way will also provide a model for practicing the art of effortlessness in everything you do.

T'ai Chi Is Not Isometrics

Most Western exercises involve some type of force or strain. T'ai Chi does not. The more effortlessly you are moving, the better you are doing it. You may catch yourself subconsciously tightening muscles because we have been taught that exercise must cause strain. Also, at first, your balance may not be very solid, and you will tighten your leg muscles a lot to hold you steady. This is normal, and over time, you'll find that you can relax your muscles more and more. As you get used to proper posture, using the vertical axis alignment, you'll need less muscle tension to hold you up. So don't be discouraged if T'ai Chi doesn't feel so "effortless" at first. We are learning how to move effortlessly, by first becoming aware of how tight we are, and then by using QiGong breathing techniques taught in Part 3, "Starting Down the QiGong Path to T'ai Chi," we begin to "let go" of needless effort as we move through T'ai Chi movements *and life*.

 Ouch!

Becoming more comfortable with your forms and using proper posture with the vertical axis allow you to relax more as you move. At first you will notice yourself losing balance as much or even more than before you started T'ai Chi. This is not unusual. Before, you probably held your balance by holding your body tightly. Now, you are learning to balance while loose.

When doing T'ai Chi warm-ups, let your mind let go of thoughts, and center on your effortless breath. Then enjoy the sensations of the muscles loosening as you move. On each breath think of letting the muscles beneath the muscles let go, letting go of each other, and letting go of the bones beneath. As we relax our muscles, the bones moving beneath provide a deep tissue massage, and the body can cleanse itself of toxins. Also, the relaxed abdominal muscles allow a gentle massage of the internal organs, which tonifies them and improves their function.

Don't force yourself to go as low or deep in your stances as your instructor. You have the rest of your life to get lower. Right now just focus on breathing, relaxing, and letting the muscles relax on the bones, again by allowing the entire body to relax as you exhale.

> ### Sage Sifu Says
>
> Don't fall into an "all or nothing" trap of self-sabotage. For example, you may have a knee problem that prevents you from rotating your knees the way the instructor does, or your asthma may prevent you from breathing as deeply or effortlessly as you would like. That's perfectly fine and natural. Do what you can in a way that feels good to you.
>
> Just because QiGong and T'ai Chi often help people lessen their reliance on pain or asthma medications does not mean you *must* give up your medication. On the contrary, use what works and helps you live better. Yet ironically, over time T'ai Chi and QiGong may reduce your reliance on the very medications that help you feel comfortable enough to move and breathe through T'ai Chi.

The knees are always bent in T'ai Chi. The depth of that bend depends on what feels good to you. Someone with knee problems may bend his or her knees only slightly at first, whereas, someone more athletic may bend more. Do not let competitiveness cause you to go any deeper than feels good. You won't win a prize, and you'll enjoy the class less because you are straining too much. The relaxed bend of the knees allows the rest of the body to be more loose and flexible, especially the hips.

Easy Does It

Again, T'ai Chi is a mind/body exercise that integrates your mental, emotional, and physical aspects. Therefore, as you learn to move more effortlessly, you will notice that emotionally and mentally you will find ways to move through life with less and less effort. This doesn't mean you will get less done. You will probably get more done because someone with calm emotions and a relaxed mind is much more creative than someone who is in constant mental or emotional turmoil.

> **T'ai Sci**
>
> Some doctors believe that our central nervous system is affected by the rhythms of our breath. This means that a restriction in a freely moving respiratory system could lead to disease, since the central nervous system regulates all other organs. The goal of T'ai Chi is to foster unrestricted breathing. By doing so, T'ai Chi may improve central nervous system function, which may reduce the incidence of disease.

As you study T'ai Chi, be aware of patterns you may have that make learning T'ai Chi more difficult. You may find that you push yourself very hard, straining at every movement. Or you may discover that you are hypercritical of yourself, or perhaps you will sabotage your progress by avoiding practice and skipping classes. All these patterns are probably something that you do in all aspects of your life, not just in T'ai Chi. By learning how to "play" T'ai Chi in a process of effortless learning, without strain, self-judgment, or self-sabotage, you will discover a new way to learn. By discovering a new way to learn T'ai Chi, you create a new, more effective way to learn in all your life's endeavors. You will become more successful and self-actualizing by becoming clearer and more self-aware of unconscious patterns that inhibit the realization of your dreams.

Round Is Cool

In Chinese, the word for "round" is roughly equivalent to the American slang word, "cool." The Chinese felt that roundness was calming and comforting, and T'ai Chi is filled with images of roundness. We often move our hands over imaginary orbs or spheres of energy that over time become tangible enough to feel. This practice, although at first a little alien, eventually becomes very soothing. It helps us become attuned to our sensations. It is like practicing "feeling." Practice makes perfect, and this is no exception.

Ouch!

Rapid expansion of the chest cavity may not efficiently oxygenate the body. However, the relaxed abdominal breathing of QiGong can be highly effective in increasing circulation of blood and Qi.

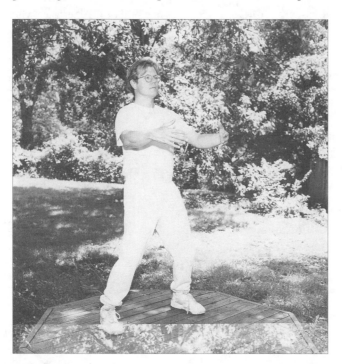

In this Moving QiGong exercise, your hands begin at groin level and circle up as if stroking a huge three-foot pearl in front of your torso. Move your hands up over and down the back of the pearl.

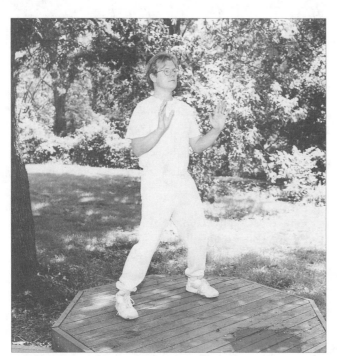

After the hands slide up and over the giant pearl, they descend along the backside until coming to rest in front of the chest, as if you were about to push someone.

Breath Is the Beginning of Everything

The essence of T'ai Chi is the breath. While doing T'ai Chi, you inhale or exhale with every movement. There is nothing more effortless in the entire universe than the release of a full breath. Therefore, T'ai Chi's ability to weave exhales with the relaxation of sinking your Qi into your weight shifts creates a powerful habit. This habit of relaxed breathing through everything we do is simple, and yet may change the way we live the rest of our lives. But again, the reason to do it is because *it feels good*.

Post-Birth Breathing

There are many QiGong breathing exercises. All QiGong exercises are breathing exercises when you get down to it. However, among all of them there are two main forms of breathing. One is *post-birth breathing*, which is pretty normal, and the second is *pre-birth breathing*, which takes a little more getting used to.

The names of these breathing forms may be based on the fact that we drew breath in through the umbilical cord prior to birth, and we draw air in through the upper body afterward. This is reflected in the way we draw air into the body during QiGong breathing, depending on which type we are doing.

With post-birth—or normal—breathing, the abdominal muscles expand out a bit as you breathe in to the abdomen, then the chest expands as the top of the lungs fills. They then relax back in as you exhale, emptying first the chest and then the lower lungs. This is how T'ai Chi and many QiGong exercises are done. However, some QiGong exercises employ pre-birth breathing.

During post-birth breathing, do not force the breath, but rather allow the body to relax as the breath enters. The following figure illustrates post-birth breathing:

Four-step post-birth breathing.

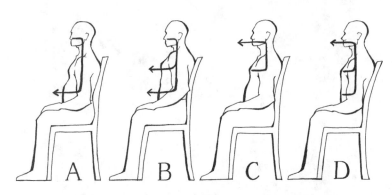

A T'ai Chi Punch Line

The Chinese believe that pre-birth breathing moves our Qi through the lower dan tien. This energy is associated with cell regeneration and sexual or procreative energy. It is therefore believed that pre-birth breathing heightens the regenerative ability of our life energy and actually slows the aging process.

1. Breathe into the lower lungs as the abdomen relaxes slightly outward.
2. Allow the lungs and upper chest to fill as well.
3. As the body relaxes with the exhale of breath, the upper chest deflates first.
4. Then the abdomen relaxes in, completely expelling the air from the lungs.

This can be repeated for 10 or 15 minutes if you like, with wonderful results for mind and body.

Pre-Birth Breathing

Pre-birth breathing is just the opposite. As you inhale, draw the abdominal muscles in gently, and as you exhale allow them to relax. Each breathing method has different qualities and will be discussed during the moving exercises in Parts 3, 4, and 5.

Pre-birth breathing is sort of the opposite of normal breathing. In pre-birth breathing:

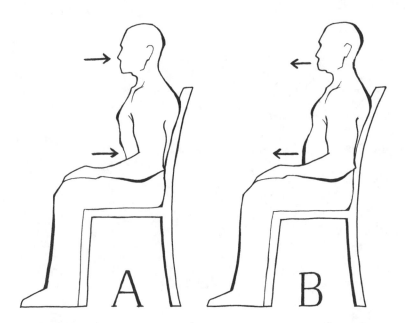

Two-step pre-birth breathing.

1. The abdomen, especially the lower abdomen, is gently and slightly drawn in as you inhale.
2. Then, when you exhale, the abdomen relaxes back out.

Pre-birth breathing involves a bit of training and some cautionary notes. It is advisable to practice normal post-birth breathing only during your exercises, unless training with an experienced QiGong instructor.

The Least You Need to Know

- Your posture is your power.
- Sinking Qi improves your balance.
- T'ai Chi practice protects your joints.
- Proper breath techniques are the most powerful health tool.

Part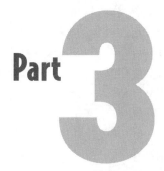

Starting Down the QiGong Path to T'ai Chi

This part details how QiGong can lubricate the way for us to fit into a new world developing around us in these rapidly changing times. Practical exercises for young, old, and everyone in between will help you breathe the breath of life and have some fun doing it.

In this part, you will also learn some QiGong history and see why some QiGong is different than T'ai Chi. Learning QiGong will make your T'ai Chi experience much richer. It is said that medicine cures, but the best medicine prevents. To that end, you'll learn not only about the personal healing powers of QiGong, but also how you can share your Qi, or life energy, with others.

This part also alerts you to some common challenges you may encounter as you begin exploring your inner self with Sitting QiGong. The Sitting QiGong exercise presented in Chapter 11 will get your Qi overflowing. In fact it will lead you through an explanation and exercise that may actually change the way you view the universe you live in. Chapter 12 exposes you to the beautiful and wonderful feeling of Moving QiGong exercises, or Dong Gong. There are thousands of them, so in this chapter you will only be able to dip your toe into an ocean of what's out there. The T'ai Chi warm-up exercises detailed in Chapter 13 are QiGong exercises that not only calm the mind, but prepare the body for T'ai Chi. These exercises alone can have a wonderful impact on your day.

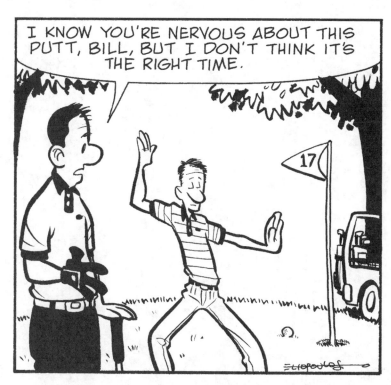

Chapter 10

Introducing QiGong

In This Chapter

- ◆ Learn why breathing is so important
- ◆ Find out how QiGong and T'ai Chi differ
- ◆ Read up on your history of QiGong
- ◆ Survive and flourish through QiGong challenges
- ◆ Discover the healing art of External QiGong

The purpose of QiGong is to let go of energy blocks by relaxing the mind, body, and emotions. Although T'ai Chi shares this purpose, there are QiGong exercises that are not T'ai Chi.

QiGong differs from standard meditations but shares many of their healing potentials. QiGong can be used as therapy for specific conditions, as well as a general tune up. Also, we can actually treat another person with the life energy QiGong fills us with.

Also, there are different types of QiGong. There is active QiGong (Dong Gong) and passive QiGong (Jing Gong). Active QiGong involves obvious movement, like T'ai Chi. Passive is where the external body is still but the awareness is directed and felt in various areas of the body, by breath, or imagery, or both.

We encounter many challenges when beginning QiGong practice. By realizing that these are common, you can begin to move past them and get all the benefits QiGong offers. These challenges to QiGong practice represent challenges we face in all aspects of our life and personal growth. Therefore, by learning to move through these challenges in QiGong, we begin to untie knots in many other parts of our lives as well.

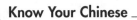

Let's Do Some Heavy Breathing

Know Your Chinese

Literally translated, **Qi** means "air" or "energy," and **gong** means "work." Therefore, QiGong literally translated means "breath work" or "energy work."

Many ancient cultures have recognized the breath as our connection with the life force, or Qi. In Chinese, the character for Qi, or life energy, is the same character used for air, as in breath. In Latin, the *spir* of *spir*it or re*spir*ate, means "to breathe." Spirit is the *breath of life*, or life energy, which is another word for Qi. So in both the East and West, breath was recognized as the key to life's energy. To breathe shallowly therefore means that you are cheating yourself out of a lot of life.

Many T'ai Chi classes begin with Sitting QiGong exercises that require us to breathe deeply. You may find this difficult because our lungs have lost capacity from lack of use, or our back and chest muscles are tight with tension. This will change. As your rigid muscles relax, you will soon discover your lungs finding new capacity.

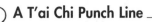

A T'ai Chi Punch Line

A corporate executive arriving promptly for a QiGong class informed the instructor, "My doctor said QiGong would be good for my heart condition, so I want to learn QiGong. But I heard about all that weird breathing you do. I want you to know, I am not into the breathing thing." The instructor responded, "We'd better hurry and get you into it before it's too late because I don't do CPR."

Some are just embarrassed to let other people hear us breathe. Maybe it's because we only think of hearing deep breathing during sex or other intense feelings, and we're taught not to show our feelings in public. After a few classes, people get more comfortable with each other and get comfortable with the idea of breathing. Then the tentative group transforms into *a wild bunch of breathing bohemians!*

A T'ai Chi Punch Line

A Chinese T'ai Chi master was asked, "Why do we do T'ai Chi?" His answer was, "To burp." He meant that T'ai Chi makes us aware of what the body needs and self-assured enough to satisfy those healthful needs. A yawn is a form of deep release, both physical and mental. To deny that release is not a healthy habit. Yawn away!

If you forget everything about QiGong except to remember to breathe deeply when under stress, you will find great benefit. Of course, that is only the beginning—the key to the door of what T'ai Chi has to offer—so don't stop there.

QiGong first of all teaches us to feel good about ourselves and to follow what our body wants and needs, like breathing deeply, *even in public*. In fact, QiGong practitioners get to where they can even yawn in public. I know that may seem pretty risqué now, but after learning QiGong, even you will be able to yawn unashamedly in public. And this ability will reflect an even deeper ability to believe in yourself enough to do what your body tells you it needs, whether it's more rest, better foods, regular gentle exercise, or a good solid yawn, even in the middle of a department meeting.

T'ai Chi vs. QiGong: What's the Diff?

T'ai Chi's goal of relaxing the mind and body to encourage the flow of energy through us makes it QiGong. However, not all QiGong is T'ai Chi (because some QiGong is sitting or lying, and all T'ai Chi is moving and standing). The mental strain of trying to figure whether you are doing T'ai Chi or QiGong will limit your ability to get the benefits. Forget about it. As you practice T'ai Chi and QiGong exercises, the differences will become obvious. *Doing* is the best way of *seeing*.

Don't sweat it; after Parts 3, "Starting Down the QiGong Path to T'ai Chi," and 4, "Kuang Ping T'ai Chi: Walk on Life's Lighter Side," you'll be an expert on the tenets of both T'ai Chi and QiGong. Remember, much of T'ai Chi and QiGong are interchangeable and synonymous anyway. As stated before, the premise of all Traditional Chinese Medicine, of which T'ai Chi and QiGong are integral parts, is that energy flows through the body, and we are likely to get sick when it gets blocked off. So QiGong's goal to allow the mind and body to release the past and fears of the future in order to live a more flowing, healthful life is also the goal of T'ai Chi.

T'ai Sci

In the Chinese Medica there are about 7,000 different breathing exercises, all gentle, all pleasant, and all QiGong. In Traditional Chinese hospitals, physicians may prescribe a QiGong exercise to help heal a problem, much the same way that a Western doctor might prescribe a drug (of course, QiGong exercises only have *good* side effects). Many Western doctors are now beginning to prescribe T'ai Chi and QiGong as well.

QiGong is a form of meditation; however, it can be more as well. QiGong can actively be used to treat a specific organ or an area of pain and discomfort by directing Qi to that area.

Like other meditations, such as za-zen or transcendental meditation, QiGong allows the mind to empty of active thought and be passively aware. In za-zen this state of mind is achieved by not thinking about anything, but just letting thoughts drift through the mind without fixing or holding onto them. In transcendental meditation, a *mantra* (a verbal utterance used in meditation), or perhaps a *mandala* (a visual meditation tool), is used to take the mind out of the problem-solving mode and into a state of free flow, whereby it "observes" rather than "thinks about" things that flow through the mind.

A T'ai Chi Punch Line

The ultimate source of Chinese medical knowledge is The Yellow Emperor's *Classic of Internal Medicine* (200 B.C.E.), which prescribed QiGong for curing and preventing illness. According to this ancient book, true medicine cured diseases before they developed. T'ai Chi and QiGong can be very effective at doing just that.

QiGong combines this passive awareness, or "letting go," with an active healing intention. If treating a headache, for example, once we think about the energy filling the muscles in our head, we have to let that thought go and then just experience how nice it feels as Qi's healing energy, or light relaxes the head. We observe the healing release in the tight muscles, and, in a way, the passive observation of our own healing becomes a mantra or mandala.

A Brief History of QiGong

QiGong is believed to be over 2,000 years old. Its roots are with ancient Chinese farmers who observed that nature's balance makes things strong. Moderation, flexibility, and constant nurturing filled crops with the life force, or Qi. These ancient observers developed exercises that mimicked that healthy way of cultivating life energy.

Know Your Chinese

The **Taoist Canon** (1145 C.E.) held all the early writing on QiGong, although at that time it was known as Tao-yin. QiGong is a fairly modern term. Taoist philosophy emphasizes being attuned to the invisible laws of nature. QiGong, or Tao-yin, was viewed as a way to connect with that deeper part of ourselves that knows what is best for us.

Welcome Back to the Future

What many Western hospitals are now considering as cutting-edge treatments for cancer, for example, can be found in the 800-year-old *Taoist Canon*. At the Simonton Cancer Center, mental imagery exercises are successfully used to help cancer sufferers live nearly twice as long as their peers who do not use imagery techniques. The *Taoist Canon* wrote of thousands of visualization techniques meant to heal various conditions.

Is Your Mind Half Full or Half Empty?

Here in the West, we have no trouble understanding and accepting that our mind can make us sick. We know that worry can cause an ulcer or that chronic anxiety can lead to a heart attack. However, we have a big problem accepting just the opposite, that our mind can also heal us.

So the world has come full circle, and what was ancient treatment in China is now the cutting edge of modern healing in the West. *Welcome back to the future.*

> **Know Your Chinese**
>
> QiGong has had other names in the past, such as **tu gu na xin**, "expelling the old energy, absorbing the new," or **tao-yin**, "leading and guiding the energy." Actually, the term QiGong is a fairly recent way of saying energy exercise.

It's an "Is the glass half full or half empty?" kind of thing. We know that our stress can cause our shoulders to tighten and our breath to get shallow and constricted, leading to hypertension and maybe a headache. But the concept of using our mind to heal us is thought of as a "weird" idea. Ponder this: We all know that recalling an argument we had a week ago or even a month ago can cause our muscles to tighten, our breathing to shallow, and our blood pressure to skyrocket. *Now, that is strange!*

So if something as abstract as a week-old memory can wreak havoc on our health, it makes perfect sense that our mind can have a healing effect on itself today. Unlocking its grip on worry and tension, the mind can allow each cell to bathe in the radiant glow of health.

Boredom? It's QiGong Time!

If you are wondering when to do QiGong, the short answer is, anytime you need it. In fact, as you practice energy work more and more, you will find that you always do it, in a way. As you open more to the feeling of energy flowing, rather than being squeezed off by stress, you will automatically sit back and breathe yourself open each time stress begins to close off your flow of Qi.

> **T'ai Sci**
>
> Western medical research has discovered that our immune system follows certain rhythms; that it is weakest at about 1 A.M. and strongest at about 7 A.M. This may partially explain why when you are sick, your cold or flu symptoms keep you from sleeping at night, and then suddenly in the morning you are ready to sleep well. Ancient Chinese doctors were not only aware of this general pattern but also began to distinguish similar cycles in specific organs.

I always remind students that after learning QiGong, they need never again be bored. Anytime you catch yourself getting anxious in a line or in a waiting room, you now can just mentally kick back and practice these wonderful exercises instead of stressing out.

Although you can practice QiGong with great results at any time of the day, Traditional Chinese Medicine has found that the energy flowing through your body is different at different times of the day. Just as Chapter 7, "Plan Ahead: Where and When to Practice T'ai Chi," explained how T'ai Chi can be performed at different times of the day for different effects, so can other QiGong exercises. Refer to Chapter 7 to see the times and related organ systems.

Mental Healing and QiGong Challenges

QiGong helps heal us mentally, emotionally, and physically, but the beginning of healing entails *becoming more aware.* This can present challenges for the novice because when we become more aware of our mental, emotional, and physical discomforts, we often think this means T'ai Chi and/or QiGong doesn't work. Many of us think a mind/body exercise like T'ai Chi means "instant and permanent nirvana," and when we discover that we have to "feel" discomfort such as tension before we know to let it go, we may mistakenly think the tools "don't work." Remember that this new self-awareness is part of a healing process, and you will get enormous benefits from your practice if you stick with it.

Bliss vs. Discomfort

T'ai Chi, QiGong, and other mind/body fitness exercises are sometimes mistakenly seen as "escapist," whereby we can use them to run away from our problems. Although T'ai Chi and QiGong can seem like a soothing vacation from our problems sometimes, they also help us heal or release the source of those problems.

For example, when doing Sitting QiGong exercises or meditations, you may feel your shoulders getting very tense. Remember the exercise is not making you tense. The exercise of sitting mindfulness is helping you become aware of a pattern or habit you have of holding tension in your shoulders. Now that you are aware of it, you can practice the release and relaxation systems presented in Chapter 11, "Sitting QiGong (Jing Gong)," to begin to let that pattern go.

As you practice T'ai Chi and/or QiGong, you may experience tension or even anxiety. Do not let that stop you or make you think you are doing it wrong. The emergence of these feelings is an opportunity to begin releasing them, using your new tools of breath and life energy.

Trying Too Hard to See the Light?

If your QiGong exercises make you feel intensely anxious or tense, it's usually because you are trying too hard to make the tools work. Ironically, the harder we try to relax, let go, and make light or life energy flow through us, the more we squeeze it off.

Life energy flows effortlessly through us when we let the mind and body let go. This is what QiGong teaches us to do. Furthermore, QiGong practice will teach you how to let your conscious mind work with the effortless power of life energy. This will take practice. You will catch yourself trying too hard to feel life energy or trying too hard to make muscles relax. Always remember that the Qi, or life energy, is completely effortless. Your mind or thoughts can direct your Qi to tense shoulder muscles, but once that thought is directed, you can and must let your mind relax, letting go of the outcome.

Chi, I'm a Healer?!

That's right, you are a healer, *master.* After practicing the Sitting QiGong exercise in Chapter 11, you will feel the Qi flowing out of your hands. Medical studies have shown that this energy can help people heal. Most nursing schools in the United States now teach a form of External QiGong called Therapeutic Touch and are finding great success with everything from anxiety reduction to facilitating healing. If someone you know has a headache, you can usually get some results even if you are a novice. Whether you completely heal the headache or not, he will likely get some relief, or at the very least, his headache won't last as long as it normally would.

Know Your Chinese

Wai Qi Zhi Liao is the term for External QiGong. Modern Therapeutic Touch used in many Western hospitals is a form of External QiGong.

In the following figures, you will see one form of an External QiGong exercise you can begin practicing today. After completing steps 1, 2, and 3, ask the recipient to describe to you how she feels, before proceeding to step 4. Your experience with these tools is the best teacher of what they offer you and others.

The giver of energy stands to one side of the receiver, with his hands extended over the recipient's heart.

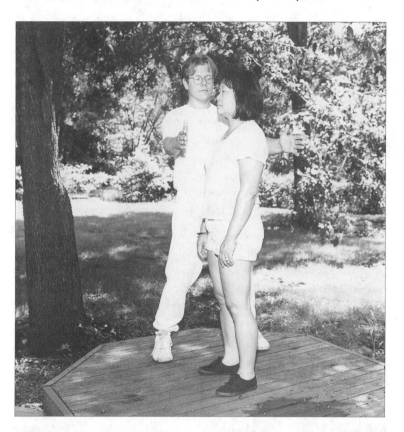

Then he slowly brings his hands over the recipient's shoulder and down her arm to allow the giver's Qi to flow from his hands into the recipient's arm.

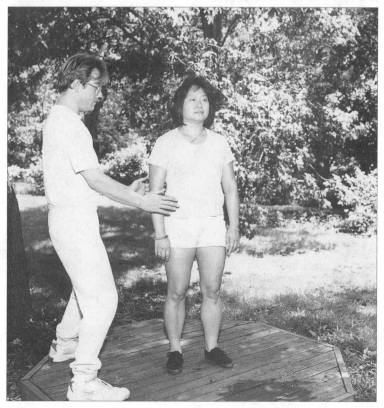

1. As you let your Qi flow through your hands into the receiver's heart, slowly bring your hands over her shoulder and down, keeping the receiver's arm between your hands so your Qi can flow into her arm.

2. Bring your hands back up to the heart and repeat three times.

3. Shake off your hands between each brushdown to let go of any stress or heavy energy you might have brushed off on the receiver.

4. Repeat this entire process after moving to the other side, so the recipient's left and right side are both brushed down.

There are many other healing exercises for various purposes. These are general cleansing treatments that will benefit anybody. However, the recipients have to feel comfortable with the process because if they feel tense, it won't work as well. Many nurses simply place their hands on patients to comfort them and then let their energy flow into the patients without their conscious awareness of it. This allows the patients to relax.

The Least You Need to Know

- If you breathe, the rest is easy. *All of it.*
- T'ai Chi is QiGong.
- QiGong is an ancient/modern healing art.
- Discomfort is information, not an enemy.
- You are a healer and a master.

Chapter 11

Sitting QiGong (Jing Gong)

In This Chapter

- ◆ Seeing and feeling Qi
- ◆ Remembering that we are made of energy
- ◆ Experiencing how Sitting QiGong lights you up

There are many ways to measure the Qi flowing through our bodies. A common way to see energy flow is through Kirlian photography. This chapter provides some examples of how Kirlian photography captures images of our energy.

QiGong practice isn't about pretending to be energy; it is about feeling what we really are, which is energy. Actually the entire universe is energy. This chapter ends with an exercise of Sitting QiGong, which will allow you to actually feel the nature of your energy, and how life energy, or Qi, feels as it flows through your body. You'll love it!

A Word About Energy Medicine and QiGong

Previous chapters explained how Chinese Medicine works by unblocking or directing the energy flowing through the body. QiGong and T'ai Chi also work to balance and unblock that energy.

However, QiGong is also about realizing that the body isn't a solid entity, but instead an open, moving wave of energy. QiGong will actually help you realize your energy nature by providing quiet sitting exercises that enable you to feel it. Over time you'll begin to feel your energy aspect in your T'ai Chi practice as well.

The Sitting QiGong exercise presented at the end of this chapter enables you to feel the Qi or energy that moves through your body. Before I get to that, however, I'd like to show you how the process works. Then, when you do the exercise, you can let your brain, and skepticism, relax and get out of the way. The energy flows easier when you are *effortless*.

So don't worry about memorizing any of these facts. Rather, sit back and be entertained by the fascinating insights into who you really are.

Ouch!

Some studies identify cynicism as our greatest health risk. This is because being constantly suspicious of the world around you triggers unhealthy stress responses. Keep an open mind and relaxed body as you learn about your energetic nature.

Kirlian Photography: Seeing Qi Is Believing

There is actually a way to take photographs of the energy aspect of our body. You may have heard this energy referred to as aura. Kirlian photography has been around since the 1950s, but it received a lot more attention as we learned about Qi and QiGong in the West. This is because Kirlian photography seems to be able to take pictures of Qi, or at least aspects of Qi.

When a Kirlian photograph is taken, the person, or leaf, or any living thing, rests on a photographic plate, and a mild electrical current is run through it. Then the camera takes an image of the energy or Qi of the plant or person.

Phantom of the Aura

When Kirlian photography was first introduced, skeptics argued that the photography captured nothing more than the electricity running through the plant or person's hand or whatever was photographed. However, this all changed with the discovery of the "phantom effect." The following figure illustrates the phantom effect, seen on a leaf.

In these front and back images, you see a leaf, but what's amazing is that the top part of the leaf that you see *isn't there!* The top quarter of the leaf has been torn off. So what looks like a leaf is actually the Qi, or energy aspect, of the top of the leaf. You can see where the leaf was torn, but still see the veins and edges of the leaf going up. This discovery changed not only the way people viewed Kirlian photography, *but also the way science began to look at what we are made of.*

This illustration represents the "phantom effect" as it appears in a common Kirlian photograph of a leaf.

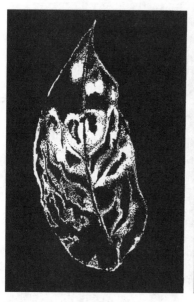 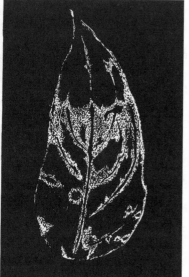

The T'ai Chi Zone, Do-Do-Do-Do, Do-Do-Do-Do

The following figure illustrates how our behavior affects our Qi, or energy. This is important for understanding the benefits of the Sitting QiGong exercise we will do later. Eating right, getting enough rest and exercise, and practicing T'ai Chi and QiGong can positively affect your energy flow, whereas behavior shown to be detrimental to health can negatively affect Qi flow.

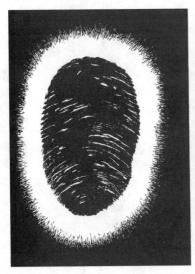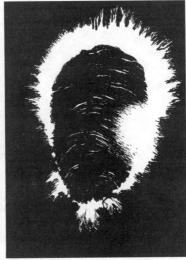

Kirlian photographs illustrate how our behavior affects our energy flow, or Qi flow, through our body and beyond.

The figure shows a woman's fingertip and the energy flowing through and around it. The image on the left shows this woman's fingertip in a normal state. The Chinese would call that Smooth Qi, or a healthful state. However, the image to the right is the same woman after she drank a cup of coffee and smoked her very first cigarette. The energy went wild! In fact, notice that in some places there seems to be no energy.

We all know how smooth Qi feels, as on those days when you wake up and everything just clicks the way it's supposed to. Every paper wad you throw lands right in the center of the trash can. In basketball, they call it being *in the zone.* So we all know how it feels when we are there, in the zone, but we might not know how to get there.

> ### T'ai Sci
> *The Tao of Physics* shows how the modern subatomic physicists' view of reality is often very close to the view held by ancient Chinese mystics. By going within themselves in QiGong meditation, these mystics somehow began to understand what modern physicists understand about the energetic nature of reality.

What T'ai Chi and QiGong offer is a way to get into the zone. As we practice our T'ai Chi movements every day, day after day, we find ourselves spending much less time frazzled and wired, like in the second image. And we find ourselves more and more in the calm center of Smooth Qi, like in the first image.

Mind Over Qi

The following figure is very important in preparing you for the upcoming Sitting QiGong exercise because it illustrates how our minds can direct energy. In this figure you see two sets of hands, both belong to the same man. In the image on the left, you see his hands in a normal state. However, in the image on the right, you see his hands when he's consciously thinking of *sending energy* out through his hands.

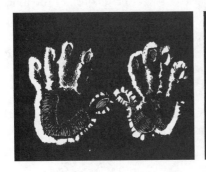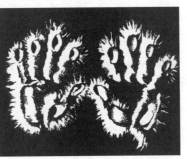

Kirlian photographs illustrate how our energy or Qi flow can be directed by thought.

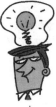

A T'ai Chi Punch Line _____

Twenty years ago, I smoked about two packs a day. It was nearly impossible for me to sit still for 20 minutes to do Sitting QiGong—because in Sitting QiGong we begin to become conscious of the energy disruption our habits cause. However, over time as my energy flowed more smoothly, I scaled back on my smoking and eventually replaced the need for cigarettes with the pleasure of my renewed energy flow.

When the man was thinking of *sending energy* out of his hands, he wasn't grunting and straining. He simply relaxed as he *let it happen*. I mention this before you start the Sitting QiGong to it remind you not to "try."

This is an important point because we often think that anything worth doing must be hard. We want to put our "shoulder to the wheel," our "nose to the grindstone," "furrowing the brow" to get something done. However, the energy work, or QiGong, doesn't work that way. The more you try, the more the muscles tighten up, and the less the energy flows through you.

So as the man was sending energy out his hands (illustrated in the previous figure), he just thought of it happening, and then relaxed and enjoyed the feeling as he let it flow out. You may experience what he felt during the Sitting QiGong exercise.

> **T'ai Sci**
>
> Harvard Medical School did studies on several relaxation response techniques and found that one thing is necessary to get the most out of any of the exercises. You have to adopt a state of mind called "passive awareness" or "effortless concentration." This means that you can't force the experience of QiGong.

The Sitting QiGong is a very effortless process. When it begins, I'll invoke images, such as a soothing flow of relaxation or light energy pouring over your head and face, relaxing all the muscles. When you read this or hear it on an audiotape (you may find it helpful to record the Sitting QiGong in your voice and then listen with your eyes closed rather than reading), you will want to imagine the shower of lightness or relaxation pouring over you. But then let go of the image and just enjoy the feeling of effortless relaxation spreading through your head and facial muscles as the lightness spreads through them.

Researchers have found that if you think of the image, let go of that mental image, and then let the lightness flow through, you will be more able to feel the pleasure of that flow.

E = MC² Means You Are Only Energy

It's easier to relax and let your Qi flow through you if you know that everything in the universe is only made out of energy, *including you*. Einstein's famous equation $E = MC^2$ means, E (energy) equals M (mass) times C (speed of light squared). Don't get an algebra attack though, because all it means is that all things, including you, are made of energy.

Actually, we are mostly just empty space. To understand just how spacious we all are consider the following. If you could take an atom out of anything in the universe, like one of your body's atoms, and blow it up to the size of a football field, the nucleus of that atom would only be the size of a BB in the center of that football field. The electrons that revolve around it would be like dust motes 50 yards away in the end zone. So everything between the BB and the dust mote 50 yards away is energy field, or empty space.

In fact, imagine if you could take all the atoms of *all the human beings on the whole planet* and somehow smush all their atomic particles together, getting rid of the empty space or energy fields we are made of. All the humans on the entire planet's smushed up atomic particles would add up to just one grain of rice. That is it!

The best image to illustrate that we are mostly open, permeable space is found in something called a "particle chamber," which can be seen in children's science museums. A particle chamber is a big glass box filled with ammonia mist. The plaque on the chamber explains that there are cosmic particles falling through space, through the roof of the building, through your skull, your body, your shoes, and right into the earth as you sit here reading this. However, the particles are too small to be seen with your eyes. So the chamber's ammonia mist wraps layers of ammonia around the particles and shines bright flood lights on them, making them big enough to see. When you look inside the particle chamber, what you see is a blizzard of these particles. The same blizzard that is flowing through us all the time.

> **CAUTION** **Ouch!**
>
> Don't feel as though you have to sit perfectly still while doing the Sitting QiGong exercise. If you need to fidget, roll out your neck or shoulders, scratch an itch, or yawn constantly, let yourself do it. Let your body be as loose and comfortable as possible. However, don't let your mind be distracted by having your eyes open. Close your eyes after reading each point, giving yourself time to experience the effects of each suggestion.

I mention all this to set the mood for the Sitting QiGong exercise. Because it reminds us that we are not solid impenetrable mass. We are mostly empty space, and the Qi or life energy can flow through our skull and brain just as easily as it flows through the air around us.

The only thing that can limit the Qi flow is a thought limitation. So if, when I invoke an image of a relaxing flow of energy pouring through your head, you think, "Hold on there, my head is solid mass," your muscles will tighten up a bit. This tightening will restrict the flow of energy that flows through you.

QiGong and T'ai Chi do not make energy flow through you. The energy flows through you every moment that you are alive. Yet as we age, we often squeeze off the flow of life energy, turning it into a dribble, rather than the river of life that flowed through us as kids. So T'ai Chi and QiGong work by allowing the mind and body to let go of fears, tensions, and grudges that squeeze off our energy flow. This Sitting QiGong exercise is about letting go effortlessly with every breath. The energy flows by itself.

Getting Started with Sitting QiGong (Jing Gong)

In this exercise you will begin to feel your flow of Qi, or life energy. The Qi will be referred to as "light" because the Qi flows right through you, like sunlight seems to soak right into your bones on a nice spring day.

Remember not to try. You are not *supposed* to see or feel anything. We are just going to have a nice relaxing experience. So, as I offer images to your mind, read them and then close your eyes and let yourself feel the result. You may want to tape record yourself reading this exercise, and then you can do it with your eyes closed. Also, you will find energy work audio tapes available for mail order in the back of this book that will guide you through this exercise.

> **Sage Sifu Says**
>
> To get better results and enjoy a wonderful experience, complete this exercise from beginning to end all in one sitting. This may take about 20 minutes. To only read this is not enough to understand Sitting QiGong. You must let your mind and body go through the different levels of relaxation to actually "feel" the results. Otherwise it would be like only reading about water and having never felt water.
>
> The Qi will move through you with no effort; the words below only initiate the process, then you can sit back and enjoy as the light or Qi moves to where your thought effortlessly directs it.

This exercise is best done sitting upright in a comfortable chair that supports good posture. Your feet should be in solid contact with the floor. Also, if your arms and legs are not crossed, the energy flows easier. When you see spaces between text divided by … (an ellipsis), give yourself a few seconds to assimilate and feel the experience before reading on.

1. Begin by placing your feet flat on the floor, with your palms flat on your legs. Let your eyes close comfortably and naturally. This exercise will be broken into sections so that you can open your eyes to read a section and then close them for a few moments to let yourself experience, or feel, the responses.

2. All T'ai Chi or QiGong exercises begin by simply becoming aware of the breath. Notice how your lungs fill and empty. Let your chest and back relax so that your lungs can fill from the bottom all the way up to the top of the lungs. Notice how as you release the breath, your lungs empty from the top, or the chest, and then empty all the way down into the abdomen, as the abdominal muscles pull in slightly.

Sit with feet flat, palms flat on thighs, and your back straight but not rigid.

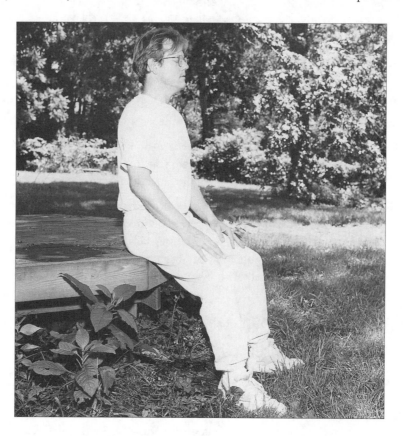

3. Let your mind relax as the muscles in your head, neck, shoulders, chest, and back relax. As the body relaxes, the breaths become not only deeper but also more effortless. Allow your awareness to relax and ride on the rhythm of that breath, as if the whole body was being breathed by the air. Let the whole body relax as you release each breath.

4. As you feel the body let go of the breath, feel the brain let go of your thoughts and worries of the day. Just as the deep exhales or releasing yawns allow the muscles to let go, the exhaled breath can also let go of mental tensions. The muscles within and around your heart likewise can hold onto fears or emotions. So as you release each breath, yawn, or sigh, allow the heart to release emotions, the body to release the muscles, and the mind to let go of worries. Each breath is a deep letting go on all levels.

5. Notice that as you let each breath out, it feels as though the atoms of the body are actually expanding away from one another. That's because they are. When we get tense, the body's atoms actually squeeze together, tightening us up. So as we breathe and allow the body to open, the atoms and cells relax away from one another … feeling as if the wind could blow right through you.

6. Now, think of the sun directly above your head. Just by thinking of an orb of lightness above your head, you may experience a subtle lift or lightening throughout your mind, or your presence. This Qi, light, or subtle energy, vibrates at a higher, more silken rate than the body's vibratory rate. Therefore, you may experience a feeling of lightness, or loosening, and a deep letting go throughout your entire being. Good.

7. Let that sun open and release a shower of clear, washing light, or silken energy, to pour over your head, body, and through your feet down into the earth below. Let go of that image and open to the feeling of deep release as you are washed by that silken energy. Like a water hose spraying through a screen door, just let the body open and be washed through, as you release each sighing exhale.

8. Be aware as a feeling of lightness expands through the tissues of the body. Notice the light spreading through the muscles in the top of your head. As the cranial muscles relax, they release their grip on the skull, allowing that permeating lightness to expand through the scalp. Expanding through the sides and back of the head, the entire scalp is lighted, as light flows out through every follicle and every hair on the head. Feel the scalp relaxing around the root of every hair.

> **CAUTION** **Ouch!**
>
> Whenever you notice that your breathing is very shallow or that you are holding your breath, make it a point to breathe deeply. Let the body relax open, allowing air down into the bottom of the abdominal region of the lungs, and let the whole body relax that breath out, as if the breath were breathing you. Do not force, just let.

9. Now allow the light to expand into the muscles at the base of the neck, then down and throughout the connected muscles in the shoulders and upper back. As they let go of their grip on the bones, experience the airy lightness permeating between muscles and bones … a deep letting go.

10. Feel as the energy expands up the back of the head and over the sides … feel the hinges of the jaw relax.

11. Now, allow this energy to expand over the forehead, the brow, down the bridge of the nose, and into the temples. Don't try to feel anything or make anything happen; just effortlessly observe as the light expands into the left eye socket … and then the right. Experience all the tiny optical muscles letting go.

12. Perceive the illumination expanding through all the soft tissue of the face, nose, mouth, and lips.

13. Experience an airy radiance expanding up through the nose into the deepest recesses of the sinus cavity. Feel that opening release as the sinuses fill with light.

14. Now, into the ears: Feel the deep skeletal muscles in the sides of the head let go as the silken energy expands into the inner ears, allowing a deep letting go in the sides of the head.

15. As the inner ears relax, the Eustachian tubes open, allowing the soothing energy to flow down into the mouth. As the mouth fills with light, the upper palate, upper jaw, gums, and even teeth seem to lighten, loosen, and let go. And now the lower jaw.

16. As you become aware of any saliva gathered in your mouth, swallow it, and experience the energy expanding down your throat, through the neck, and into your chest, shoulders, and back.

> **Sage Sifu Says**
>
> Do not rush through this. Be sure to close your eyes between each instruction point, allowing yourself to sit back and savor the experience of each image. Don't rush through it. Enjoy. Breathe. Breathe.

17. The heart itself can begin to lighten. If you catch yourself trying to feel or make something happen, let all that go. Be willing to feel absolutely nothing as you passively observe the lightness expanding through your heart and chest, permeating all the fibrous tissues of your lungs.

18. This allows every beat of the heart to carry lighted oxygen to all the extremities of the body; in fact, every cell begins to be lighted as the energy moves through the liquid systems of the body. Let the body open to that lightness, even in the tightest places.

19. Allow the light to expand through the abdomen, lighting the stomach … the liver … intestinal tract … kidneys … and lower back.

20. Now, think of the sun above your head again. Think of it opening and releasing an even greater flow of light over and through the body. Once you think the thought, let go of it, and experience the feeling of expanded release … as the bones themselves begin to lighten, the deepest skeletal muscles begin to release their grip on the bones.

> **Sage Sifu Says**
>
> The light or Qi heals and lifts without any effort on your part; let go of those tight head muscles and enjoy the feeling of release.

21. As the skull becomes permeated with light, the soothing energy expands right into the brain, illuminating the left frontal lobe and then the right frontal lobe, and expanding into the forebrain, above and just behind the eyes, into the midbrain and temporal lobes, and on into the brainstem, or old brain, in back.

22. Experience as all the billions of brain cells open up to that silken effortless radiance. It's as if the brain were a muscle that we've held clenched very tightly for a long, long time. And now as we allow the light to expand through the brain, we are finally allowing that muscle to let go, to expand open, and to light.

23. Now let the energy expand through the spine to the entire nervous system. Any nervous tension on the frayed nerve endings can now be released into that silken healing lightness now passing through all the nerves to the furthest dendrites in the skin.

24. Experience the light flowing down to the tip of the tail bone and radiating out, filling the pelvic bowl, and expanding on down through the legs and feet. Now think of the feet opening to allow this river of cleansing energy to pour right through into the cleansing pull of the earth.

25. Let the whole body open to be washed through as the feet release any loads or heavy tensions down into the earth's cleansing pull.

26. As you allow yourself to be washed through by this radiant cleansing shower, you may become aware of blocks in the flow. Tight spots, tensions, anxiety, feelings of restlessness, or thick drowsiness may appear. Any discomfort you feel is due to a block in the flow of energy. Note where you may feel those blocks or discomforts. Take a deep breath, and as you close your eyes, let the breath out. Think of the light expanding in the center of that tightness or blockage. Experience the opening release.

27. This enables the light to expand in the center of the blockage, allowing that area to open up. Release the blockage into the cleansing shower that pours through you to wash the blockage away and release it out through the feet into the earth. Breathe and release yet a bit deeper with every exhale, as if the bones themselves could let go of the load they carry.

28. Sit in this cleansing downpour for a while, enjoying the release. As any thoughts, worries, or tensions surface in your mind or heart, release them into the cleansing shower of washing light. Breathe, release, and enjoy.

29. Now, think of the feet closing. Instantly that happens, with no effort. By closing the feet, you may experience a sensation of back-filling energy on the soles of your feet as the light fills the feet and the field around, like a silken cocoon of light, coming up over the feet, ankles, knees, legs, and torso, and spilling over the top of your head to fill the field around you.

Sage Sifu Says

Our thought directs energy, and once directed, it moves there without any effort on our part. Having our eyes closed allows us to experience this within ourselves, to enjoy the cleansing release. This is effortless. The light, or Qi, moves with no effort. Once you think the thought, let it go, and sit back and enjoy your responses.

30. With the eyes closed, lift your hands in front of you, as if you were holding a giant beach ball between your palms (see the following figure). Think of the palms and fingers opening, and effortlessly the back-filling energy in your body now flows out through your palms and fingers.

31. Take a few deep-cleansing breaths to release all the muscles in your upper body, even though your hands are raised. It's the letting go that allows the energy to flow through more powerfully.

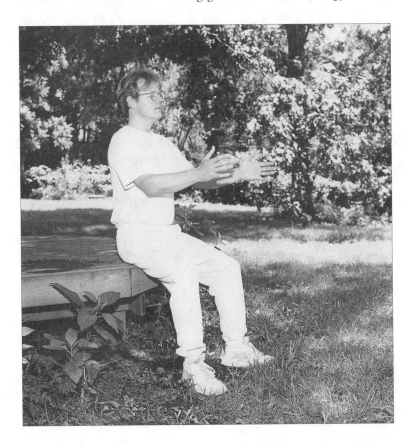

Be sure to let the upper body relax, even though the hands are raised. Slowly move them together and, with eyes closed, open to experience the sensations of Qi in your hands.

32. Slowly, begin to move the palms of your hands toward one another, opening them to the experience of the energy you've begun to gather, not only within and around you but between your palms as well. Move them toward one another, until they are almost touching … and experience.

33. Good, now slowly move your hands apart until they are about three or four feet away from one another, feeling the difference as they move apart. (Repeat moving hands in and out two more times.)

34. Now, gently place your palms back down on your thighs. With each releasing breath, let all that go, relaxing a bit more into your chair with each exhale.

35. As you let go of that experience, re-open yourself to the downpouring light washing over and through your head and body. With the feet closed, the body is saturated with light. Allow it to spill over the top of your head, quickly filling the field around you.

36. Soon it will feel as though you are floating within a limitlessly expanding ocean of light. With every exhale, allow yourself to be floating more effortlessly within it. Sit back and enjoy this feeling.

37. In doing so, you can begin to feel any remaining loads or heavy energy squeezed within the muscles or other tissues being magnetically lifted up and out of the body in all directions.

38. You can literally begin to feel burdens being lifted up and off of the shoulders, just by breathing and being willing to let go. Any worries and concerns are lifted off the temples or brow, again just by being willing to let go, and then observing the release. The deep facial muscles release tensions they've held onto during the day.

> **Sage Sifu Says**
>
> After learning and regularly practicing the soothing exercise of Sitting QiGong, you will become very adept at it. So when waiting in line at the supermarket, rather than being bored or anxious, just pretend to be staring at the latest tabloid scandal and open yourself to a soothing flow of life energy as it fills and permeates all the areas where your body is holding onto tension.

39. Now any heaviness or angst around the heart begins to be lifted up and off your chest. As the body continues to release these loads, you become aware of your entire being filling with a limitless permeable lightness, refreshing and absolutely effortless.

40. This process of release, cleansing, expanding, and enlightening will continue throughout the day. Even when you're not consciously aware of it, the rhythm of breathing and the willingness to let go will allow you to be lifted into the lightness of this ocean of silken energy. Here your stresses and loads can continually be released into the cleansing light, and your cells and surrounding field will be bathed in its effortless healing.

41. Let yourself sit within this ocean of light, assimilating and soaking in the light. Let go. There is no need to hold onto the light, for the more we let go, the more there is.

42. After assimilating the light for a few minutes, very slowly and very gently, when you're ready … open your eyes.

The Least You Need to Know

- Qi is scientifically observable and measurable.
- QiGong is effortless.
- Practice Sitting QiGong everyday to supercharge your strength, calm your attitude, and improve your health.
- QiGong is a way to program each cell to let go of stress at the earliest indication of blockage.
- QiGong programs the mind and body to radiate health.

Chapter 12

Moving QiGong (Dong Gong)

In This Chapter

◆ A word about mindful movements and mindless exercise

◆ Practicing Bone Marrow Cleansing

◆ Becoming elegant with Mulan Quan

◆ Learning to make walking a meditation

◆ Tonifying kidney function with Carry the Moon

The Sitting QiGong presented in Chapter 11, "Sitting QiGong (Jing Gong)," is a prerequisite for the simple, yet powerful, Moving QiGong exercises in this chapter. Remember, "mindfulness" is the act of observing, experiencing, and perhaps enjoying, rather than analyzing the world around us *or within us*. Sitting QiGong's effortless mindfulness of truly experiencing yourself from the inside is a big part of how Moving QiGong works its magic.

In this chapter you will experience how Moving QiGong can help treat illnesses and organs. QiGong can enhance immune system responses by cleansing the bone marrow of stress.

The following Moving QiGong exercises promote elegance and grace in your movements, while also promoting a calm and peaceful state of mind.

Mindful Movement vs. Mindless Exercise

Like Sitting QiGong, the goal of Moving QiGong is to let the mind initiate physical, mental, and emotional releases throughout the body. The more we let go, relax, and open, the more easily and healthfully the energy flows through us.

Much exercise is not very thoughtful. We strain and pound our joints and tissue running on pavement or in other high-impact exercises without paying much attention to the toll it can take on your body. Or for that matter the toll on our mind, as we often listen to loud music or watch the news while scurrying through our exercises. Studies have shown that loud noises and excessive TV watching can actually elevate damaging stress responses.

Moving QiGong, like T'ai Chi, is different. When you practice these exercises, let yourself take a break from the rat race, the noise, and the endless demands of the day. Practice QiGong in silence, hearing only your breath and the motion of your body. Let your mind be filled with the experience of letting go of *everything*.

Bone Marrow Cleansing

Some Moving QiGong exercises have a specific purpose, such as the Bone Marrow Cleansing. As you go through these gentle motions, the energy is encouraged and allowed to flow through the body, even the bone marrow, to cleanse this tissue of frantic energy. The tissue can function at a higher, clearer level when not burdened by old stress.

What follows are the instructions for a Bone Marrow Cleansing QiGong exercise. These instructions are broken into sections. Each section is preceded by a photograph that captures a key step in the exercise.

Hands at chest in prayer position.

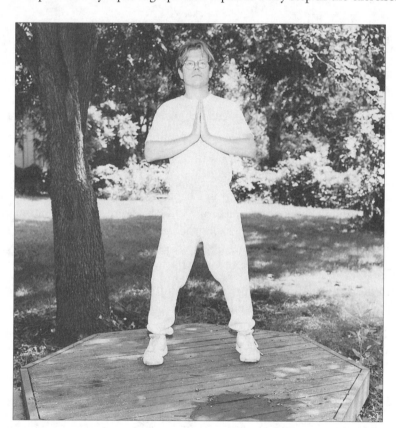

The following two instructions help you practice the movement presented in the previous figure:

1. Bone Marrow Cleansing begins with the feet about shoulder width apart and the knees slightly bent. Your hands are relaxed at your sides.

2. Bring your hands up in front as if lifting a one-foot ball to chest level, then letting the hands come together at the sternum.

T'ai Sci

TMany centuries ago before modern microscopes, Chinese health professionals understood that blood and bone marrow were associated with the immune system. They studied exercises like Bone Marrow Cleansing, not by viewing another's cells with a microscope, but by practicing the exercise and then observing their own internal health responses.

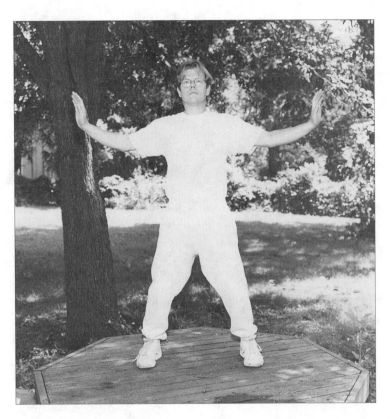

Arms out to sides, palms turned outward to universe.

The following two instructions are step-by-step supplements to the previous figure:

1. Lower your hands now back down to your sides, and then slowly raise your arms out to the sides.

2. Turn the palms outward. Think of opening the body to absorb the energy of life from the universe. Allow the body and mind to become open and porous.

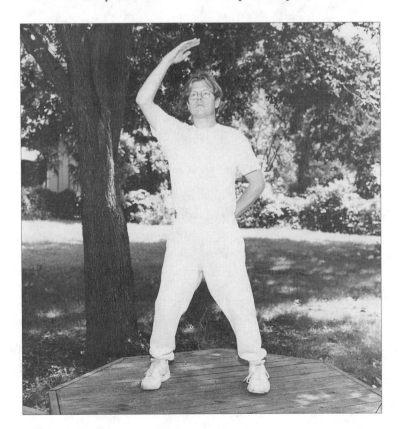

One hand overhead with palm down, and the other hand with back of hand on small of back.

The following four instructions guide you through the movement depicted in the previous figure:

1. Allow your arms to slowly descend to your sides.

2. One hand now floats up and outward away from the body until eventually it is above your head, with the palm turned down toward the top of your head. Meanwhile, the other hand drifts to settle the back of the hand on the small of your back.

3. As the palm above your head turns palm down, allow the energy to pour over and through the head and body. As the hand descends down in front of the body, the body fills with energy, washing through the bones and bone marrow, cleansing the body of any toxins, which are carried right down into the earth through the feet.

4. Repeat this on the other side, each hand now doing what the other did before. Repeat on both sides three times.

*Palms above forehead down,
similar to Grand Terminus.*

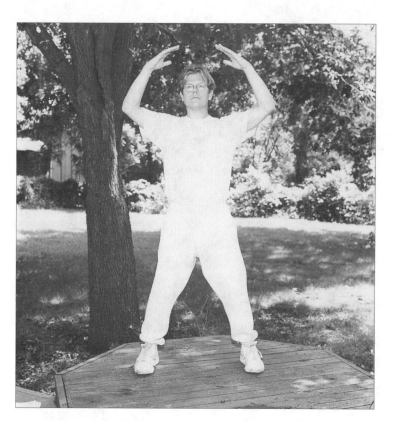

The following three instructions guide you through the last section of the Bone Marrow Cleansing exercise:

1. With both arms relaxed at your sides, begin lifting both palms up toward the sky.

2. Push your hands up toward the sky above your head, then turn the palms over facing downward.

3. As the palms float down in front of the body, let the energy pour through the bones and other tissues, carrying any impurities or dense energy right out through the feet into the earth.

A T'ai Chi Punch Line

Sometimes in classes, students express their concern for the environmental repercussions of releasing their heavy or toxic energy down into the earth. Look at this like our physical human waste, which becomes fodder or nutrients to the earth. Heavy energy the body releases is transmuted and lifted back into a healing force, just like trees breathe our carbon dioxide to create new oxygen. All things balance.

The Elegance of Mulan Quan

Mulan Quan warm-ups incorporate several lovely moving QiGong exercises. These promote elegance in movement and carriage, but also have healing effects as well.

Spread Wings to Fly

Spread Wings to Fly is a Moving QiGong exercise that specifically helps with upper limb disorders and to loosen tightness in the shoulders. This is a wonderful exercise to perform during breaks at work to release job tension.

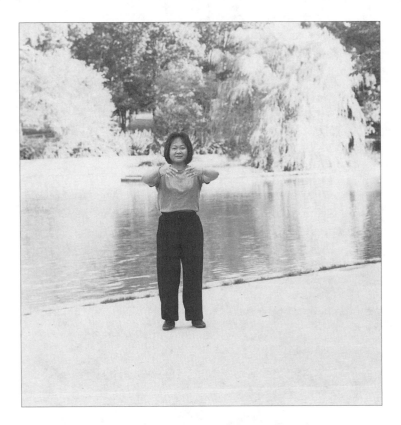

Hands out in front of chest.

These are the instructions for Spread Wings to Fly:

1. Begin with your hands out in front of your chest (as shown in the previous figure). Relax your shoulders and breathe naturally with the tip of the tongue lightly touching the roof of your mouth.

2. Begin a long slow inhalation of breath as you gently pull your arms back around to your sides (as shown in the following figure), until the shoulder blades touch in back, while simultaneously turning your head slowly to the left.

3. Begin exhaling as your arms slowly circle back down and around (rolling out the shoulder sockets) to the start position in front of your chest, while turning your head back to the front.

Ouch!

Although all Moving QiGong is likely an excellent addition to any physical therapy you may be involved in, you should use common sense and not force yourself into positions that you are not ready for. Always consult your physician or physical therapist before beginning any new exercise program.

Arms back till shoulder blades touch.

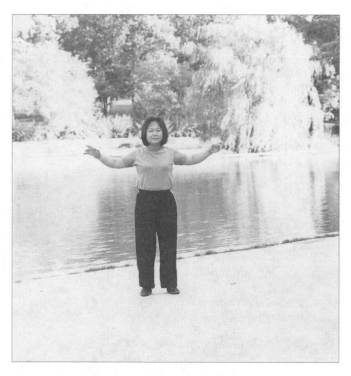

4. Repeat the entire process with your head turning to the right this time.

5. Repeat the process alternately turning your head to the left and then the right until completing eight forms (four with the head turning to the right, and four with the head turning to the left).

Tupu Spinning

Tupu can be therapeutic for movement limitations of the back, buttocks, legs, knees, and ankles. Here are the step-by-step instructions for this exercise:

Form fists held at the waist with elbows tucked in and knees slightly bent.

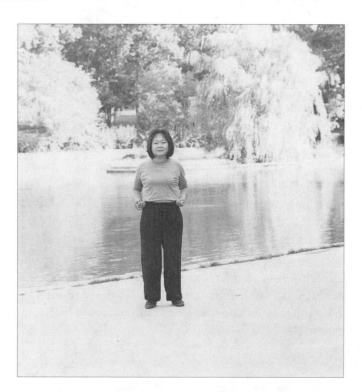

1. Begin by forming fists held at the waist, with your elbows tucked in and your knees slightly bent (as shown in the previous figure). Breathe normally and easily, yet fully.

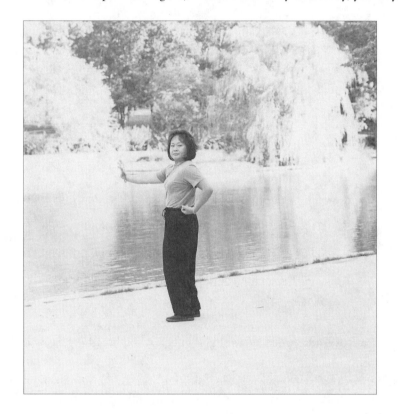

Look left, extend right arm out, left shoulder pulling back.

2. Inhale as you extend the right shoulder forward and as your right hand pushes out in front of your body (as shown in the previous figure). Simultaneously the left shoulder and elbow pull back as you turn your face to look back over your left shoulder. Exhale as you reverse this, pulling your right hand back to square off your shoulders, thereby returning to the start position.

3. Switch, extending your left shoulder out as your left hand pushes, and your right shoulder pulls back as you look back over your right shoulder.

4. Repeat on both sides four times each.

> **Sage Sifu Says**
>
> It is very difficult to fully comprehend how to perform QiGong by reading it from a book. If live classes are unavailable to you, there are many fine QiGong videos available. The Mulan Quan QiGong described in this section is available on the *Mulan Quan Basic Short Form* video listed in Appendix C, "Audio-Visual Resources."

Bring Knee to Chest

This movement not only feels great; it also helps with any pain in the legs and buttocks and is therapy for functional disorders of the leg involving bending and extending. Follow these instructions for the Bring Knee to Chest exercise:

Hands at sides relaxed, knees bent.

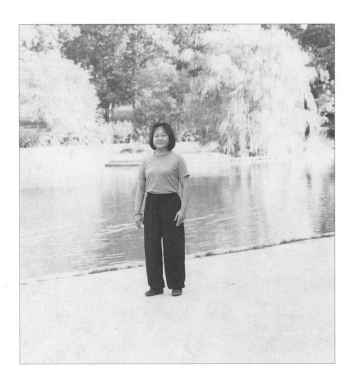

1. Begin with your hands relaxed at your sides, your knees slightly bent, while breathing easily and naturally.

2. Now begin inhaling as you step forward with your right leg, shifting your weight to the right leg as your arms swing upward and back in great round arcs (as shown in the following figure).

3. As the arms' arcs begin to swing down and toward the front, the left leg begins to lift.

Step forward with your right leg, swing arms backward.

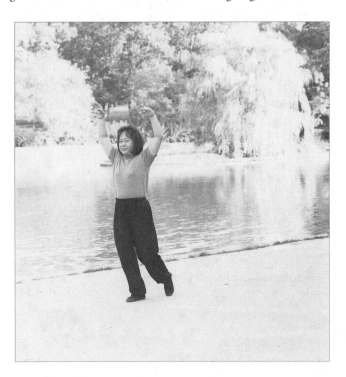

4. Lift up your left knee in front, pointing the toes of the left foot down, and wrap your hands around your knee to help it stretch up gently (as shown in the following figure).

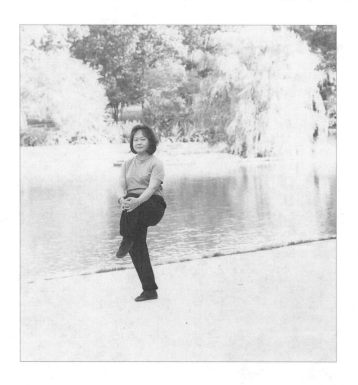

Lift left knee, wrap hands around knee.

5. Now exhale. As the left leg is released, the arms begin to swing down and back.

6. Place your left foot behind you and shift the weight back onto the left leg as your arms swing from the back over the top toward the front (as shown in the following figure).

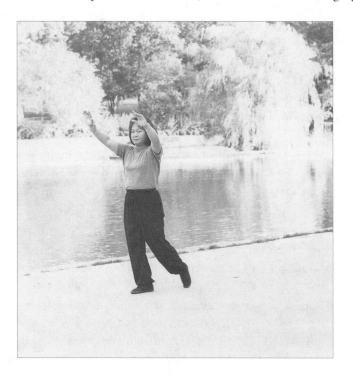

Left leg steps back behind as arms swing up and over.

7. Allow the right leg to come back even with the left, as your hands descend, returning you to the start position.

8. Repeat with the left leg stepping out this time. Repeat the entire process alternating sides (four times on each side).

Zen Walking in the Old Soft Shoe

Zen meditations involve a mindfulness that simultaneously allows your mind let go of the worries of the world, while attuning yourself to the world in a clear and healing way. Zen walking is a common T'ai Chi exercise. It teaches us how to let our movement fill our mind, while improving our balance and dexterity. Follow these instructions to Zen walk like the masters, and remember to breathe easily and naturally when Zen walking:

Zen walking resembles the way Groucho Marx used to walk.

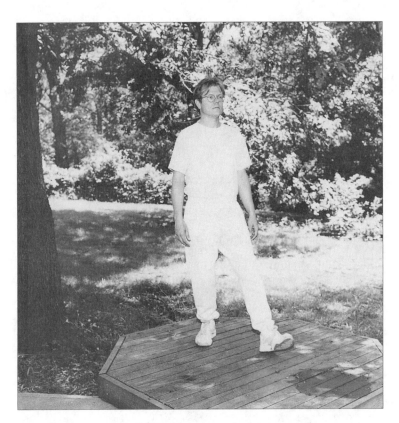

1. Place the heel of one foot outward at a slight angle, while maintaining balance over the back foot (as shown in the previous figure).

2. Slowly shift your dan tien, or weight, up toward the front foot, while slowly rolling the foot down onto the ground.

3. The back foot stays flat until your vertical axis, or dan tien, is settled over the front foot. Now let your heel lift up, then the foot, and now bring that foot up near your weight-bearing foot, before placing it out in front at a slight angle just like in the beginning.

4. Repeat many times, all the way across your living room or backyard. The goal is to Zen walk enough so that you forget about everything in the world except the soles of your feet, the ground they contact, and the shifting tissue in your body.

CAUTION **Ouch!** _____

Although QiGong may help with premature hair loss, it works best as part of an overall healthful lifestyle. So if you are in a high-pressure job you hate, aren't getting enough sleep, and smoking too much, the benefits of QiGong will be limited. QiGong practice may help you sleep better and eventually quit smoking. Therefore, QiGong should be viewed not as a cure-all, but as a stairway to a healthier lifestyle.

Carry the Moon

As discussed in Chapter 3, "Medical T'ai Chi: The Prescription for the Future," QiGong can treat specific organs, or systems, in the body. Carry the Moon is great for keeping the spine supple and can also tonify kidney function. It has been said that this may also help reduce premature baldness. This may be because, as with all QiGong and T'ai Chi, it promotes circulation, but in the case of Carry the Moon, especially in the scalp.

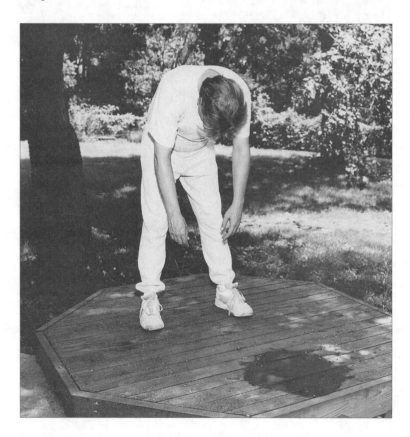

Leaning over with hands hanging down to about knees.

1. Begin with letting your hands and head simply hang loosely over as you bend effortlessly forward (as shown in the previous figure). Do not try to strain, as if attempting to touch your toes. Just let yourself hang comfortably, with your hands at about knee level or higher.

   Breathe naturally and easily.

2. Form a circle using the thumbs and forefingers of both hands. As you slowly rise up the hands ascend up above your head (as shown in the following figure).

3. Let the hands go up and slightly back behind as you gently arch your back to look up through the circle your hands form.

4. Hold this position as you breathe effortlessly and naturally for a few moments, then let yourself hang forward again, and begin again. Repeat several times.

With hands above head forming a circle between thumb and forefingers, looking through it.

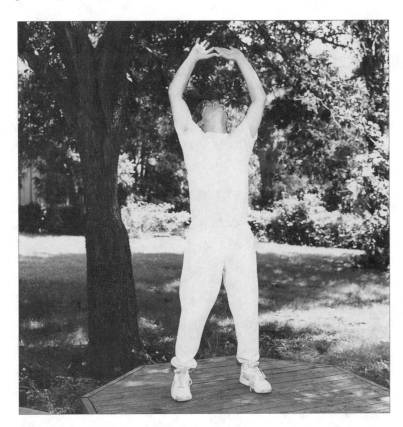

The Least You Need to Know

- Sitting QiGong prepares you for Moving QiGong.
- Breath and mindfulness is important in QiGong.
- QiGong can improve all organ functions.
- QiGong may slow premature hair loss.
- Use QiGong as a launch pad to a healthier you.

Chapter 13

Warm-Up Exercises

In This Chapter

◆ Using warm-ups to calm and center

◆ Loosening the body and the mind

◆ Healing your joints while perfecting your balance

◆ Cleansing your tissues and your mind

T'ai Chi warm-up exercises are not only meant to warm the muscle and other tissues but also to center the mind. You cannot listen to the radio or watch TV while warming up for T'ai Chi.

Unlike the way many of us were taught to "stretch" out our muscles when warming up by using straining stances, T'ai Chi warm-ups start from the very center of our being. We begin by becoming self-aware of that center and then relaxing ourselves from the deep skeletal muscles outward. We prepare ourselves for fluid and effortless movement by allowing our body to relax around our breathing lungs, and then all the muscles relax on top of the moving skeleton.

Each warm-up is a form of QiGong and promotes health and healing on many levels. These warm-ups are a beneficial exercise program even without T'ai Chi, but T'ai Chi offers so much more.

Dan Tien Takes Us for a Ride

When we start our Sitting QiGong, warm-ups, or T'ai Chi movements, our mind is usually scattered. We are thinking about what we need to do at work, what we need to do to prepare dinner tonight, and so on. So the first task of warm-ups is to center our mind, and the center of our being is, as you know, the dan tien.

Breathing Our Way to Center

There is nothing more calming and centering than hearing and feeling your own breath. Therefore all T'ai Chi–related exercises begin by simply closing your eyes and feeling the rhythm of your own breathing.

◆ Let your eyes close easily and naturally as you stand comfortably with feet fairly close together and knees slightly bent.

◆ Notice how your lungs fill and empty. Think of breathing into the bottom or abdominal part of the lungs, then letting the top or chest area fill.

◆ As you breathe, allow the muscles in your head and torso to let go. This allows the breaths to become not only deeper but also more and more effortless, almost as if the breath were beginning to breathe you.

◆ Let your awareness or mind relax, riding on the rhythm of your own breath.

◆ Now, think of breathing down into the dan tien area. You can experience the slight expanse of the upper pelvic muscles as you breath in, and how those muscles relax in as you release the breath.

◆ You may experience a feeling of air expanding down into that area. Of course the lungs don't go down that far, so you are feeling the Qi, or your awareness, expanding through the dan tien area.

> **Sage Sifu Says**
>
> When doing all T'ai Chi warm-up exercises, let your eyes close so that your awareness can relax within. Enjoy the sensations of loosening and breathing. Breathe fully, but don't force yourself. Breathe easily and naturally.

Let the Dan Tien Do the Driving

The breathing exercises help your awareness expand in the dan tien area, which prepares you to let the dan tien be the movement. This may sound a little odd at first, but after playing the following exercises for a while, it'll be quite natural and will dramatically improve your focus, balance, and movement. The first two T'ai Chi warm-up exercises employing hip rotations help you to practice this.

> **Sage Sifu Says**
>
> If you are in a wheelchair or have an injury or condition that requires you to sit, let the most inner part of your upper pelvis go into motion and be aware of that motion, allowing the body to relax as much as possible around that motion. If you are paralyzed, let the internal rotation begin in the center of the body at the lowest point your physical awareness begins.

Feet together, rotating hips in hula-hoop fashion.

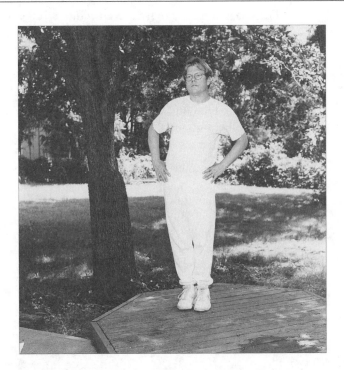

Follow these instructions to kick off your warm-up exercise:

1. With your feet close together, let the dan tien, or hips, begin a counterclockwise rotation, sort of like a hula hoop motion. If you were looking down at a clock face beneath your feet, you would be going counterclockwise.

   Notice that the dan tien begins to move effortlessly like a gyroscope in motion, allowing you to let your muscles relax while the dan tien moves the skeleton underneath. The shoulders do not move too much; most of the motion is in the dan tien, or hip area. However, don't be rigid about this. The goal is to get loose.

2. Repeat the counterclockwise hip rotations 32 times, if that feels good to you, and then repeat 32 in the opposite direction, clockwise.

   Close your eyes as you rotate the dan tien. At first this may challenge your balance, but you'll get better. With eyes closed your awareness can go within. You will notice areas of the body loosening as you rotate and breathe. Think of letting the muscles let go of bones and other tissue, allowing the body to just generally loosen on top of the skeleton. You will notice the lower back vertebrae loosening as the muscles around them begin to let go. You will also notice this loosening spreading up the back through the lumbar region, up through the dorsal vertebrae between the shoulders, and into the neck and back of the head. Basically, anywhere you let your light of awareness shine within, your body, mind, or heart can begin to loosen as you breathe effortlessly and move effortlessly in these dan tien rotations.

3. Now, repeat the hip rotations both ways (first counterclockwise and then clockwise), with your feet about shoulder width apart, and again knees slightly bent. Relax and enjoy the sensations of movement. With the feet farther apart and eyes closed, you will notice that you can very tangibly feel the top of the femur or hipbone rotating in the hip socket. Slow the rotations down, and you will feel the hipbone rotating all the way around the inner rim of the hip socket.

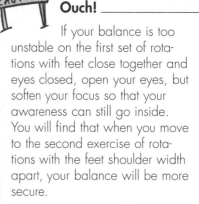

Ouch!

If your balance is too unstable on the first set of rotations with feet close together and eyes closed, open your eyes, but soften your focus so that your awareness can still go inside. You will find that when you move to the second exercise of rotations with the feet shoulder width apart, your balance will be more secure.

Enjoy the deep-tissue massage that the rotating bones give, as the deep hip muscles begin to let go of the tensions built up there. As you breathe and let muscles relax on top of the moving skeleton, you can enjoy this loosening through the back, legs, and rest of the body.

The enjoyment of this internal loosening helps us almost "see inside ourselves." Practicing this pleasant internal vision is a powerful health tool. By becoming aware of how good effortless motion feels inside, we also become aware of tensions or "diseases" at a very early stage before they actually become diseases.

Sage Sifu Says

We are a very shallow-breathing society. Therefore, you may catch yourself breathing very shallowly or even holding your breath as you move. Let your lungs fill effortlessly all the way down to the abdominal region and up to the top. Allow the entire body to relax that breath out, as if every cell of the body were letting go at the deepest level with each breath. Each breath lets us practice living effortlessly. There is nothing more effortless than the release of a breath.

Lengthened, Not Stretched

In T'ai Chi warm-ups, we don't strain to stretch out muscles. We allow ourselves to "lengthen" until we begin to ease up against strain. The tension we become aware of indicates a block. Then, we take a deep breath, and as we exhale, we allow light, or Qi, to fill the area of tension or restriction, which lets the block begin to let go. You can actually feel the lightness or release spread effortlessly through a tight or restraining muscle as you let the breath out. Our mind's awareness of the block directs the Qi, or energy, into the center of the block as we let the breath relax out of our body.

Fingers interlaced, stretching upward.

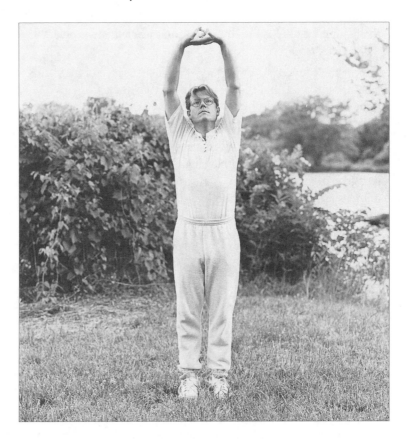

Follow these instructions to continue your warm-up:

1. With fingers interlaced, extend your hands up over your head.

2. Don't stretch, but allow your body to be effortlessly lengthened, as if the hands were being lifted up toward the sky.

3. As you release each sighing exhale, think of letting the muscles beneath the muscles let go.

4. Enjoy the feeling of effortless release through the back, shoulders, neck, head, and down into the hips and legs. As you breathe and let go, the entire body gets a bit of a stretch.

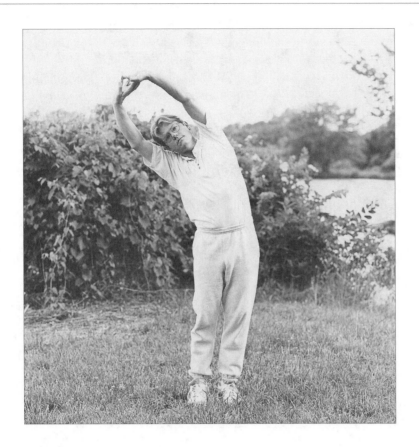

Hands extended, but now stretching over sideways.

Continue your exercise with these instructions:

1. Now stretch out to either side, but rather than thinking of stretching, think of the hands being drawn out and upward toward the sky out to the left and then the right. First the hands are drawn outward and up off to the right side of the body, and then easing back upward and over to the left side.

2. Go back and forth. Do not stretch so far to the side that it is a big strain. Rather, go just far enough that you can savor the sensation of the muscles stretching across the back, between the shoulders and through the neck. Again, as you loosen, the entire body gets a bit of a soothing effortless stretch.

Back bent flat, with hands hanging down.

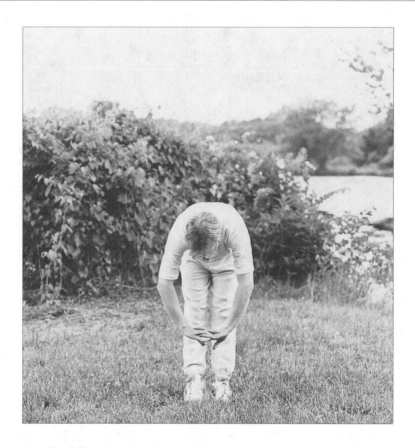

Now relax into this effortless posture by following these instructions:

1. Now, lengthen straight up again before stretching out and forward. The back should be fairly straight, bending from the hips and letting the arms just hang down.

2. Do not strain to touch your toes. That's not the point. The point is to feel an effortless lengthening through the upper body as you simply let go.

3. Enjoy that feeling of effortless elongation through the shoulders, neck, and back of the head. Notice that with each releasing exhale you can let go even more. With each releasing breath the muscles in the head can let go even more, showing you that relaxation is not a destination, but an endlessly enriching process of letting go.

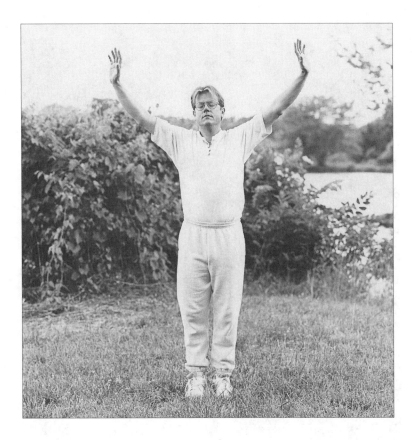

Hands descending to the sides.

Now follow these instructions to deeply let go:

1. Slowly and gently straighten back up to the original position of the figure above, with hands high over the head interlaced.

2. With eyes closed, take a deep breath and on the sighing exhale, allow the hands to descend to the sides so slowly that you can feel the air passing between the fingers. As the hands arc down from above the head out to the sides and the breath relaxes out, experience the different muscle groups letting go through the head, face, jaw, neck, shoulders, torso, arms, legs, and even into the hands and feet.

3. Let each exhale trigger a deep letting go from the very center of your being, as if the bones themselves could let go. Let every cell in the body relax those breaths out.

4. As you stand with your eyes closed, let go of all the muscles with each breath, and also let go of the heart. Just as the muscles release tensions with each sigh or yawn, the heart can let go of tensions or loads that it has squeezed in the heart muscle or muscles around the heart.

5. Think of the brain or mind letting go. Just as the cranial muscles let go of their grip on the skull, the mind can release worries and mental tensions with each releasing breath.

6. Realize that each breath can trigger a deep cleansing on many levels, mental, emotional, and physical. With each exhale, experience a deep letting go.

Filling the Sandbags, Sinking the Qi

Settling down into the Horse Stance is sinking your weight down into both feet as if you were sinking down into a saddle on a horse. Again, the tailbone drops as the pelvis tilts slightly up, and the head is drawn upward toward the sky, while the chin is pulled slightly in. This causes the spine to lengthen, which is great for the back, releasing a lot of the pressure daily stress puts on it.

Moving from the Horse Stance not only improves posture and balance, but it can also preserve your joints and make you more powerful.

Moving from the Horse Stance

Once you settle in the Horse Stance, let the dan tien flow back and forth from one leg to the other. Picture yourself sitting on an office chair with wheels, rolling from side to side. Or as if you were sitting on the back of a park bench, sliding your bottom from side to side. Notice that the head and shoulder never lead the way, nor do the hips stick out from side to side. The upper body stays stacked above the dan tien as it flows back and forth.

Note that the knees in the Horse Stance are slightly bent, and the upper body is stacked above the dan tien, erect but relaxed and not rigid.

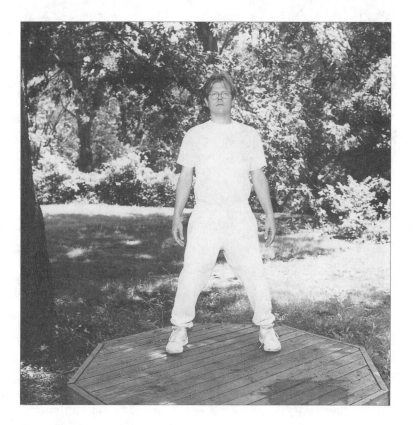

As you become aware of discomfort or tension—the fatigue you may feel in the muscles above the knees, for example—play the following game.

1. Let yourself feel the tension or discomfort, wherever it is in your body.
2. Experience how it feels and where you feel it.
3. Now, as you let the next breath out, think of letting the light, or Qi, expand right in the center of that feeling.
4. Let your awareness sit back and enjoy whatever responses you experience. Often you will experience a lessening of the discomfort or even a pleasure of the expanding lightness.

Sinking the Qi

In T'ai Chi, the upper body does not lean; it stays stacked up above the dan tien, just like in the Horse Stance. The dan tien flowing toward one leg fills that leg with the Qi, or energy (or the weight of your body). Simultaneously, the leg that the dan tien moves away from is emptying of Qi, or weight. In T'ai Chi, you rarely ever pivot a leg that has weight on it because it makes your balance precarious. More important, it damages the knees to pivot feet that bear weight. So this Moving from the Dan Tien exercise teaches you to shift your weight from one leg to the other. This simple exercise is the most important T'ai Chi warm-up because this is what T'ai Chi is. All of T'ai Chi's elaborate forms are based on the dan tien moving from one leg to another.

CAUTION Ouch!

Do not feel as though you must do all T'ai Chi warm-ups. Whatever warm-ups fit your abilities are the ones you should do. However, you may be able to modify exercises to fit your ability. If you are in a wheelchair or must sit while performing T'ai Chi, develop upper-body stretches you can perform.

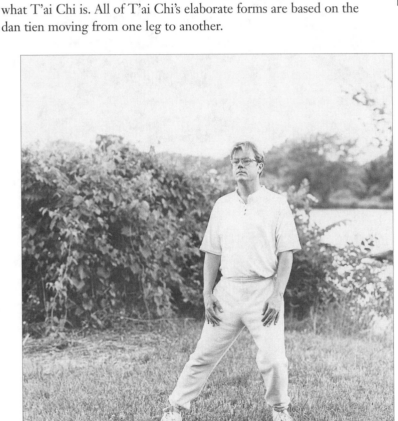

Flowing upper body to the other side.

Deep-Sinking Your Qi

If your mobility permits and you feel adventurous, you can practice a deep sinking of the Qi exercise, illustrated in the following figure.

Note that as the dan tien drops deeply down into one leg by bending that knee, the back is not bent over. As always, you do not bend, keeping the upper body stacked up above the dan tien.

Deep bending of one knee with back straight.

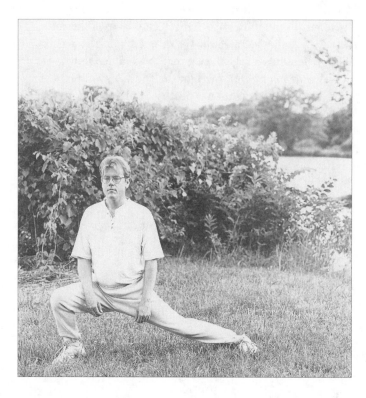

The Chinese Drum's Kaleidoscopic Sensations

The Chinese Drum mimics the motion of those little toy drums with the two swinging beads. When the drum is turned from side to side the beads twist and drum alternately on each side. This is how your relaxed arms and hands will gently strike your body, as you follow the instructions below and refer to the next two figures.

1. Now stand up with feet about shoulder width apart and knees, as always, slightly bent. Gently turn, swinging arms out. The lead arm swings across the back to strike the flank or lower back, as the trailing arm swings across the front of the body to strike the shoulder.

2. As the hands strike the shoulder and flank in back, close your eyes and enjoy the physical contact. The gentle slapping begins to massage the muscles, as you turn back and forth, alternately slapping each flank and shoulder in turn.

3. Let your mind release any analytical or problem-solving thoughts and simply open to the pleasure of the motion.

4. With each turn and releasing breath, allow the body to let go even more.

5. Let the mind relax into the pleasure of that letting go, allowing the mind to experience the tens of thousands of sensations throughout the body.

6. With eyes closed, you can attune yourself to the sensations of the pads of the feet shifting on the floor, the interactions of bones and muscles throughout the body, and the releasing pleasure of each breath. Feel the wind on your skin as you turn through space.

7. Even with closed eyes, patterns of light and shadow flow across your eyelids, and sounds both internal and external flow over and through you.

8. Do not try to hear, feel, or see. Rather, let your mind relax and allow sensations, images, and sounds to pour over and through your mind the way clear mountain water pours over a waterfall.

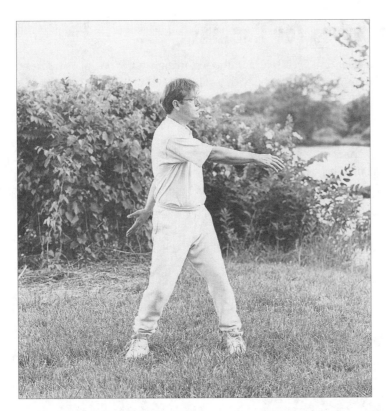

Turning and arm swinging out from body.

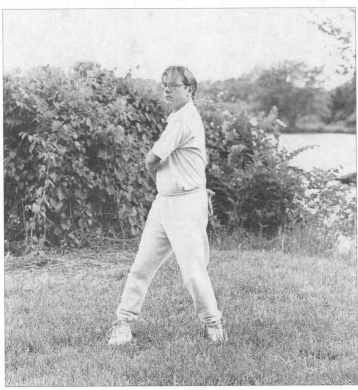

Hands striking body in back and shoulder.

Let the mind give up straining to function or reaching out to the world, but rather allow the world to flow to you in a soothing experience of effortlessness. Think of your mind releasing its grip on the dock of logical thought and floating down a river of kaleidoscopic sensation, carried on the beauty of existence, savoring the ability to breathe, flow, and experience sensation … effortlessly.

Deep-Tissue Cleansing Leaves You Radiant

QiGong provides many deep-tissue cleansing exercises, and the following is only one of them. It contains two parts that should be practiced gently and, as always, with awareness of your own mobility range.

Flinging Off and Breathing Out Toxins

Most tensions that we carry around are energy we've squeezed in our mind, heart, and the muscles in the body. You know this is true because on days when you feel heavy and weighted down by the world, if you get on a scale you don't weigh any more than usual. Therefore, we can simply fling off much of the loads we lug around.

Hands up high ready to swing out and down.

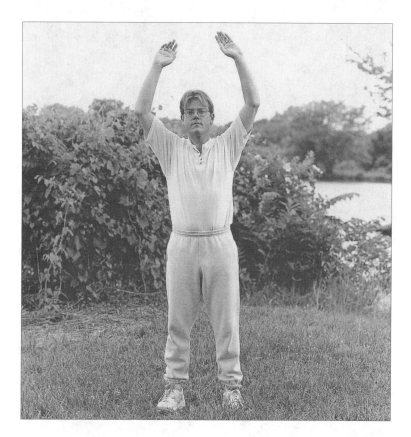

1. Begin with hands above head and then simply swing them gently outward and downward, flinging off the weight of the world you've held in your body.
2. Think of letting the bone marrow itself release the load it's holding on to, which, of course, it can release.
3. As the hands fling toward the ground, think of the hands and feet opening to release that load to fly out of you into the cleansing earth. As your hands swing out and down, exhale deeply to facilitate the release.
4. Breathe in as you raise the hands back up over the head, and again release all as you swing the hands out and down again. Repeat several times.

Elvis Impersonations Cleanse the Soul—*Baby!*

This tissue-cleansing exercise looks very much like an Elvis impersonation.

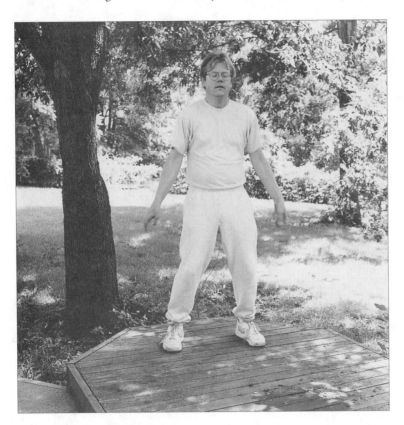

Let yourself go as liquid and limp as you can, with eyes closed, enjoying a loosening throughout your being.

1. With feet about shoulder width apart, eyes closed, and knees slightly bent, just shake. Gently let the arms and entire body go liquid and shake. Do not jolt the joints, but allow a liquid rippling to wave through every muscle and joint.

    Experience the skeletal muscles jiggling on the bones, from the top of the head to the pads of the feet. It's very slight and very subtle, but as those muscles loosen, they begin to cleanse the body of deep toxins. Think of the brain and heart loosening as well, letting worries, angst, and tensions evaporate out of the body with each yawn or sighing exhale.

2. Have one last good series of shakes while taking in a nice full breath. On the long sighing exhale, stop shaking and just feel the body awakening. Notice how every cell fills with an effortless lightness, clear, clean, and alive. Wherever you notice remaining tension or block, with each releasing breath allow the light to expand with that area as if the body were expanding endlessly outward, releasing any heavy loads to evaporate in that endless lighted expansion.

> **T'ai Sci**
>
> There are blood lactates, or lactic acids, which accumulate in the deep skeletal muscles during times of anxiety. Studies also show that these acids produce anxiety. Therefore, T'ai Chi and warm-ups like the Elvis Impersonation or Tissue Cleansing allow the body to release these long-held anxieties and to cleanse itself of them.

The Least You Need to Know

- ◆ The dan tien makes all movement effortless.
- ◆ Let warm-ups loosen your entire being.
- ◆ Moving from the Horse Stance is the most important warm-up exercise.
- ◆ The Chinese Drum cleans your mind and body.
- ◆ Let the exercises be a sensory amusement park.
- ◆ Doing warm-ups with eyes closed helps the mind relax within.

Part 4

Kuang Ping T'ai Chi: Walk on Life's Lighter Side

Part 4 introduces the Kuang Ping Yang Right Style's 20-minute long form. Chapter 14 helps you prepare mentally for the physical experience presented in Chapter 15. You will learn how T'ai Chi movements aid certain organs, and what T'ai Chi has in common with the ancient Chinese *I Ching*, or *The Book of Changes*. Chapter 15 illustrates the 64 postures of the Kuang Ping Yang style's forms in detailed sketches that help you analyze and study each move individually, as well as how they *flow together*. The text accompanying the images further details how movements are performed. Many of these forms can be seen performed in other styles of T'ai Chi as well. So the explanations of the benefits each movement provides and the T'ai Chi principles and insights explained can also benefit those practicing other forms.

Yet no matter how you learn your forms, once your entire 20-minute form is learned, it becomes a gateway to another state of mind. The constant effortless focus on the pleasure of movement and relaxed breathing, coupled with the concentration demanded by gravity and balance, brings your mind, heart, and body to a place of tranquil calm. As you learn and practice T'ai Chi, you will constantly ask yourself one recurring question, "How did I ever get along without this?"

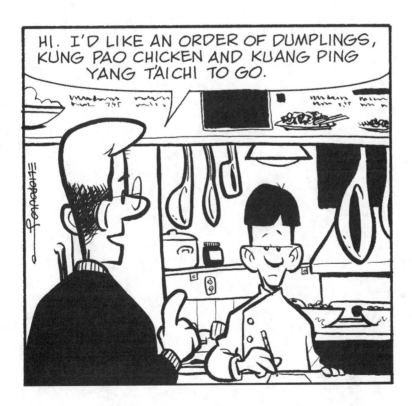

Chapter 14

Introducing the Kuang Ping Yang Style

In This Chapter

- ◆ Uncover T'ai Chi's ancient roots
- ◆ Learn how T'ai Chi became a philosophy of life
- ◆ Absorb the advantages of the T'ai Chi long form
- ◆ Find out why the Kuang Ping Yang has 64 movements
- ◆ Discover how the historical roots of medicine and T'ai Chi intertwine

The Kuang Ping Yang style of T'ai Chi has a rich and colorful history, as do all the ancient styles. The history of T'ai Chi is a great way to better understand its benefits and why it is so perfect for our modern harried lives.

This chapter discusses the roots of all T'ai Chi and explains how Kuang Ping Yang and the more extant Yang style became different. You will also learn why some styles offer shortened versions and why Kuang Ping has not developed a short form.

Understanding some of the historical or ancient tenets of T'ai Chi may actually help you get many more and endlessly richer benefits from its practice. The more your mind believes in your therapy, the more powerfully it heals.

The Snake and the Hawk

According to legend, T'ai Chi was born from an observation of nature. A martial arts master observed how a snake slowly evaded a crane's attack by moving away each time the crane's sharp beak struck. What may have been mortal combat became a gentle exercise that left the exhausted crane flying off for easier prey.

> **CAUTION**
>
> **Ouch!**
>
> If the idea of learning a long T'ai Chi form that may take 8 to 12 months to learn is daunting, remember the following: The journey of a thousand miles begins under one's own feet.

This example of yielding to the brute force of the world has created not only a powerful martial art but also an extremely healthful philosophy for surviving the stressful onslaught of an accelerating future. If this crane's attacks are compared with today's rapid changes, we may be much smarter to bend and yield to that change than to dig our heels in and fight it. The snake's yielding was much less stressful than a head-to-head fight with the larger, sharp-beaked crane.

> **Sage Sifu Says**
>
> Master Henry Look, one of the original students of Master Kuo Lien Ying of China, says there are seven important principles to T'ai Chi:
>
> - Centering
> - Quiet movement
> - Quiet breathing
> - Focus
> - Quiet smile
> - Quiet mind
> - Coordination

The Shao-Lin Temple: Where It All Began

The Shao-Lin Temple that was featured on the famous television series *Kung Fu* is actually where T'ai Chi began. An 18-movement stretching exercise that eventually grew into T'ai Chi was taught to the monks by a man known as Ta Mo around 400 C.E. The purported founder of modern T'ai Chi, however, was a monk named Chang San-feng, who lived about a thousand years later. It was Chang San-feng who is said to have watched the snake yield and avoid the crane's harsh attacks.

From the Temple to the West

The Chen family, founders of the Chen style of T'ai Chi, created one of the earliest family styles. The Chen style was taught to a young martial artist named Yang Lu-chan, who was the founder of today's Yang style.

The Yang family taught a style of T'ai Chi while residing in the city of Kuang Ping. Here the founding master Yang Lu-chan's eldest son, Yang Pan-hou, was made an offer he couldn't refuse to teach T'ai Chi at the imperial court and become the emperor's personal teacher. Since Yang could not refuse the emperor, he decided to create a lesser version of the family style to teach him, one that was inferior to the real Kuang Ping Yang style, which was practical, powerful, and a highly effective self-defense system.

> **Know Your Chinese**
>
> Chinese names begin with the family name. Therefore **Yang Lu-chan,** founder of the Yang style, would be called Lu-chan Yang in the West, as Yang is his family name.

This Kuang Ping Yang style was passed down from Yang Pan-hou to his student Wong Jao-yu, who taught master Kuo Lien Ying who eventually migrated to the United States and taught this to students who have since spread this style all across the United States.

This can be about as difficult to sort out as the cast of a soap opera, so don't worry about these details. It's just important to remember that the tools you are about to enjoy are the fruits of centuries of study. I include these stories not to confuse but to acknowledge and to thank these people for making available all that T'ai Chi has to offer.

T'ai Chi Becomes a Philosophy

Around 1500 C.E., the Taoist philosopher Wan Yang-ming began to blend the gentle centering philosophical concepts of Taoism into the equally centering physical concepts of T'ai Chi. This gave practitioners a real way to live a more healing, nonviolent life—not just preaching it or thinking about it, but actually training their mind and body how to live that way through T'ai Chi's gentle mind/body fitness program. The modern styles now widely practiced—Yang, Chen, Wu, Mulan Quan, and others—all incorporate the beautiful personal growth concepts of Taoist philosophy.

The philosophy of T'ai Chi is based on the idea of the balance of nature, both internally in our health systems and externally in our relationships with the natural world. Therefore you will see nature imitated in many of the T'ai Chi form names, such as the following:

- Wave Hands Like Clouds
- Wind Blowing Lotus Leaves
- White Crane Cools Its Wings
- Retreat to Ride the Tiger

> **A T'ai Chi Punch Line**
>
> T'ai Chi styles have been created with the same fluidity to the world's demands that T'ai Chi encourages its practitioners to have. For example, the Wu style was created by Wu Quan-yu, a palace guard in the Imperial Court who designed a system of T'ai Chi that could be performed in the restrictive clothing of an imperial palace guard's uniform.

The poetic quality of these names does more than just remind us how to perform the movements. On a subliminal level, they make us feel more at home in the natural world, somehow more attuned to our connection to the whole of life.

T'ai Chi movement names can also help us remember our multidimensional nature. We are all physical and mental beings, of course, and T'ai Chi integrates these aspects of ourselves well, but it connects our minds and bodies with our spirit or energy nature as well. This connection is reflected in movement names, such as:

- Strike Palm to Ask Blessing
- Focus Mind Toward the Temple

T'ai Chi reminds us that we are part of the universe, and that in fact we are made of the same energy that stars and everything else are made of. T'ai Chi is meant to open us up to the limitless supply of energy within us, in the earth we walk upon, and from the universe our world hurtles through. That universal connection is also reflected in movement names:

- Step Up to Form Seven Stars
- Grand Terminus

Grand Terminus, the final movement, opens us up to the limitless energy of the universe around us.

Short Forms vs. Long Forms

Today, there are several short versions of the original long forms of T'ai Chi. Although these shortened versions serve useful purposes, such as enabling a student to acquire a practice system more quickly, there may have been a reason for the average 20-minute length of some of the long forms. The value of a 20-minute-long form is now borne out in modern medical research.

> **Sage Sifu Says**
>
> Most short forms of T'ai Chi take between 8 to 10 minutes. If you practice a short form, simply loop it twice so that you can exercise for 20 minutes and get more benefit. However, if you ever get an opportunity to learn the long form of your style, do it. The complexity of 20 minutes of different movements keeps your mind in a state of relaxed focus, even more so than repetition of the same movements does.

We now know the original ancient forms, which usually took a minimum of 20 minutes to complete, were that length for a good reason. In his groundbreaking book *The Relaxation Response*, Dr. Herbert Benson notes that a 20-minute relaxation response exercise seemed to evoke the optimum benefits. Apparently, the first few minutes of a relaxation therapy are used by the mind to just wind down; the remaining time truly allows the deep alpha state relaxation these therapies are known for. It is highly advisable, therefore, to take the time to learn a long form of T'ai Chi.

Why Sixty-Four Movements?

While the more extensive Yang form names 108 movements, the Kuang Ping Yang style long form claims 64 movements.

There may be more to this than just chance. The number 64 has profound philosophical meaning. The Chinese classic *I Ching*, or *The Book of Changes*, is an ancient text of divination and philosophy that attempts to explain how the universal forces of yin and yang ebb and flow, combine and disintegrate, and rise and fall to create the dance of existence. The central premise is that all things are in a constant state of change, including our lives and us. T'ai Chi's goal is to help us flow with the change and not be compulsively attached to the old *or the new*, using what works and discarding what is no longer useful. As if you were a surfer riding the changing waves of life, let go of old waves as they recede, to ease onto the mounting power of the new wave.

The *I Ching* uses Trigrams, or figures with three lines (pictured in the following figure to symbolize the changes in life). When two Trigrams are combined, 64 possible combinations are obtained. These 64 hexagrams are said to represent all possible states of change in the universe. Therefore, Kuang Ping Yang's 64 flowing movements symbolize, and in some ways physically help us to flow through, all the possible changes and challenges of life those changes entail.

Trigrams are combinations of three lines, which can be broken in half or be whole, making eight possible combinations.

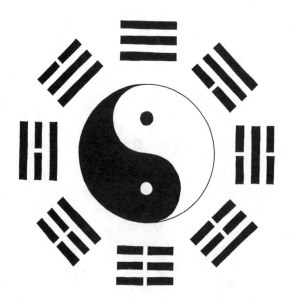

That Kuang Ping Yang style T'ai Chi forms involve 64 movements may have deeper reasons than we know. The complexity and powerful healing qualities that T'ai Chi offers are only now beginning to be discovered by modern science. There may be many other details of how and why T'ai Chi does what it does that will be uncovered in years to come.

T'ai Chi and Chinese Medicine

As I discussed in Chapter 3, "Medical T'ai Chi: The Prescription for the Future," Traditional Chinese Medicine uses the Zang Fu system of understanding how organs interact. Each of these organ systems is represented by one of the five elements of the earth, according to ancient Chinese physics.

- ◆ Metal = Lungs and large intestines
- ◆ Wood = Liver and gall bladder
- ◆ Water = Bladder and kidney
- ◆ Fire = Heart/pericardium/small intestine/triple warmer
- ◆ Earth = Spleen and stomach

T'ai Chi movements are described with this same system, and the motion of the body that T'ai Chi promotes may have a healing effect on those systems. The directions of movement each correlate to one of the earth elements.

Movement Directions Relative to the Body:

- ◆ Metal = Advance
- ◆ Wood = Retreat
- ◆ Water = Left
- ◆ Fire = Right
- ◆ Earth = Center

Movement Directions Relative to Earth:

- ◆ Metal = West
- ◆ Wood = East
- ◆ Water = North
- ◆ Fire = South
- ◆ Earth = Center

> **T'ai Sci**
>
> Some T'ai Chi movements look very similar to modern physical therapies. For example, Dropping the Duck's Beak, which is an extension of the fingers bending down to touch the thumb, is the same as a Carpal Tunnel prevention exercise used in many corporations. Could it be the therapy for modern repetitive stress disorders had been discovered centuries ago?

> **CAUTION** **Ouch!**
>
> It is not important to mentally calculate what movement or direction benefits what system of the body. It is more important to simply allow the mind and body to enjoy the exquisite pleasure of effortless breath and movement as you do T'ai Chi. Rest assured that each aspect of your mind, heart, and body is being nourished and healed by the life energy T'ai Chi practice promotes.

The 64 postures of the Kuang Ping Yang style take about 20 minutes to complete. The movements flow in an unending progression from one to the next until the final movement, the Grand Terminus. The movements will move the body outward and backward in all the directions previously described. There is also a meditative quality to that motion that cannot be described or conveyed in print.

Chapter 15, "Out in Style: Right Style, That Is," however, provides detailed sketches of each of the 64 Kuang Ping Yang style movements, numbered in sequence. They explain many of the benefits of each movement, complete with pointers on correctly performing them and cautionary notes to help your T'ai Chi experience be both healthy and profound. If live classes are unavailable to you, you may want to check out the video listed in Appendix C, "Audio-Visual Resources," for further details.

The Least You Need to Know

- ◆ T'ai Chi teaches us to yield when life attacks and advance when opportunities open.
- ◆ Twenty-minute-long forms have advantages over short forms.
- ◆ The 64 Kuang Ping movements ease the mind and body through changes.
- ◆ T'ai Chi movements have healing abilities we've yet to completely understand.

Chapter 15

Out in Style: Right Style, That Is

In This Chapter

◆ Learn the Kuang Ping Yang style long form

◆ Adjust T'ai Chi to fit your body

◆ Breathe through life's challenges

◆ Use T'ai Chi to help prevent repetitive stress injuries

◆ Relax into "complexity" and tap into universal, limitless energy

This book will greatly enhance your T'ai Chi experience, no matter what style you practice, by offering you value that you may not get otherwise, by fleshing out how and why each movement can benefit you, and by understanding the internal mechanics of posture, weight shift, and Qi flow. Since T'ai Chi is constant movement, video instruction and/or live classes may help you fill in the gaps. Appendix C, "Audio-Visual Resources," lists an instructional video and DVD, by the author, teaching this long form in a step-by-step lesson-based, real-time, format, just as you'd learn in a live class. This video provides an added dimension of the timing of breath, imagery, and relaxation.

The explanations and instructions you find in this book are *unparalleled* and will provide *profound* added benefit to even video or live classes. Each movement will be broken down in a series of sketches, to help you see both external and internal aspects of each movement. The movement sketches and their accompanying text include …

◆ **Directional arrows.** Arrows show how your limbs or body move from *the previous* "ghost image" position into the current position. Taking all the guesswork out of how you get from one pose to another.

◆ **Markers.** "L" and "R" marked on the figures so you can see at a glance whether the "left" side or "right" side of the body is depicted.

◆ **Shading.** The leg the weight is on, or the *filled leg*, will be shaded to a darkness level reflecting just how much weight is shifted on to it. When both legs are shaded, weight is evenly distributed.

- ◆ **Posture line.** A line indicating your *vertical axis* or postural alignment centered over the dan tien.
- ◆ **Emphasis.** Occasional *italicized* text explains what *sensations* and *internal awareness*, releases, and benefits you may be experiencing *within* as you go through the motions.
- ◆ **"Ghost" images.** Most of the sketches will have a *ghost* image indicating what the previous posture was, helping you see transitions.

A couple of the sketches will also reflect how the Qi or life energy flows outward through the hand or the foot. This is only shown in a few figures, as too many graphics would be distracting. As a general rule, when you are physically moving an empty foot to a new location on the floor, *an in-breath is being taken in.* When the weight (vertical axis) is shifting over/into/onto a leg and foot, *the breath is being exhaled, as you sink into the leg,* allowing Qi to flow down through your relaxed "filling" leg and out the extending arms and hands. This illustrates why the practice of Sitting QiGong is such a critical element to a powerful and effective T'ai Chi form (no matter what style you do), as it enables you to practice "feeling the Qi," or relaxation flowing through your arms and body.

The Kuang Ping Yang style long form takes approximately 20 minutes to complete. Before beginning the movements, to understand why the vertical axis and filling illustrations are so important to your T'ai Chi practice, try this simple exercise:

1. Standing comfortably in the Horse Stance, close your eyes and breathe while relaxing the entire body, and standing in your proper vertical axis with the head stacked up above the lower dan tien.

2. Lean your head forward, noticing how the muscles tighten to hold you up. As the head goes back into vertical axis alignment, notice how effortless the stance becomes. The same thing happens when you lean back slightly.

Moving in vertical axis posture will make everything more effortless. Practicing T'ai Chi with this awareness of effortless versus effortful movement will easily and naturally change the way you move through life. T'ai Chi and life, should be mostly effortless, and strangely when it is, is usually when we are getting *the most accomplished.*

As you go through this exercise, note that the movement names offer two tools. One is they evoke healthful and soothing mental/sensual images to calm the mind and heart. Second, they offer visual mental images to help us remember how to move. Part of the calming effect results from T'ai Chi's left-brain/right-brain integration of "feeling" and "thinking."

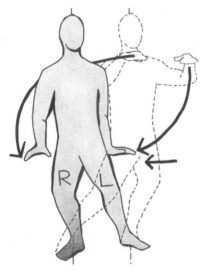

15-1a

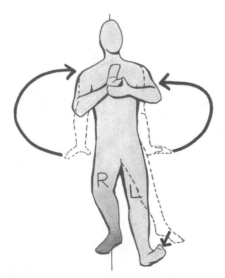

15-1b

15-1c

Strike Palm to Ask Blessings, #1

15-1a: Breathe in deeply and lift your palms as if circling them up in front of you over a large three-foot ball, shifting weight toward the left foot.

15-1b: As the palms pull back over the sphere, ending up in front of your chest as though you were going to push something away, the weight shifts back to the right foot, sinking the Qi, or filling the right foot, as palms drop to sides of hips.

15-1c: From palms down position, palms pull out and behind a bit to rotate out the shoulders. As empty left foot comes out in front, place left heel lightly on the ground. Continue circling arms around in front of body as if hugging a large tree, and left heel touches just as your palms meet. The left palm is lateral as in the sketch, while right palm is vertical. Although the movement is called Strike Palm, the palms don't actually strike; pretend there is a soft energy sphere the size of a honeydew melon between your relaxed, rounded hands.

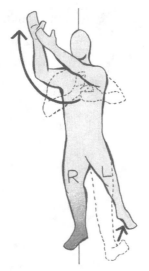

15-2a

Grasp the Bird's Tail, #2

15-2a: From completed Strike Palms, reach up with your arms, reach up and out to the right as your left toe reaches out to the left and back.

Sage Sifu Says

Strike Palm, Grasp Bird's Tail, and Single Whip are all wonderful for loosening the daily stress from tight shoulders.

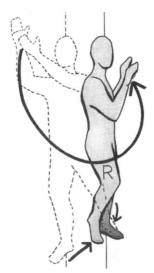

15-2b

15-2b: With your right hand palm down on top of your left hand palm up, stroke the bird's tail as your arms pull down and back. Your weight shifts back to the left foot behind.

Your hands stroke down to the groin, releasing the bird's tail. Turn palms away from your body with your elbows at your sides while your hands continue to circle up in front of your face. Your right foot pulls back touching your right toe near the left instep.

15-2c: Now, turn your dan tien and torso to the right at a 45-degree angle (front/right), while your arms follow around and in front of your chest, ready to push out diagonally to right.

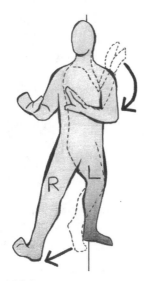

15-2c

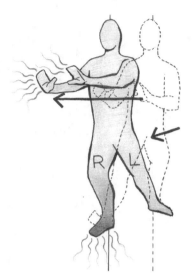

15-3a

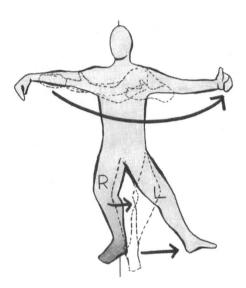

15-3b

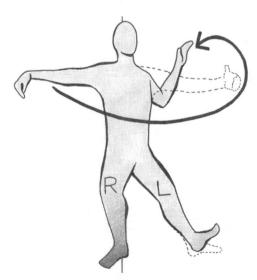

15-3c

Single Whip, #3

15-3a: Step out with your right heel, pushing your hands forward as the weight shifts onto the right foot (rolling onto the heel first and then the rest of the foot goes flat). Notice how Qi flows through the relaxed body, out pushing hands and down through the filling right leg into the earth. At first you simply relax and ex-hale, then over time a feeling of "empty flow" will settle through you, and in time you'll perceive a soothing flow of energy.

Your arms stretch out to your right side, as the fingers on the right hand bend down touch-ing right thumb (forming a duck's beak).

15-3b: Your left fingers stroke the inside of the right arm. Your left palm pulls across your body in a great half circle toward the left side as the body follows, turning at the dan tien, as shown in the following sketch.

15-3c: Your left palm continues over to the left side, as if circling a globe on its axis, until your palm is near your shoulder …

T'ai Sci

T'ai Chi's a uniquely right-brain/left-brain experience. Our analytical mind follows detailed forms, while sensory mind enjoys a sense of being carried through motions, almost being massaged by the process effortlessly. Book instruction is left-brain, while video/class is more right-brain.

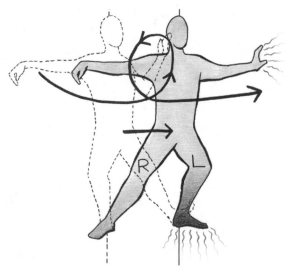

15-3d

15-3d: … and then your left hand pushes the imaginary globe away to the left, while the weight sinks onto the left heel and then the rest of the left foot. Again, note how the Qi or life energy flows through the relaxed body, out the hand and down the leg into the earth.

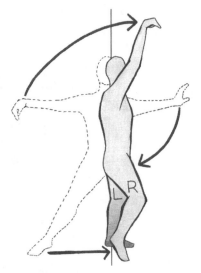

15-4a

White Crane Cools Its Wings, #4

15-4a: Your weight shifts to the left leg as the torso turns to the left. The left arm drops down to your side, the palm facing the ground, as the right arm circles from behind up above head.

T'ai Sci
Place the tip of the tongue lightly against the roof of the mouth while performing your movements, and fully fill and empty the lungs from bottom to top on each breath, allowing the torso to "relax" around your breathing. Studies show that long, relaxed abdominal breathing oxygenates the body much more effectively than rapidly inflating the chest.

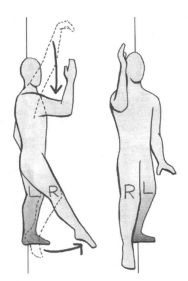

15-4b

15-4b: Note that these two sketches show the same pose, so you can now see it from a frontal angle as well. The right arm comes straight down as the right foot sticks out a few inches in front.

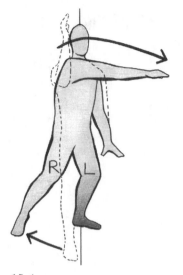

15-4c

15-4c: Step out to the right side with your right toe, as the right elbow circles to the left side, to prepare, by winding up, for upcoming elbow strike. (Both palms face down, in their respective positions.)

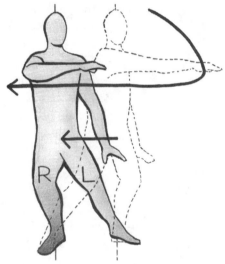

15-4d

15-4d: Now, shift the weight to the right foot as the right elbow pulls across in an elbow strike, allowing the sinking dan tien to pull the elbow strike across.

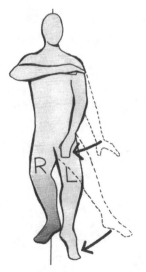

15-4e

15-4e: Lift the left foot and place it out in front, as the left hand moves slightly to the front.

Sage Sifu Says

Remember that the "ghost" images in most of the instructional sketches represent the "previous" posture, included to help you see *transitions between positions.*

Brush Knee Twist Step, #5

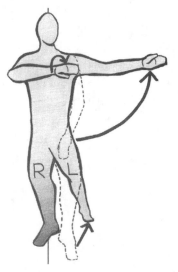

15-5a

15-5a: The left hand extends out 45 degrees to the left of front, as the left foot steps back behind slightly. The right forearm twists a bit so that the "back" of the right hand is facing the chest, and the palm faces out.

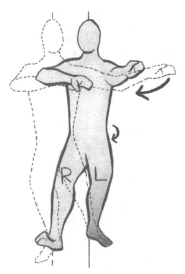

15-5b

15-5b: Now, the weight sinks back into the left foot as the left arm brushes to the center of the body as if slapping an imaginary wall in front of you. Exhale and allow the body to relax as the weight, or dan tien, sinks back on each Brush motion.

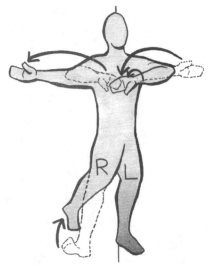

15-5c

15-5c: With the weight back on the left foot, the right empty foot steps slightly back as the right hand extends out 45 degrees to the right, and "back" or left hand is placed in front of heart.

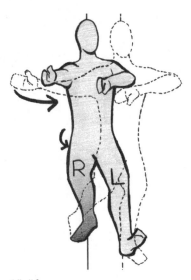

15-5d

15-5d: Just as you did on the left side, now shift your weight back to the right, brushing the right hand toward your center.

Repeat once more on both sides, as in Figure 15-5a through 15-5d. As you finish the last brush, shift to the right foot and brush across the body with the right hand.

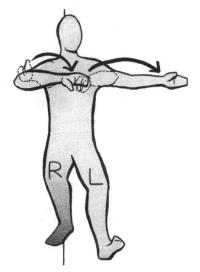

15-5e

15-5e: Move the left hand out 45 degrees to the left, but do not move the left foot this time.

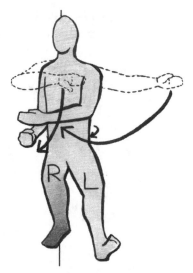

15-5f

15-5f: Brush the left hand across the body, and let the left arm circle out in front as the right hand forms a fist by the right hip.

CAUTION **Ouch!**

If any of the movement descriptions cause pain, alter them to suit you. For example, if you have a bad knee share some weight on the empty foot as well.

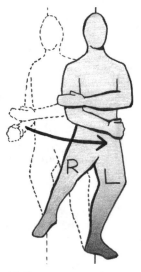

15-5g

15-5g: Now, shift your weight 60 percent onto the left foot and throw the right fisted punch out in front beneath the left arm circling out in a defensive posture, or parry.

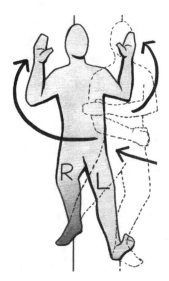

15-6a

Apparent Closing, #6

15-6a: From the parry and punch position, the palms turn down, then hands open and come back to the temples, as your weight shifts back onto the right leg and the left foot rolls back on its heel.

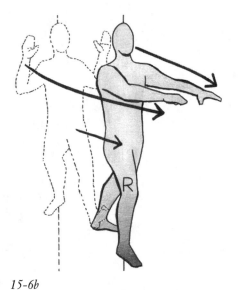

15-6b

15-6b: Push out as the weight rolls forward onto the left leg. Step through with the right foot, and then shift your weight to the right leg as you push out to point with flat hands.

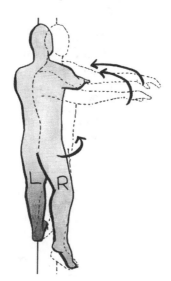

15-7a

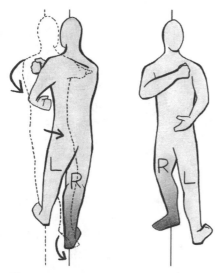

15-7b

15-7c

Push Turn and Carry Tiger to Mountain, #7

Carry Tiger to the Mountain, as other movements, reminds us of our connection to nature, as we mimic the grace of noble beasts.

15-7a: With your weight on the right foot and your hands pushed out flat, your weight comes off the left foot until only the toe is touching as your pushing hands circle flatly (as if on a table top) to the left as the left foot pivots on the toe.

15-7b: At ¾ of the hands circling to the left, your weight begins shifting to the left foot as the empty right foot pivots on the toe.

15-7c: With the 180-degree turn complete, your weight settles back on the right foot. Only the left heel touches, as your left toes come up off the floor, and your right fist rests over the thumb of your open left hand in front of your abdomen. Note the two figures in this sketch depict the same posture, only shown twice so you can now view it frontally.

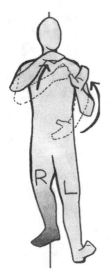

15-8a

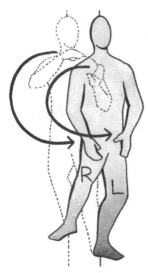

15-8b

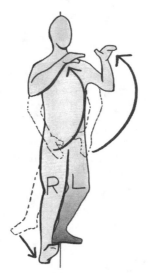

15-8c

Spiraling Hands to Focus Mind Toward the Temple to Parry and Punch, #8

This movement encompasses the spiritual image of Focusing Our Mind Toward Our Temple, which is the heart, while providing a protective shield for the vital/vulnerable areas of the body.

15-8a: With your hands open, the palms should be parallel to one another and pointing straight as the left heel lifts (your weight is still on the right leg) and the left heel lightly retouches the ground.

15-8b: Your weight slowly shifts up to the left foot as your hands begin a clockwise corkscrew downward. (Keep your hands relaxed at the wrists so that they pivot facing straight.)

15-8c: As your weight shifts completely to the left foot, your hands begin the upward part of a clockwise rotation, lifting the right foot up from behind, as if a string were attached from your hands to your feet, and reaching the top as the right heel touches the ground in front of you.

Remember not to "bob up" as you shift up into the front leg. In T'ai Chi you always stay "down" in a slightly bent knee stance.

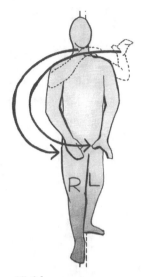

15-8d

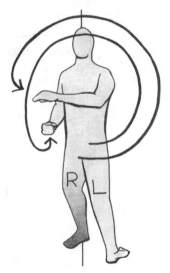

15-8e

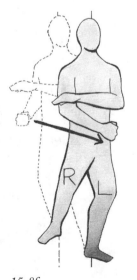

15-8f

15-8d: Repeat this stepping/ shifting/spiraling hands with the right foot out this time, and repeat left foot out, and then right foot out (for a total of five times stepping forward on this Spiraling Hands Movement, alternating feet each time, of course).

15-8e: However, on the fifth step, which is with the left foot out, do not shift your weight to the left foot. Leave it out and empty as the hands corkscrew one last time all the way around.

Then allow the right hand to fall to your side, forming a fist as the left circles in front to parry.

15-8f: Now, parry and punch with your weight shifting about 65 percent onto the left foot.

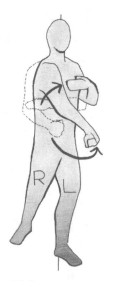

15-9a

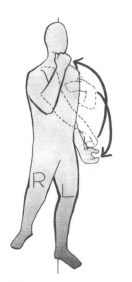

15-9b

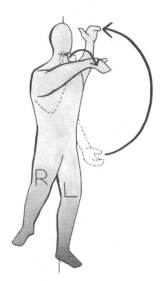

15-10a

Fist Under Elbow, #9

15-9a: With your weight still mostly on the left foot (in the punch parry position), drop your right fist down under your left elbow.

15-9b: As right fist is pulled up with the palm facing your chin, left parry hand drops to the palm up position to rest at left hip.

Repulse the Monkey, #10

Repulse the Monkey can be a powerful martial arts tactic of blocking an incoming blow, yielding to the opponent's force, and allowing that force to carry the opponent flying off to your side. However, it also fosters a very healing exchange of energy that Traditional Chinese Medicine (TCM) calls "Long Qi" when the open palms pass one another in front of the heart chakra, an energy center called the "middle dan tien." According to TCM, this has a supercharging effect, opening the body to the healing force of Qi, and practitioners feel this sense of opening release through that area of the body each time they practice.

15-10a: Without moving your legs, the left hand (palm up at your waist) begins an outside arc up to the left ear, as if stroking out and away over a large orb at the side of the body.

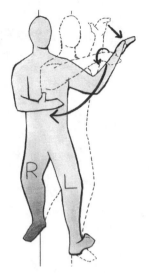

15-10b

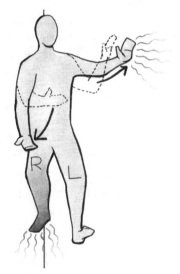

15-10c

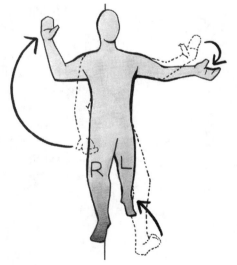

15-10d

15-10b: Now the right hand palm up pulls back to the right side of your waist, while the left hand palm facing front pushes outward from your chest; simultaneously, as weight sinks back into your right leg.

15-10c: Now, the weight shifts back to the right leg. Notice how your relaxed torso and body allow Qi to flow out of your relaxed left shoulder, arm, and hand as it also flows down and through your sinking back into the right leg.

15-10d: Prepare for the next three moves by moving the opposite leg back as your palm at waist circles up near the ear, poised to push when the other hand pulls back as you shift back.

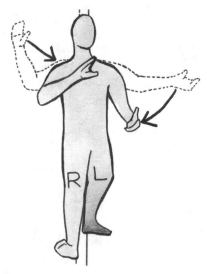

15-10e

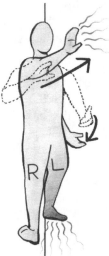

15-10f

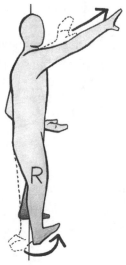

15-11a

15-10e: Repeat with the right hand pushing, the left hand pulling as you sink back.

15-10f: Shifting back to the left leg, Qi flows out of your relaxed torso, right shoulder, right arm, and right hand.

Repeat with the left hand pushing, the right hand pulling, shifting back to the right leg (see Figures 15-10b and 15-10c).

Repeat with the right hand pushing, the left hand pulling, shifting back to the left leg (see Figures 15-10e and 15-10f).

Stork Covers Its Wing/Sword in Sheath, #11

15-11a: After completing last Repulse with the right hand pushed out, the weight back on the left, back foot, the right foot now pivots on the heel to follow the extended right arm out to point diagonally 45 degrees to left/front.

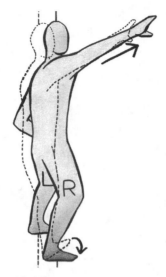

15-11b

15-11b: Upon completing the pivot, the weight shifts to the right foot, while pivoting on the left ball, and dropping the left heel in toward the right foot a bit.

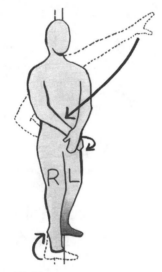

15-11c

15-11c: Now, as the left palm up turns into a sheath (palm turns in to face body), the weight shifts back to the left leg, and the right extended hand pulls back into the left hand's sheath between the left palm and the left hip. The right toe simultaneously pulls back to rest at the left instep.

Slow Palm Slant Flying, #12

Slow Palm Slant Flying is one of the most beautiful and uplifting movements in the entire series.

15-12a: The right heel goes out diagonally.

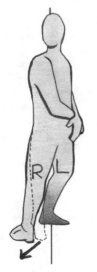

15-12a

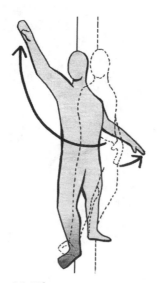

15-12b

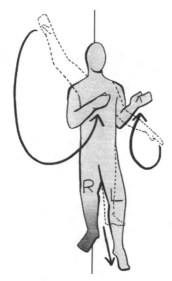

15-12c

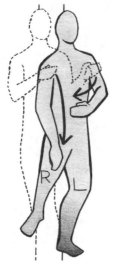

15-13a

15-12b: As weight shifts to right foot, right palm extends slowly outward from left hand's sheath as left hand extends back to opposite corner.

15-12c: Extend arms fully with weight totally on right leg; right arm begins a great arcing circle around a bit behind your body, while open left palm arcs up from behind until both open palms meet in front of chest. Lift left foot to place the left toe lightly a couple of inches in front of body below parallel palms.

Raise Right Hand and Left: Turn and Repeat (Part I), #13

Although each movement has powerful martial applications, the goal of T'ai Chi is to "soong yi dien," to loosen up the mind, heart, and body. This movement loosens up the abdominal area, and back and shoulders, by performing Long Qi. The palms passing one another healthfully stimulated the dan tien energy centers within the body, also relaxing the solar plexus.

15-13a: Now, left heel extends forward, as left arm curls around (as if hugging a tree), and as in the figure the weight continues rolling up onto left foot, as heel of right wrist begins descent (a soothing Long Qi experience can be felt in the abdomen as the right palm passes the left palm as the right hand drops). Now, right hand forms a Duck's Beak and begins to lift upward.

15-13b: The right hand's Duck's Beak rises, as if pulling a string attached to the right foot, it pulls the back right foot up in front to touch the toe, and when the Duck's Beak is above the head, the palm opens.

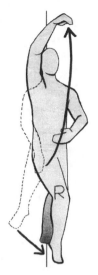

15-13b

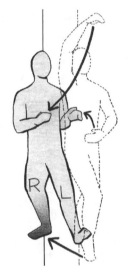

15-13c

15-13c: Now the right hand drops down as the right toe reaches back behind, until the right and left palms are once again parallel facing one another in front, and the weight has shifted back to the right foot, only left heel touching.

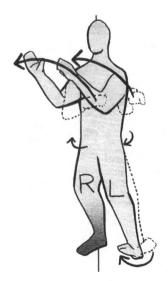

15-13d

15-13d: Turn to the right, pivoting on the (empty) left heel, palms arcing across in front of chest still parallel facing one another.

Ouch!

While moving, remember to breathe deeply into the diaphragm, but also easily and naturally. This conditions us to breathe through life's changes just as through T'ai Chi's changing postures.

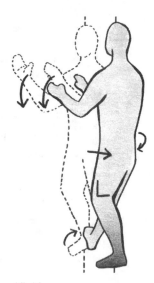

15-13e

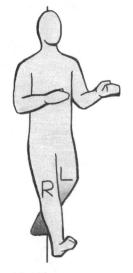

15-13f

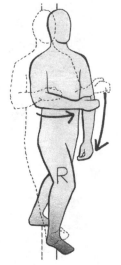

15-13g

15-13e: As 180-degree turn/pivot completes, the weight sinks completely back into the left leg, and hands fall again parallel in front of chest.

15-13f: This sketch merely gives you a frontal view of 15-13e, for easier viewing.

15-13g: Now, the left wrist will begin its descent as the right arm parries, as if hugging a tree, and the weight begins shifting up onto the right leg.

> **T'ai Sci**
>
> T'ai Chi can accomplish the seemingly paradoxical goal of fostering deep relaxation *and* martial arts training, simultaneously. Teaching that effectiveness in all aspects of life can be effortless.

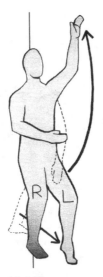

15-13h

15-13h: The left hand forms the Duck's Beak, pulling the imaginary string up bringing the left toe to touch in front as left hand raises overhead and weight completely shifts to right leg.

Although this movement is very soothing to the upper body and therapeutic for the hand and arm, it's martial application is powerful. As the right hand blocks a punch, the left hand lowers to block a kick. The left hand then rises to strike opponent's face or nose, as the left knee rises to kick the groin. Ouch!

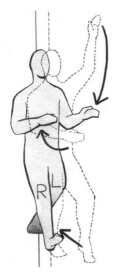

15-13i

15-13i: As the left hand opens and descends the left toe reaches back, weight shifts back to left foot as palms face parallel in front of chest (right heal touching in front).

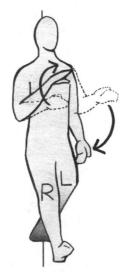

15-14a

Wave Hand Over Light/Fly Pulling Back, #14

15-14a: With palms parallel facing each other, they rotate as if over a ball, so that the right palm is over the left palm.

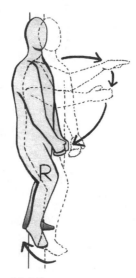

15-14b

15-14b: Right fingers extend straight out from chest level at shadow opponent's throat level, as weight shifts forward onto right leg. Right palm curves around downward as if it has gone over and now curving back under a sphere of light, to rest in front of the dan tien cradled in the left palm, as right toe pulls back to rest by left instep.

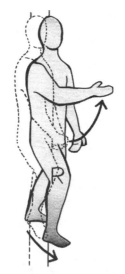

15-14c

15-14c: Right heel extends out front, as right palm circles this time from "beneath the sphere of light" …

15-14d: … and continuing up and over the back of the sphere of light, until the back of the right hand rests in front of the chest. As right hand is completing the circle, the left foot pulls up to rest toe at right instep.

Fly Pulling Back extends your Qi forward and out in an expressive motion and then relaxes your Qi, sinking back into a retreat.

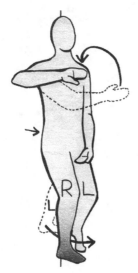

15-14d

> **Sage Sifu Says**
>
> As you extend or strike, the upper body torso muscles relax and loosen as you exhale. A cadence of breath timing can be further refined using video or live class instruction, but the figures help you see very precisely where your weight shifts occur.

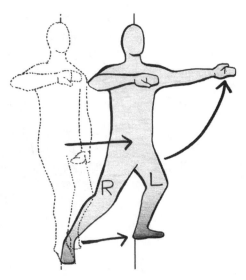

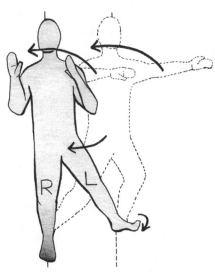

15-15

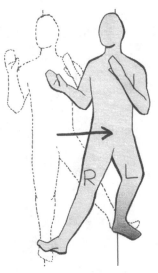

15-16a

15-16b

Fan Through the Arms, #15

15-15: With the back of the right hand facing chest, and open left palm in front of the dan tien, the left palm arcs outward to left at shoulder height, weight shifts 60 percent to left.

Left fanning arm relaxes away from body as weight shifts toward left leg. Dan tien carries the arm outward, as it sinks over left leg. Arm moving out and up like a clock hand moving from 6 to 3 o'clock, as you relax and exhale.

Green Dragon Rising from the Water, #16

15-16a: Weight shifts back to right foot, as left foot pivots on heel to point left toe cattycorner toward your right, and left arm follows so entire body is turned cattycorner to left now.

15-16b: With right and left palms falling parallel in front of chest, weight settles back onto left leg, and right foot comes to heel, as right toe comes up.

Sage Sifu Says

Each time weight settles or *sinks* into a leg, exhale and let every muscle "let go" of whatever tension it had unconsciously squeezed within it. This conditions mind and body to stop straining through life, getting things done in a healthy, effortless way.

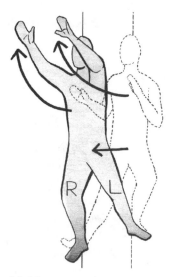

15-16c

15-16c: Lift right heel slightly and replace it to extend out more cattycorner to right, then reaching open palms upward and outward while shifting weight about 65 percent up toward the right foot.

This Green Dragon move teaches us to push, and lift, from the dan tien, keeping the back heel planted down, thereby reducing back pressure. This creates more power and less chance of injury in performing daily tasks.

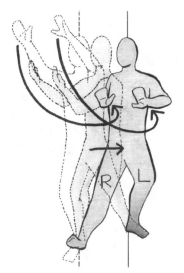

15-16d

15-16d: As if the hands are pulling a sphere of light back down into your heart, the weight settles back onto left leg and right toe pulls back to touch at left instep.

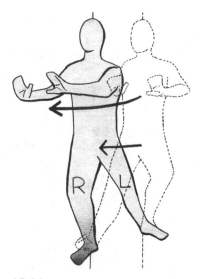

15-16e

15-16e: Then right heel goes out and hands push out from the torso.

Weight shifts on up to right leg as you complete push, then hands turn to right side, where the Duck's Beak begins for Single Whip.

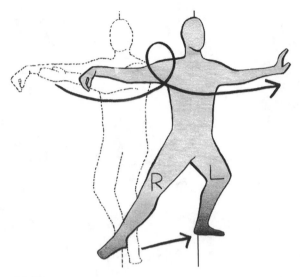

15-17

Single Whip (Part II), #17

15-17: Right hand is in a Duck's Beak (fingers touching right thumb), left fingers stroke the inside of right arm, the left palm pulls across body. (Refer to the Single Whip #1, Figures 15-3b through 15-3d.)

On the Duck's Beak, all the fingers on the right hand extend down to touch the right thumb. Modern carpal tunnel prevention exercises include movements like these. So among its many benefits, T'ai Chi appears to be an ergonomic carpal tunnel prevention exercise as well.

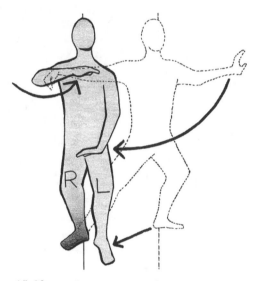

15-18a

Wave Hands Like Clouds (×3), #18 (Part I, Linear Style)

T'ai Chi connects us with nature as we rise up from the water to Wave Hands Like Clouds.

15-18a: As hands draw in from Single Whip extension, turn both palms to face down. Shift weight to right leg, bringing left toe out to touch in front, as right hand comes parallel to ground at shoulder height to center chest, and left hand comes down to arrive at center dan tien level.

15-18b: As left toe goes straight out to the left, both hands reach straight out to the right at shoulder level.

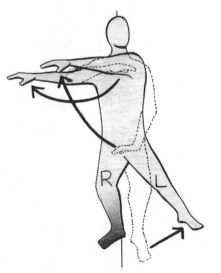

15-18b

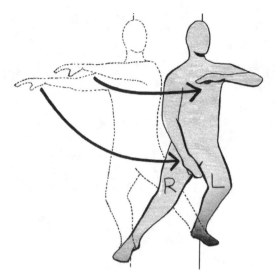

15-18c

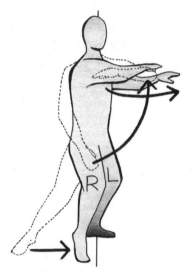

15-18d

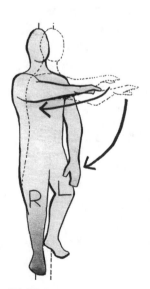

15-18e

15-18c: As weight shifts back to the left leg, the right hand drops to dan tien center, while the left hand pulls parallel to the ground across the center chest.

> **CAUTION**
>
> **Ouch!**
>
> You'll know you are doing movements correctly if they feel good. If you feel undue strain in a knee, leg, or the body, you are probably forcing the position. All T'ai Chi positions are designed to enable you to relax into the position. If you feel lower back pain in Wave Hands, or other moves, it's usually because your lower back is overarched. Make sure as you exhale you allow the tail bone to *relax* down.

15-18d: Weight shifts to left leg, as right leg is drawn toward left leg, and as hands reach out to left at shoulder level.

15-18e: Weight shifts to right leg as hands come to center (right at chest, left at dan tien).

Though obviously martial, there's also a soothing quality of imagining hands waving like clouds. The thought unlocks an effortlessness flow throughout mind and body.

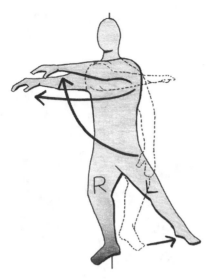

15-18f

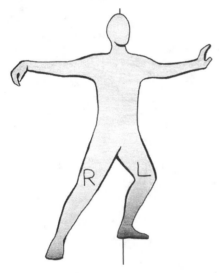

15-19

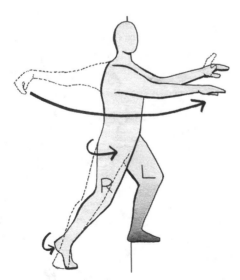

15-20a

15-18f: As left toe goes straight out to the left, both hands reach straight out to the right at shoulder level.

Repeat Figures 15-18b through 15-18f two more times (for a total of three repetitions for Wave Hands Like Clouds). However, on last repetition you leave off the action from Figure 15-18f, because you will be going right into a Single Whip from there. All Wave Hands Like Clouds (and there are four of them in this style) begin and end with a Single Whip.

Single Whip (Part III), #19

15-19: Refer to the first Single Whip (Figures 15-3b through 15-3d) for sketches and details if needed, although if you are this far, you should know the Single Whip by heart by now. If not, go back and review. It's not a test, only a game. Enjoy!

> **Sage Sifu Says**
>
> T'ai Chi is taught in three stages. First, the movements are learned. Second, the breath is incorporated into the regimen by learning an inhalation or exhalation that is connected to each movement. Third, a relaxation element or awareness of the flow of energy through the body is learned. Although the first step offers many benefits from the first day, the benefits get richer and deeper with each level you learn.

High Pat on Horse/Guarding the Temples, #20

15-20a: From the Single Whip pose, the torso rotates to the right, and the arms begin to curve into a horseshoe shape in front of

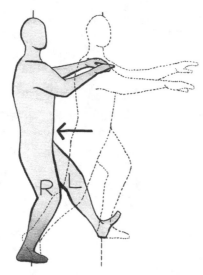

15-20b

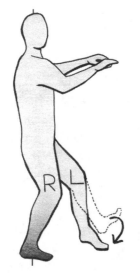

15-20c

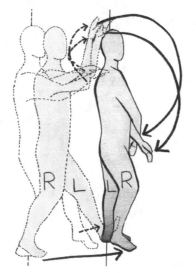

15-20d

the body. While the torso turns you pivot on the ball of the right foot.

15-20b: The weight now sinks back on the right leg, as left toe comes up (left heel down), arms settling in front of the chest.

15-20c: With weight settled on the right leg, raise left foot a bit and then touch left toe in front, palms patting downward a little as if patting a pony's hind quarters.

15-20d: While shifting up into left leg, turn palms outward each palm arcing up to the side of the temples of the head as if protecting from a side blow, then arcing down to form low block by crossing right wrist over left in front of dan tien. The right foot comes up to touch empty by left instep.

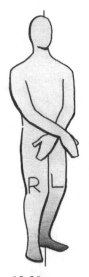

15-20e

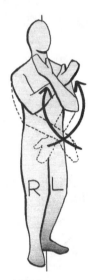

15-21a

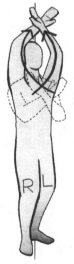

15-21b

15-20e: This sketch shows the front position of Figure 15-20d.

Lower Block/Upper Block, Separation of Right Foot; Lower Block/Upper Block, Separation of Left Foot, #21

15-21a: Wrists crossed at dan tien in previous figure, now lift to be crossed at mid chest block (palms still facing in toward chest).

15-21b: Now arms continue rising as palms turn out, causing wrists to twist forming an up block (with palms facing out). It takes a seven count to go from the low block to the up block and kick that follows.

CAUTION Ouch!

Remember that there is no correct height to kick at. Your kick may be only a few inches off the ground, or, if you're a soccer player, your kick may be two feet higher than in the upcoming figure. There is no wrong or right, the only rule being to relax and enjoy.

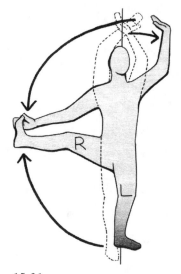

15-21c

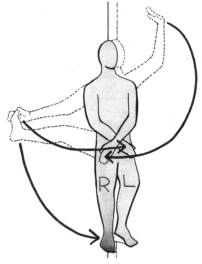

15-21d

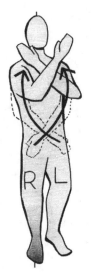

15-21e

15-21c: Kick right foot up/out to right side, as right hand chops down to meet foot (at whatever height is comfortable, don't force; your kicks will get higher over time). Catch the foot on its descent and slowly settle descending right foot down by left foot.

Your hand may not touch the kicking foot at first. That's okay; just kick as high as is comfortable.

15-21d: Weight shifts back into right foot as left wrist crosses over right this time.

15-21e: Begin low/mid/upper block, left leg preparing for separation kick.

A T'ai Chi Punch Line

During an explanation of how one movement fights off attacks from four different directions, one student wisely explained, "I know where those attacks are coming from—mostly between here and here" (pointing fingers into each temple). *We are often our own worst enemy.* As T'ai Chi promotes peace within, the world around us often becomes more peaceful as well.

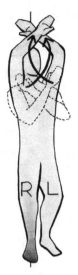

15-21f

15-21f: As up block completes, the left hand begins to slip sideways to left, as left foot prepares to kick out and up to the left.

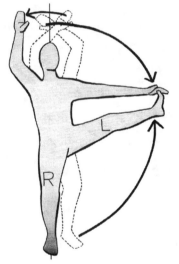

15-21g

15-21g: Kick left foot out and up to left side, as left hand chops down to meet foot (again, kick only as high as is comfortable), and catch left foot as it drops to slowly settle "behind" right heel.

Turn and Kick with Sole, #22

15-22a: As left foot settles behind right heel, the body turns a quarter turn to the left. The left leg fills and the right leg empties as you complete the quarter turn.

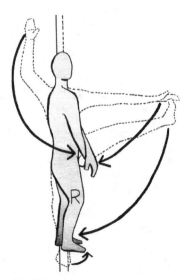

15-22a

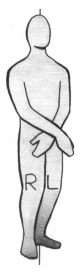

15-22b

15-22b: This sketch presents a frontal view of the pose in Figure 15-22a.

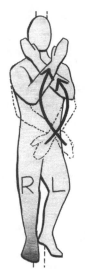

15-22c

15-22c: Weight shifts into right leg as low block rises to mid block.

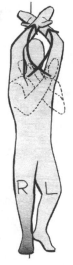

15-22d

15-22d: Weight sinks fully into right leg as mid block rises to high block as palms twist out.

A T'ai Chi Punch Line

T'ai Chi breath is fully exhaled from chest to abdomen, with the tip of tongue lightly touching the roof of mouth. So that a *full inhalation* accompanies preparations, and full *exhalations* with shifts, kicks, or punches.

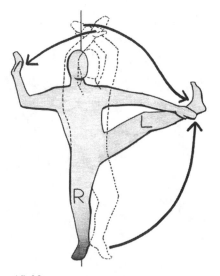

15-22e

15-22e: Kick left leg up and out to left as left hand swings out in front and around to side to slap instep of left foot (or inside of left leg) as right hand chops out to right slightly.

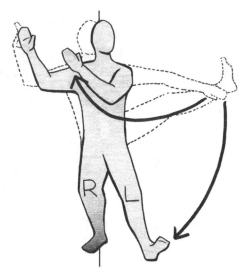

15-23a

Wind Blowing Lotus Leaves (×4), #23

This is an exquisite move. It is artistically beautiful and feels fantastic because it loosens the entire torso. It also helps the body learn to push the lawn mower or perform other tasks with much less pressure on lower back. Correct T'ai Chi movement shifts strain from lower back to thighs, which are much stronger and less delicate than our back's vertebrae.

15-23a: After left hand smacks instep or inside of left leg, it pulls back to head just off the right ear, and right hand pulls behind that, as if holding a beach ball off to right side of head. Placing left heel down at a 45-degree angle to left/front.

15-23b: Weight shifts forward onto your left leg as the front/left arm drops down in a circular motion blocking groin area as the torso turns to shift over the left leg, right hand still by the right shoulder to push as body shifts forward. Exhale as you shift forward, relaxing.

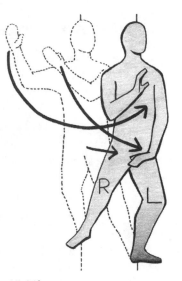

15-23b

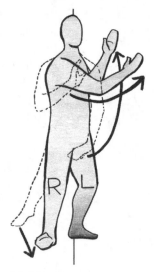

15-23c

15-23c: Now, imagine holding the beach ball off to the left side of your head (right hand forward of the left this time), as your right heel goes out 45 degrees front/right.

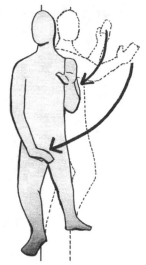

15-23d

15-23d: Weight shifts forward onto your right leg as the front/right arm drops down in a circular motion blocking groin area, torso turning slightly to shift over right leg, left hand still by left shoulder. Exhale as you shift, relaxing.

Shift forward, as the breath seems to relax out of every cell. As your Qi sinks into the earth, its power also flows through you and out your hands. The dan tien pulls your relaxed body forward.

Repeat 15-23a through 15-23d.

Block Up/Fist Down, #24

15-24: Begin similar to Figures 15-23a and 15-23b. However, this time your right hand forms a fist and rises up and over to deliver a downward hammer-fist. Your left hand doesn't stop down at a groin block, but continues circling up in front to a high block protecting your forehead, left palm down in Down Block and as the block arcs out and up in front of the body the palm continues to face palm away from the upper body even as block is completed.

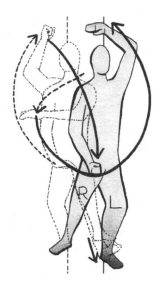

15-24

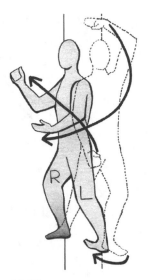

15-25a

Turn and Double Kick, #25

15-25a: Turn 180 degrees to prepare for the Double Kick by shifting weight back on right leg and pivoting on "empty" left heel as body turns to the right.

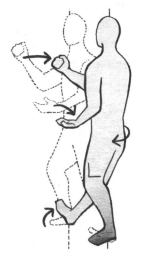

15-25b

15-25b: Sink back into left leg as pivot completes, allowing right toe to come up pivoting on right heel. Left open palm rests at left hip facing up, right fist swings out in front of right shoulder.

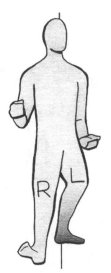

15-25c

15-25c: This sketch shows a frontal view of preceding figure.

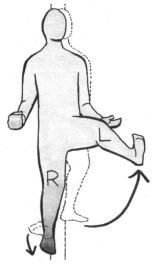

15-25d

15-25d: From sunken down on right leg, shift forward and kick left leg up and out for a left front kick.

Remember that your kick does not have to be as high as illustrated.

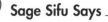

Sage Sifu Says

The complexity and variety of movements may seem daunting at first, but just relax and learn the move you're learning today. You'll get it, one move at a time. *A lesson for life.*

15-25e: Then place left leg out in front and shift up into left leg …

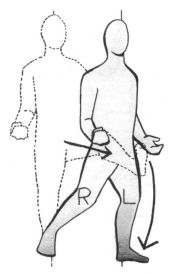

15-25e

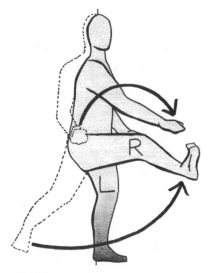

15-25f

15-25f: … kicking right leg up and out front while opening right fist and smacking right palm down on top of kicking right foot (or leg).

As the right leg kicks up, the right palm turns over and smacks down to slap the top of the right foot, or calf, or knee, or wherever your hand comfortably slaps without leaning forward.

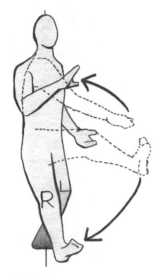

15-25g

15-25g: Place right foot down in front after kick, heel first.

Parry and Punch, #26

15-26a: Step forward with left foot, while preparing right fist near right hip, and dropping left parry.

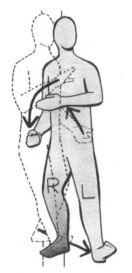

15-26a

15-26b: Then parry and punch as weight shifts onto left front foot about 60 percent forward. Again, do not lean forward as you punch. The body or vertical axis always stays stacked above the dan tien.

As punch is thrown and Qi sinks into forward left leg, breath is released in an easy sigh. This action is a wonderful stress release for both hips and upper body. Tension can be allowed to pour out left foot into earth, and upper body tension can be released out the punching fist.

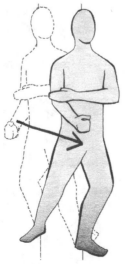

15-26b

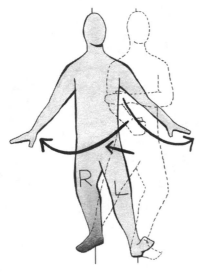

15-27a

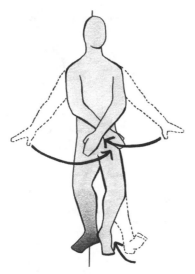

15-27b

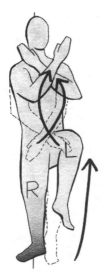

15-27c

Step Back/Lower Block/Upper Block; Kick Front, #27

15-27a: Shift weight back to right leg, rolling up off left heel, as hands drop out to the sides.

15-27b: Bring hands back down to center (left wrist crossing on top) as left foot comes back to touch at right instep.

15-27c: Low block rises to mid block as left knee rises up.

T'ai Sci
Timing on all low, mid, and up blocks is a seven-count, but over time the rate of your relaxed breathing will become your timer. Breath and motion become one, allowing effortless flow to fill and sooth our mind ... as healing soothing motion expands Qi and circulation through every relaxing capillary ... cell ... and atom of our being.

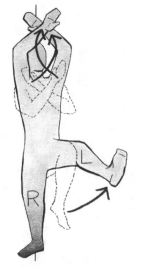

15-27d

15-27d: As mid block becomes upper block, palms twist out and begin to strike up and out to sides, as left foot kicks out front.

This kick is great for balance. You do not have to perform the kick this high. You may begin much lower. Go as high as is comfortable, without leaning backward out of your vertical axis. As with all movements it is done very slowly, placing the foot out in front as you breathe. Observe your balance as you do this.

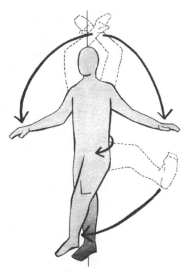

15-27e

15-27e: Hands slowly lower to sides, as left foot slowly lowers to rest flat on right side of right foot.

CAUTION **Ouch!**

A relaxing exhale always accompanies the weight sinking into a leg to end a pivot. Let your motions become effortless as the breath relaxes out of you, and the muscles beneath the muscles "let go." Over time it will feel almost as if the exhale were turning you effortlessly.

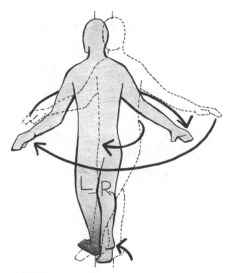

15-27f

15-27f: Pivoting clockwise, shift weight slowly to left foot, pivoting on right ball (we are working to achieve a ¾ turn pivot).

Shift weight to right foot as ¾ turn continues to right.

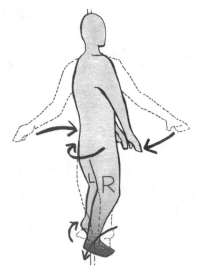

15-27g

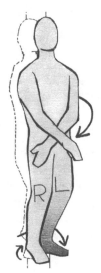

15-27h

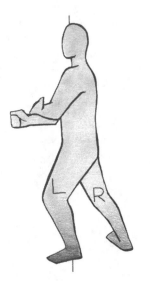

15-29a

15-27g: Pivot on left ball as ¾ pivot is completed.

15-27h: This is a frontal view of the previous figure, not more turning. See that weight shifts back to left foot as right wrist crosses over left.

Lower Block/Upper Block Separation of Right Foot, #28

Perform a lower/mid/upper block with right wrist crossed on top and weight on left foot, so you can separate right foot kick. Refer to earlier lower/mid/upper block separation right foot kicks if you need a refresher, see Figures 15-20e through 15-21c before proceeding on to this parry and punch.

Don't psyche yourself into thinking this isn't for you. It's perfect for you. If you are in a wheelchair, this movement will involve your hand arcing down. If you are paralyzed to the waist, you'll give the right side abdominal muscles instructions to extend upward toward the arcing right hand, and this intention of motion will exercise and coordinate mind and body, relieving tension.

Parry and Punch, #29

15-29a: When Separation Right Foot completes, place right heel out to the right side and shift into it, proceeding in to a Parry and Punch. Refer to earlier parry and punch instructions if you need a refresher.

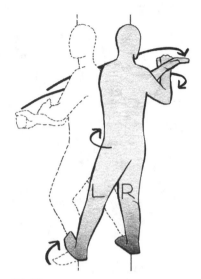

15-30a

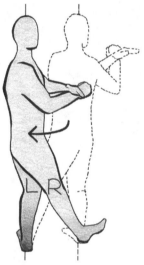

15-30b

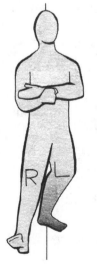

15-30c

Chop Opponent with Fist (Pivot and Rotate Fist [×3]), #30

15-30a: When turning, you must empty a leg before pivoting on it. That way, you do not damage the knee. Once a foot is pivoted to desired position, then weight can be returned to it. From Parry and Punch position, weight shifts back to right leg, as torso pivots 180 degrees toward right, and "empty" left leg pivots on heel to right.

15-30b: Sink back into left leg, as empty right leg pivots on heel, toes coming up, to result in a completed 180-degree turn.

15-30c: Note that this figure is simply a frontal view of 15-30b.

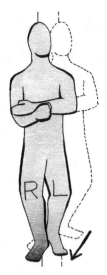

15-30d

15-30d: Dan tien sinks forward over right leg, empty left leg comes up to place empty left foot by right instep.

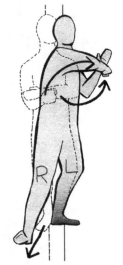

15-30e

15-30e: Weight now shifts onto left leg, placing empty right foot out heel first at 45-degree angle, front/right, simultaneously drawing right elbow back to left to prepare for upcoming strike.

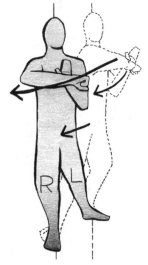

15-30f

15-30f: Now, shifting forward into right leg, throw out right elbow strike, exhaling and allowing body to relax into strike.

Sage Sifu Says

Allow your mind to empty as you exhale and strike. This lets the pleasure—of the relaxed muscle and tissue being gently massaged by the body's motion—fill your empty awareness.

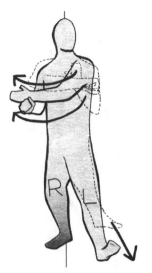

15-30g

15-30g: Weight continues shifting onto right foot with left foot placed out at 45-degree front/left angle.

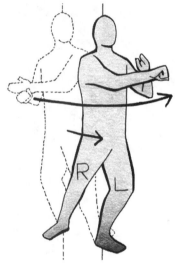

15-30h

15-30h: Weight shifts into left foot as right fist strikes punch out to left/front.

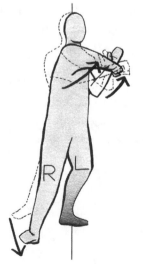

15-30i

15-30i: Right foot comes up to touch near left instep and continues on out at 45-degree angle front/right.

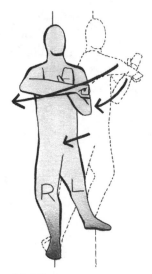

15-30j

15-30j: Sinking weight forward to right foot, and throwing another right-elbow elbow strike.

To recap, Chop Opponent involves an elbow strike stepping to the right, a punch stepping to the left, and an elbow strike stepping to the right. Over time this movement, although martial in appearance, becomes soothing, healing, and almost dancelike in the way it lifts your mood to do it.

Sink to the Earth/Backward Elbow Strike, #31

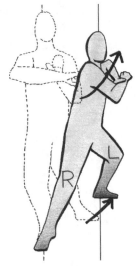

15-31a

15-31a: Now dropping weight back to left foot and throwing elbow strike out left/behind. (Don't look back, it's supposed to be a surprise.)

The depth of this strike is all in the bend of the left knee. If your knee only feels comfortable with a slight bend, then that is perfect for you, it will get deeper in time, no rush.

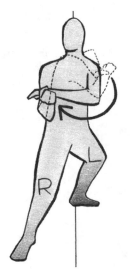

15-31b

15-31b: Before coming up out of back stance, turn to right and aim right forearm to front/right 45-degree angle.

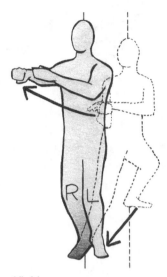

15-31c

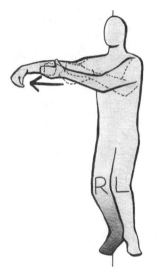

15-32a

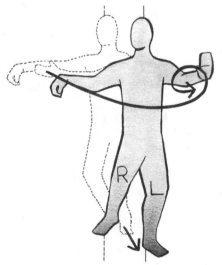

15-32b

15-31c: Now right fist punches upward and weight springs forward to settle over right foot, left wrist still crossed over right fist, but then turning to follow right hand to prepare for Single Whip.

> **Sage Sifu Says**
>
> Many of our problems come from mindlessly forcing ourselves to live in ways that do not feel good to us. T'ai Chi teaches us to move in the ways that feel good to us. Listening to what *feels right* is the most powerful thing we can do for ourselves and our world. It's T'ai Chi's essence.

Single Whip, ³/₄ Single Whip (Part IV), #32

15-32a: Begins like normal Single Whip.

15-32b: However, the left foot doesn't go all the way out to the left, but heel touches out left/front at 45-degree angle, and then hand pushes out at that same left/front angle.

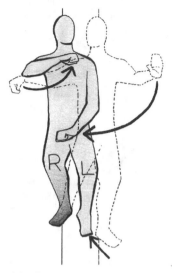

15-33a

Partition of Wild Horse's Mane (×4) and Single Whip, #33

15-33a: Eyes keep looking straight ahead (ideally). Right arm/fist settles back from Single Whip at chest level, left hand dropping down to groin level, and left toe touch in front of body. Much like preparing for Wave Hands Like Clouds position, except with fists.

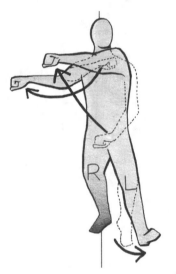

15-33b

15-33b: Now, as left heel extends out front/left 45 degrees, fists begin to roll back behind/right. Left elbow rises as right fist lowers. Again, this is much like the hand motion you learned for Wave Hands Like Clouds, except with fists, and Wave Hands Like Clouds steps sideways, while Partition of Horse's Mane steps out at 45-degree angles forward.

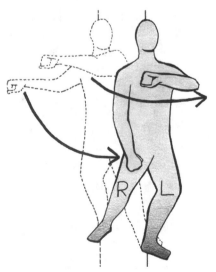

15-33c

15-33c: As weight shifts up into left leg, left elbow strikes out.

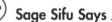 **Sage Sifu Says**

Just as in Wave Hands, in Partition of Wild Horse's Mane (and all moves, really) the dan tien actually *pulls* the relaxed body and limbs into positions effortlessly, as the dan tien sinks into/over the filling leg.

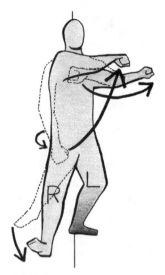

15-33d

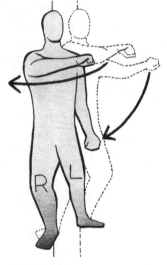

15-33e

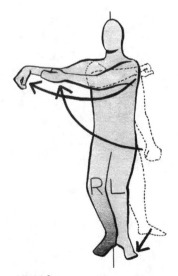

15-33f

15-33d: Now, with left leg full, right leg extends out front/right 45 degrees, arms rolling back to the back/left this time.

15-33e: Right elbow strikes out as weight shifts up to fill right leg.

15-33f: Repeat Figures 15-33b, 15-33c, 15-33d, 15-33e (and a total of four elbow-strikes, left, right, left, right strikes in Part Wild Horse's Mane). End after the last right-elbow strike by stepping up to form a Single Whip.

When striking forward, the "back" heel should stay down on the floor until the vertical axis is "completely" over the front filling foot. Also, remember never to lean into a strike, maintaining upright posture.

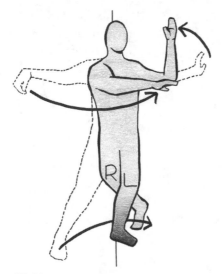

15-34a

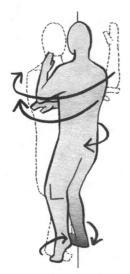

15-34b

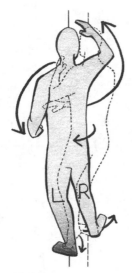

15-34c

Fair Lady Works at Shuttles, #34

Fair Lady Works at Shuttles is actually a shadow boxing routine involving blocks and punches used to spar with four opponents coming from four different directions.

15-34a: From a completed Single Whip position, the right toe reaches back to behind the left heel. Left forearm points up to the sky, and right arm comes across to rest right open hand (palm down) just below the left elbow.

15-34b: Now, fill the right foot, as the left pivots on the ball of the left foot. Both the body and the left foot are now pivoting toward the right for a ¾ pivot.

15-34c: As pivot completes, sink weight back on left foot pivot as right toes come up pivoting from right heel. Left hand drops beside waist to form a fist, as right hand arcs up to form an up block (palm out).

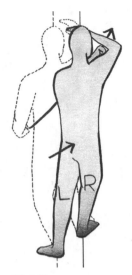

15-34d

15-34d: Shifting weight forward about 60 percent into right leg, left hand punches out at about nose height, punching out front just beneath and beyond the blocking right forearm.

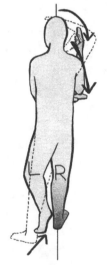

15-34e

15-34e: To prepare for the right hand punch, you first empty the left leg, bring it up to touch left toe by right instep, as open left hand (palm down) touches under the right elbow, and right forearm points up to the sky.

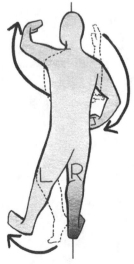

15-34f

15-34f: Now left heel extends out front/left at 45 degrees, left arm rising in arc to up block (palm out), and right fist drops to right hip preparing for a punch.

Ⓒ CAUTION Ouch!

On all pushes, strikes, and punches, the back foot stays down until the front foot is completely full and the push or punch is complete. If you raise the back foot as you strike, the only thing behind that strike is a wobbly little ankle. However, if the back foot stays down, you have the whole planet behind it.

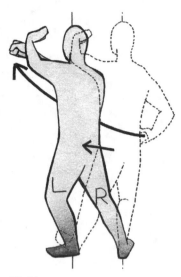

15-34g

15-34g: Weight shifts 60 percent forward into left leg as torso turns to left slightly to deliver the right fist punch, beneath the blocking left arm.

Repeat movements shown in Figures 15-34a through 15-34g (except, of course, beginning from this punch position, not from a completed Single Whip [as in 15-34a]).

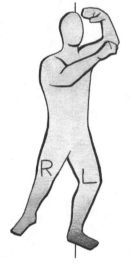

15-34h

15-34h: Again, note that the back foot remains down flat until the punch is complete. The body in a state of "song" or relaxation, allowing the force of the earth to flow up through your body.

This sketch presents a frontal view of Figure 15-34g.

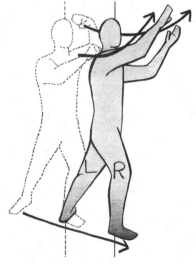

15-34i

15-34i: To proceed from punch in 15-34g to Grasp the Bird's Tail, you continue on through punch stepping "forward out to left catty-corner" with your right foot reaching hands up into Grasp the Bird's Tail.

Grasp the Bird's Tail (Part II), #35

15-35a: Notice this figure is simply a frontal view of the previous figure. Refer to earlier Grasp the Bird's Tail instructions if you need a refresher (see Figures 15-2a through 15-2c).

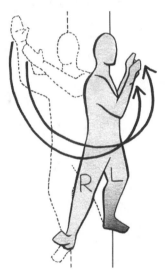

15-35a

15-35b: This is the same as the first Grasp the Bird's Tail, except to get in position you step forward from the last punch of Fair Lady Works at Shuttles with your right foot out to grasp bird's tail.

Caressing the Bird's Tail, Waving Hands Like Clouds, and so on, all can return upward cosmic experiences to the solid roots of earth, and it feels great!

15-35b

Single Whip (Part V), #36

15-36a: From Grasp Bird's Tail, push out to prepare for Single Whip, left leg coming forward as push completes.

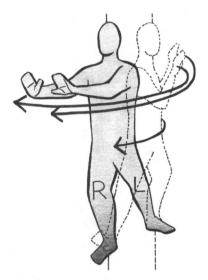

15-36a

Sage Sifu Says

As you push out on Single Whip's you can enjoy a nice "cat stretch" feeling through the shoulders and back, while at other times more of a "deep letting go" feeling. Each time you do a movement you can enjoy different sensations.

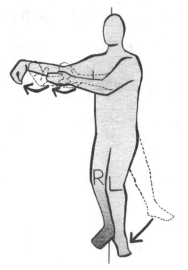

15-36b

15-36b: Refer to the Single Whip instructions in Figures 15-3b through 15-3d if you need a refresher on Single Whip details.

Wave Hands Like Clouds (Part II, Linear Style), #37

Refer to Wave Hands Like Clouds Part I if you need a refresher (see Figures 15-18a to 15-19), but end with Single Whip "Down" as in next figure.

Incorporate breath with each movement. This slows down the movement and makes it a relaxing and centering exercise, of and by itself. Be absorbed and loosened. Enjoy!

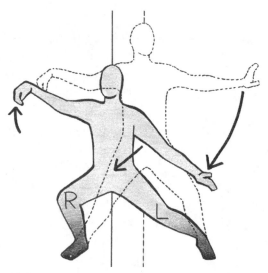

15-38

Single Whip Down; Return to the Earth (Part I), #38

15-38: Single Whip Down's are performed just like regular Single Whip except step out left farther and on ball of left foot rather than heel. Note: You do not have to go as low as shown in this figure. Go to your comfort level.

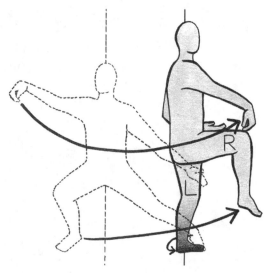

15-39a

Golden Cock Stands on One Leg (×4), #39

15-39a: From Single Whip Down pose, shift weight over to right leg a bit more to empty left leg completely so you can drop left heel in slightly toward body. Now shift your weight up into the left leg, and bring the right leg/knee up, while forming Duck's Beak with right hand and sliding it down the top of right thigh. Left hand falls palm up to side of left hip.

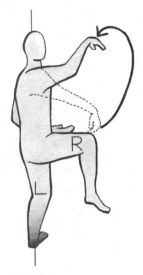

15-39b

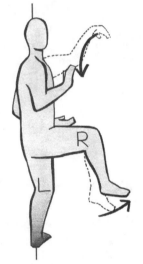

15-39c

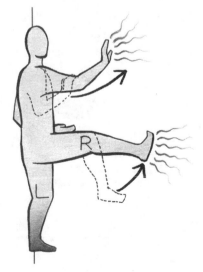

15-39d

15-39b: Slide right hand Duck's Beak off the end of right knee, up in a circular motion and around back toward body. Left palm up still rests next to left hip.

15-39c: Hand completes circle down to chest, with palm open and ready to push away from body.

15-39d: Then both right hand pushes out as right foot kicks straight out in front kick simultaneously. Note: You don't have to kick as high as the figure, just as high as is comfortable and balanced. You'll get higher in time, so just relax and enjoy.

This movement may look tough if you are leafing through the book, but learning the previous movements changes your body and mind in ways that will now make this movement feel easy. As always, each of us does it in our own way.

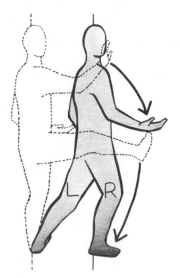

15-39e

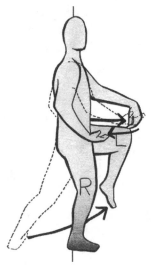

15-39f

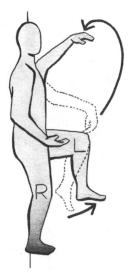

15-39g

15-39e: After kick, place right foot down slightly out in front of body, and now weight begins shifting toward right leg, as palm up right hand begins dropping down to waist level, and left hand now forms Duck's Beak.

> ### T'ai Sci
>
> Emory University's study found T'ai Chi to be *twice* as effective in improving balance as other therapies. By the time you get to this move, your balance is much improved!

15-39f: Now shift your weight completely into the right leg, and bring the left leg/knee up, while forming a Duck's Beak with left hand, which now slides down the top of left thigh.

15-39g: Slide left hand Duck's Beak off the end of left knee, up in a circular motion and around back toward body.

> ### T'ai Sci
>
> Neurologists referring patients with balance disorders to T'ai Chi note that practitioners gain increased self-confidence and lose the fear caused by being "out of control."

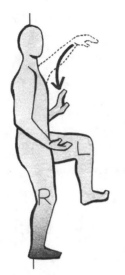

15-39h

15-39h: Left hand completes circle down to chest, with palm open and ready to push away from body.

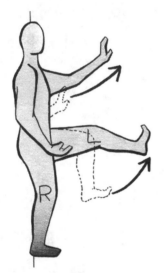

15-39i

15-39i: Left hand pushes out as left foot kicks straight out in front kick simultaneously. Kick only as high as is comfortable and balanced, it'll get higher in time. Relax, enjoy!

From here repeat both right and left kicks again as in Figures 15-39a to 15-39i, but as you finish last front kick with left leg, put the left leg behind you and right hand will circle up from right side to put you in position for Repulse the Monkey.

Repulse the Monkey (×3) (Part II), #40

15-40: This Repulse the Monkey series begins with right hand pushing out, so it's only three repetitions, not four as in first one. Again, enjoy the soothing "Long Qi" as palms pass one another, allowing a "loosening" of the back and shoulders.

Movements #40 Through #44

The next four movements are repeats of movement series 11

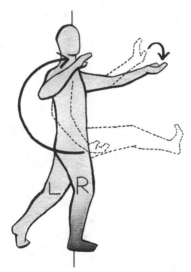

15-40

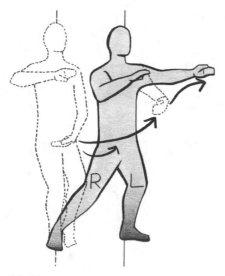

15-45

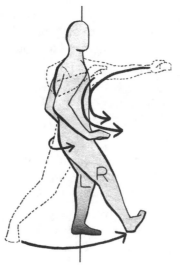

15-46a

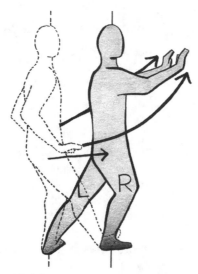

15-46b

through 14. *You already know them!* But go back for refresher, if needed. The movements are …

♦ Stork Covers Its Wing/ Sword in Sheath (Part II), #41.

♦ Slow Palm Slant Flying (Part II), #42.

♦ Raise Right Hand and Left: Turn and Repeat (Part II), #43.

♦ Wave Hand Over Light/Fly Pulling Back, #44.

Fan Through the Arm (Backhand Slap), #45

15-45: This Fan Through the Arm doesn't come up in a rising arc to left (as the first one did in 15-15a), but swings out front and then to left side like a back-handed slap. As always, dan tien turning left throws slap/blow. Let the body loosen and relax the slap out from dan tien up through the relaxed body and out the hand.

Step Push/Box Opponent's Ears/Cannon Through Sky, #46

This series, a powerful advancing attack involves three consecutive blows and three leg lunges forward, toward the opponent.

15-46a: After Back Hand Slap, weight shifts totally to left leg. This movement begins with the right foot stepping forward, as the hands begin to drop, preparing you to push away in front.

15-46b: Dan tien now shifts over front/right foot as you push out. Back heel stays down until push is complete.

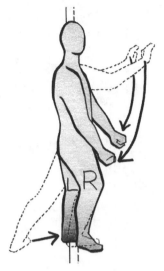

15-46c

15-46c: Weight completely fills left leg, so empty right leg can come up. Now right heel touches out front as hands drop down and back, forming fists.

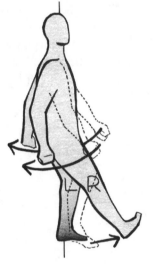

15-46d

15-46d: Weight shifts toward right leg while fists begin to fly out and forward.

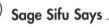 **Sage Sifu Says**

Notice on each of these advancing attacks, the hands drop back into a preparatory position as the heel touches out front. This is like cocking a crossbow, before the trigger is pulled.

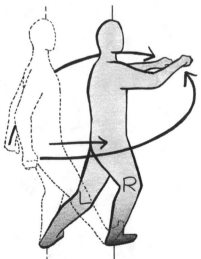

15-46e

15-46e: Fists arc around to drive into shadow opponents ears or temples, carried forward by force of dan tien shifting up completely into the right leg.

Just as Fanning Through the Arm allows deep tension releases through the hips, Box Opponent's Ears can foster releases through the spine, shoulders, and head.

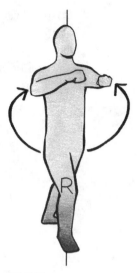

15-46f

15-46f: This is simply a frontal view of pose in Figure 15-46e.

Sage Sifu Says

Allow the blows or strikes to flow through your relaxed body, enabling the power of the earth, beneath your back heel, to pour through your hollow frame. T'ai Chi wisely recognizes "we" are not powerful, unless we "let go" of the illusion of our own "power and control."

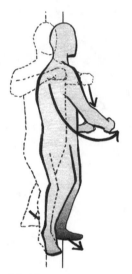

15-46g

15-46g: Left toe comes up to touch at right instep, as fist drops down below waist in front (slightly to the left of body), and weight shifts into left leg.

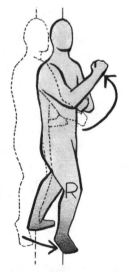

15-46h

15-46h: With right heel touching out, front fist now circles up and out to drive forward as weight settles up into right foot.

Make sure not to "lean" into your opponent as you box ears, push, or strike. Remember all punches come from shifting the dan tien forward, rather than from a lunging upper body.

Single Whip (Part VI), #47

15-47: Finishing right fist punch of Cannon Through Sky, step up with back/left foot, turn fist into a Duck's Beak for Single Whip, which begins next Wave Hands Like Clouds sequence.

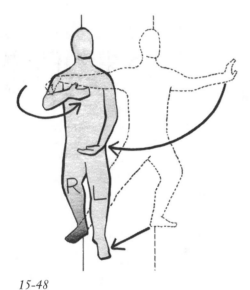

15-47

15-48

Wave Hands Like Clouds (Round Style; Part I), #48

15-48: Round Style Wave Hands is nearly identical to original Wave Hands except hands are held palm up (bottom hand) and palm in (upper), as in this figure. You already know Wave Hands, but if you need a refresher, see Figures 15-18a through 15-19.

Beware of "creeping butt syndrome" as you do this exercise. Any lower back pain is likely caused by your sacral vertebrae (or butt) creeping out behind you, causing an overarch in your lower back. As your breath relaxes out of you, allow lower back muscles to relax and tailbone to drop. Don't force it—let it relax down.

Single Whip (Part VII), #49

15-49: As always, Wave Hands Like Clouds begins and ends here with a Single Whip.

15-49

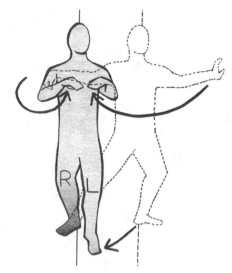

15-50

High Pat on Horse (Part II), #50

15-50: From the Single Whip, the left hand stays in place as the right arm circles around. Once the right arm is around, both arms bend and relax like a horseshoe, before patting the horse's behind in front. Shift your weight back to the right foot, as the left toe touches out front. (If you need a detailed refresher, refer back to first High Pat shown in Figures 15-20a through 15-20c.)

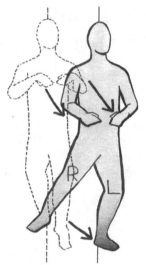

15-51a

Cross Wave of Water Lily Kick (Part I), #51

15-51a: From High Pat on Horse, left heel steps out, then weight begins to sink into it.

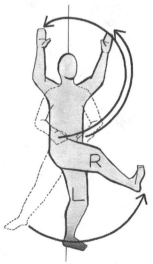

15-51b

15-51b: Then right leg kicks up and out to left side of front, as hands begin a clockwise circle up and out to left of body. Right leg is then pulled back across the body in an arc toward the left, where the now descending hands circle to touch the foot or leg as it passes underneath, hearing a "pat-pat" sound as they lightly connect in passing. Note that your "pat-pat" sound may come from tapping your shin or thigh rather than your foot. That's fine, don't force it, you'll gain flexibility over time.

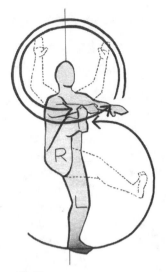

15-51c

15-51c: After the "pat-pat" of hands lightly striking kicking foot or leg, palms continue on out to left as arcing leg continues on to right, passing by one another.

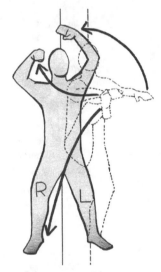

15-51d

15-51d: Place right foot down in a normal horse stance, as palms rise upward above head to form right fist and a left up block, preparing for next movement.

Parry Up; Downward Strike, #52

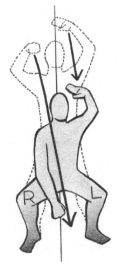

15-52

15-52: Right fist strikes down, left palm faces outward from forehead. As you punch downward, try not to bend your back over. Again, we always maintain our vertical axis, aligning the three dan tien points vertically.

Now, you'll step forward at a 45-degree left/frontal angle to Grasp the Bird's Tail.

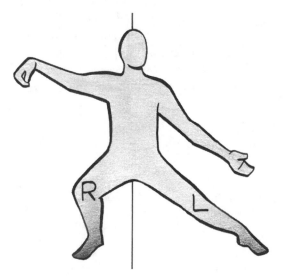

15-57a

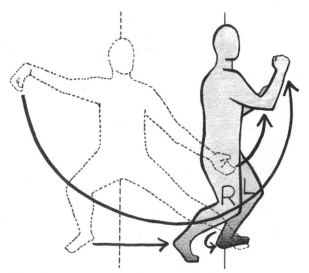

15-57b

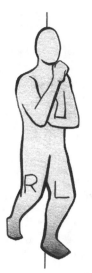

15-57c

Movements #53 Through #56

Movements #53, #54, #55, and #56 are a repetition of movements #35, #36, #37, and #38 with one exception: This time around, Movement #55, Wave Hands Like Clouds, is "circular/round" rather than linear (see Movement #48 for hand placement on Round Style Wave Hands, if you need a refresher). *Wave Hands is a deep loosening of torso muscles and tissue when done well, and each time you do it your body opens more deeply to be permeated by the expanding Qi energy.*

Step Up to Form Seven Stars, #57

Form Seven Stars and the remaining movement's complexity is at first a bit mind-boggling. However, as that complexity is absorbed into our being, we grow from it, and that growth feels great! We learn to breathe and relax through seeming chaos, which stretches our mind's capacity to comprehend, absorb, and function. This ability carries over into all aspects of our lives.

CAUTION

Ouch!

Step Up to Form Seven Stars does not have to be done with knees bent as much as in the figure. The height of stance or depth of knee bend as always is determined by your comfort. Many do this with only a slight bending of the knees, standing almost erect.

15-57b: From Single Whip Down, shift up into left foot, forming a fist from the Duck's Beak, and swinging it down and up into a groin punch.

15-57c: This is a frontal view of Figure 15-57b, to help you see the

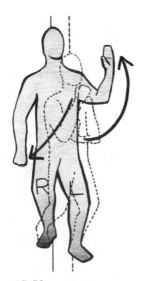

15-58

next move's details better. Note: You can bend knees more for a lower strike, or higher if your knees "ask you" to bend them less. "Listen" to your knees and body—this is the essence of T'ai Chi, working with your body rather than riding roughshod over it with harsh demands.

Retreat to Ride the Tiger, #58

15-58: Right foot steps back flat, so weight is about 50-50 on both feet, as left hand swings to left in an out block (palm out, away from body), and the right hand drops back and down to form a Duck's Beak.

Slanting Body/Turn the Moon, #59

15-59a: Weight sinks fully into left leg so that empty right foot can pivot on toe as body turns to the right for a ¼ turn.

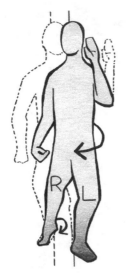

15-59a

15-59b: Completing ¼ turn as weight settles back on right leg.

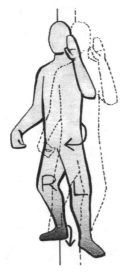

15-59b

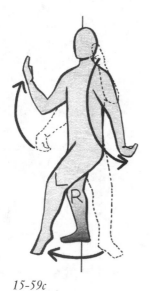

15-59c

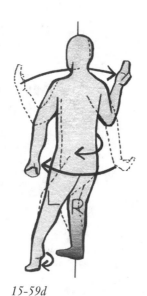

15-59d

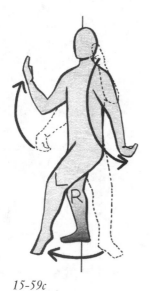

15-59e

15-59c: Arms exchange positions, right going up (palm in)/left going down (in Duck's Beak), as left toe touches out in front.

Although these blocks have very direct martial applications, they are soothing to the upper body. Breathe easily and enjoy the circular movement of the right arm blocking up and out, while the left hand arcs easily down to form the Duck's Beak behind. As you memorize the movements, such as this one, the silken flowing will be more and more soothing each time you perform it.

15-59d: Left foot raises slightly and as body pivots, left foot is pivoting on empty left toe left heel dropping in to the left (moving toward a 180-degree pivot).

15-59e: Pivot completes as weight sinks back into left foot and right toe comes up pivoting on right heel.

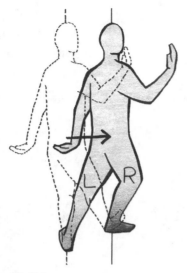

15-59f

15-59f: Weight shifts up into right leg.

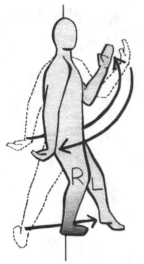

15-59g

15-59g: With weight fully into right leg, the arms again exchange places, left swinging up (out block, palm in facing body), and right swinging down (side/down block), as left foot touches the left toe out front.

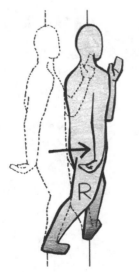

15-59h

15-59h: Weight sinks back up into left leg.

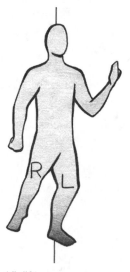

15-59i

15-59i: This is a frontal view of Figure 15-59h, to help see the transition to next movement.

Cross Wave of Water Lily (Part II), #60

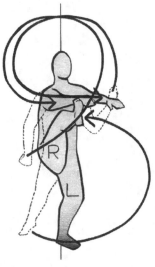

15-60

15-60: From Cross Wave Kick, hands keep going out left for Stretch Bow to Shoot Tiger.

This movement is a repetition; see movement #51 for details if you need a refresher.

Stretch Bow to Shoot Tiger, #61

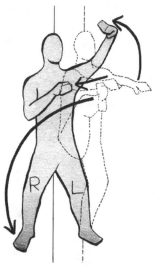

15-61a

15-61a: Imagine you are stretching a bow string back with the right hand, while the left hand (palm out away from body) aims the bow out to the left at a 45-degree angle.

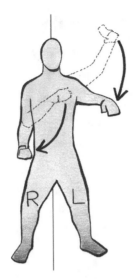

15-61b

15-61b: The right hand settles at the right hip.

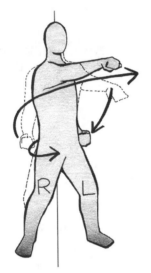

15-61c

15-61c: Now your right fist punches out and around to punch out directly in front of your chest.

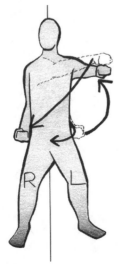

15-61d

15-61d: Then the left hand punches out and around, while the right hand returns to the hip.

Punch three more times, right, left, right. Both hands punch and return for five punches total, beginning with the right fist and ending with the right fist.

As one hand punches, the other draws back to act as a pulley system. The hand pulling back adds power to the hand punching out. Stay loose; this is where your power is maximized.

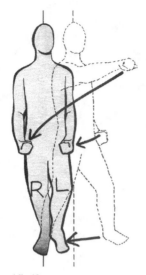

15-62a

Grasp the Bird's Tail (Right Style), #62

15-62a: From the last right fisted punch, bring the fists down to the sides, and the left foot over to touch by the right instep.

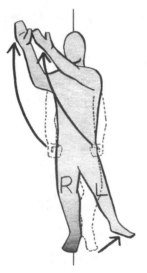

15-62b

15-62b: Then go into Grasp the Bird's Tail by dropping the left foot back and reaching up to the right. Complete Grasp Bird as shown in Figures 15-2a through 15-2c.

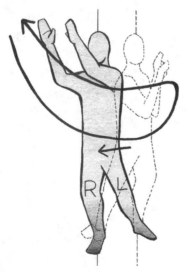

15-62c

15-62c: After drawing back the bird's tail, shifting back to the left leg, you then shift forward to the right leg performing a movement just like Green Dragon Rises from the Water, as in Figures 15-16b through 15-16d.

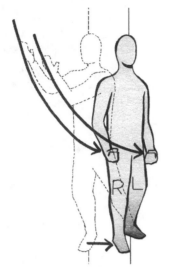

15-62d

15-62d: Complete the Green Dragon move by drawing the arms back and bringing the left leg back, to now stand on both legs with fists at sides.

Grasp the Bird's Tail (Left Style), #63

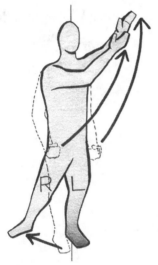

15-63a

15-63a: This and the next figure mirror the Grasp the Bird's Tail and Green Dragon–like movement just done in the preceding figures, except as you'll see, with opposite sides.

Reach up with hands out to left (with left hand on top for this left style movement, and right hand palm up underneath), and right foot goes out behind.

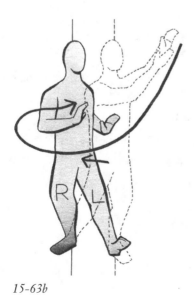

15-63b

15-63b: Draw bird's tail back, then pushing up into the Green Dragon type movement to the left/front this time.

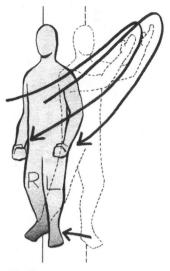

15-63c

15-63c: Complete left style motion before drawing back to start point (as shown in Figure 15-62a), and now begin Grand Terminus, the very last movement.

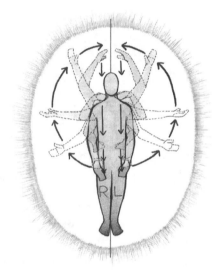

15-64

Grand Terminus; Gather Heaven to Earth, #64

15-64: Congratulations! You deserve a great deep bow. Upon completion of learning the entire 64 posture series of the Kuang Ping Yang style form, you are now about to do the most wonderful movement of all, Grand Terminus.

This final move cleanses and reinvigorates the body, leaving you feeling about as terrific as a kid could feel, or as Dave Letterman might say, "Feeling better than people should be allowed."

1. From Grasp the Bird's Tail Left Style/Green Dragon movement, return to feet-together/fist-at-sides pose to start Grand Terminus.

2. The hands reach out and slightly back, extending the arms back and outward.

3. As you stretch up, the knees straighten for the first time throughout the entire 64 posture series.

4. Gathering the Qi from all around, the light pours over your relaxing body as the palms turn down.

5. Slowly, the palms descend, invoking the cleansing light to wash through every area as the palms pass through.

6. As the hands descend back to your sides, just bask in the soothing healing of this ocean of light washing over and through. Experience effortlessness.

"Experience the Light!"

This movement is meant to gather all the light, or Qi, we have generated through the 64 movements. As the hands turn downward at the top of their arcs, allow the light to spill, washing over and through your entire being to cleanse any heavy loads or toxins. Let the feet open to release any loads right down into the earth's gentle pull. Continue to allow the light to wash over and through you throughout the day.

A T'ai Chi Punch Line

Grand Terminus is not only the last T'ai Chi movement, it is also the name of that popular yin/yang symbol you see on jewelry. The white wave interacting with the black wave symbolizes a balance of all things, hard and soft, force and yielding, concentration and empty awareness. Each time you complete your T'ai Chi forms, you will have integrated all aspects of yourself. You will have centered yourself in all ways. The Grand Terminus is a completion of renewal and a gateway to greater and greater adventures. As you learn to move smoothly and effortlessly through an increasingly meaningful life, an ancient friend called T'ai Chi will always be there to console and inspire, no matter what life throws at you.

The Least You Need to Know

- Practice movements with full, easy abdominal breaths.
- Relax each breath out of the entire body, allowing Qi to flow into and through limbs as weight shifts or sinks.
- Allow yourself to become T'ai Chi's natural elegance.
- Feel at one with the world when practicing. Each movement learned and practiced transforms you.
- Push from your dan tien, not your shoulders or back. T'ai Chi's powerful self-defense moves can be soothing and teach you to lift groceries correctly.
- T'ai Chi is *effortless*, showing that most battles are fought in our own minds and hearts.
- Adjust movements to fit your mobility. No matter how expansive or limited your mobility, T'ai Chi extends it. Don't force it.
- Pushing and punching with the back foot planted and the body relaxed guides the force of the earth through you.
- T'ai Chi connects you to the heaven and earth.
- T'ai Chi practices letting go of what's inevitable, and diving into what's changeable.

Part 5

T'ai Chi's Buffet of Short, Sword, and Fan Styles

About a mere 30 years ago there was almost no T'ai Chi available to Westerners. T'ai Chi was a Chinese secret. However, today we are fortunate to live in interesting times, as the Chinese would say.

In most cities today you can find a variety of T'ai Chi styles, including not only basic forms, but the more artistic and challenging sword and fan styles, as well. Feast your eyes on just a sampling of the wide variety of short forms, sword style, and fan style T'ai Chi now available to you, and then choose an adventure to embark upon.

Push Hands closes this part, explaining how this ancient aspect of T'ai Chi is not only a sparring technique, but even more important, a way to observe our state of mind and the way we may *unconsciously* interact with the world around us. Interestingly T'ai Chi helps us understand the world by more deeply exploring our own internal state, while Push Hands' *external*/engagement exercise inspires a deeper awareness of our *internal state*. T'ai Chi and Push Hands team up to illuminate every aspect of our nature, so we can grow endlessly with eyes, mind, and heart, *wide open*, and ready for adventure!

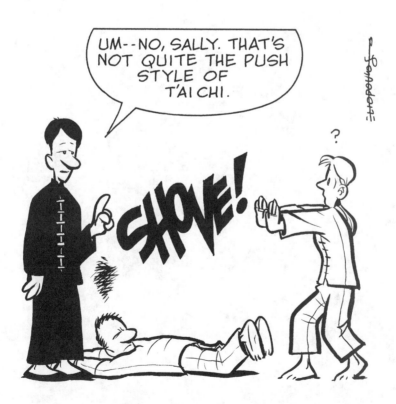

Chapter 16

Mulan Quan Basic Short Form

In This Chapter

- ◆ Discover Mulan Quan style T'ai Chi
- ◆ Learn how Mulan Quan promotes grace, beauty, and health
- ◆ Find out what Mulan Quan can do for your heart

If Mulan Quan's main benefit could be put into one word, it would be "self-esteem." The artistry of its forms and the mental healing of its practice expands and enhances our self-perception. Mulan's elegant promotion of grace and agility make it perfect for women, yet great for men, too.

Mulan Quan is a rather modern form of T'ai Chi, but it is derived from an ancient, nearly extinct form of Hua Chia Quan (*Hua* is flower, *Chia* is frame, *Quan* is fist, meaning "beautiful boxing style"). The Mulan Quan T'ai Chi short form comprises 24 powerful yet delicate movements that flow one into the other. This chapter introduces the first 10 movements of the Mulan style of T'ai Chi. To learn the rest of this beautiful style and to supplement the information in this chapter, please refer to the *Mulan Quan Basic Short Form* video, listed in Appendix C, "Audio-Visual Resources." Again, it is difficult to convey in still photographs the multidimensionality of T'ai Chi's flowing motions.

Mulan Quan Promotes Elegance and Health

The physical elegance of *Mulan Quan* gives the practitioner a regal appearance that is mesmerizing. The practice of its forms has a wonderful impact on the self-esteem of its practitioners. However, the mental healing is just the beginning because this vehicle enhances our physical beauty, as well as our physical health.

- ◆ **Mulan beauty treatment.** Mulan Quan is a highly effective beauty regimen for women. Its ability to simultaneously instill a sense of deep personal power and elegance in motion literally changes the practitioner's personality and outlook on life. This living embodiment of power, grace, and artistry actually transforms the practitioner. No external cosmetic can come close to the beauty treatment Mulan Quan offers. However, with a more beautiful being within, anything you adorn yourself with externally will be very effective.

Know Your Chinese

Mulan Quan translated literally is "wooden orchid fist," which means "strong, beautiful, fist." *Mu* is wood, *lan* is orchid, and *quan* (chuan) is fist. This style is named after the brave young woman, Mulan Fa, who selflessly took her aging father's place in the war to save his life. Her story was made famous by Disney's epic animated feature, *Mulan*.

◆ **Mulan the healer.** Mulan Quan is recommended for many ailments and chronic diseases, including obesity, heart diseases, insomnia, and lower back problems. (Chinese T'ai Chi masters often say, "You are as young as your spine is flexible.") Reports from Chinese hospitals indicate Mulan Quan has been very useful in stroke rehabilitation treatment and as an adjunct therapy for cancer patients. The Beijing Cancer Center used Mulan as a physical therapy for patients, who then saw improved appetites, weight gain, and better overall health.

Step East to Lotus

This series of movements rotates both upper and lower body joints, while promoting a deep sense of tranquility. These movements improve your balance and promote an expressive attitude of elegance. The insights in this chapter go deeper than a video or live class could, due to the time limitation of classes and video. However, moving instruction offers a right brain quality that adds a soothing and hands-free learning dimension. If you want to augment the instruction in this chapter with a video dimension, refer to the instructional video of this beautifully feminine style in Appendix C.

Step in the Eastern Direction

Stepping in the Eastern Direction helps you relax into your forms. This initial motion's liquid quality places the mind in a pool of tranquility as it prepares the body for what's to come.

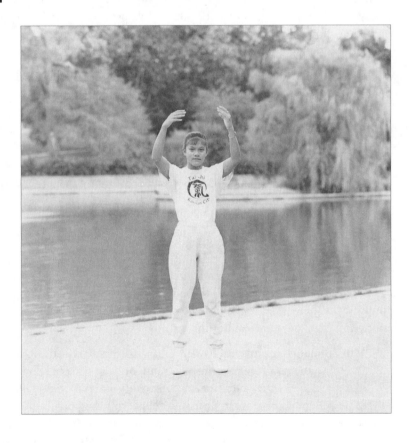

Spread Wings on Lotus

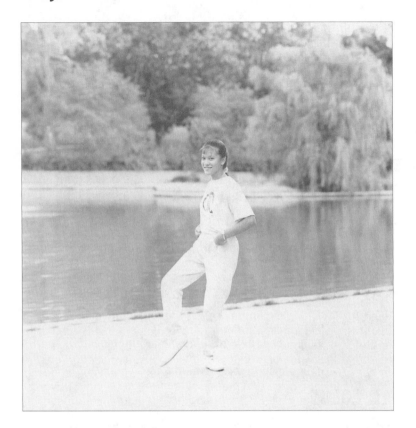

This motion fully rotates the shoulder joints, which can begin to loosen some of the daily stress we tend to accumulate there. This movement challenges and improves your ability to balance, as it carries you through a transitional move toward the next movement.

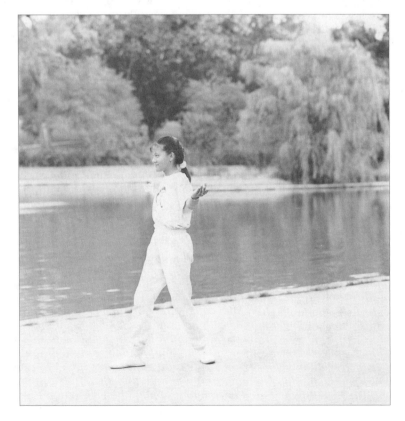

This is the preparatory movement leading to lifting the left leg.

Elegance and balance are the hallmarks of this form. This movement rotates and begins to release deep tensions in the hip sockets and surrounding tissue.

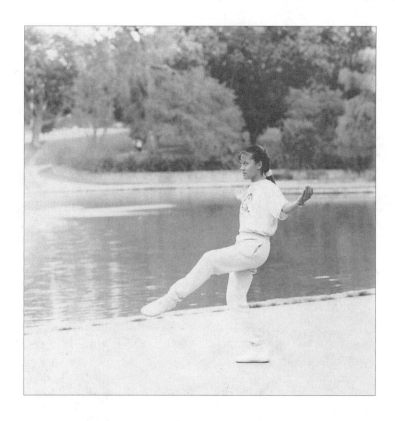

Float Rainbow to Golden Lotus

This series begins with deep loosening throughout the upper body and out to the fingers. Yet it continues to open Qi's flow throughout the entire lower body as well.

Floating Rainbow

This beautiful extension lives up to its lovely name. Floating Rainbow tones the body and exercises the shoulder, elbow, wrist, and finger joints.

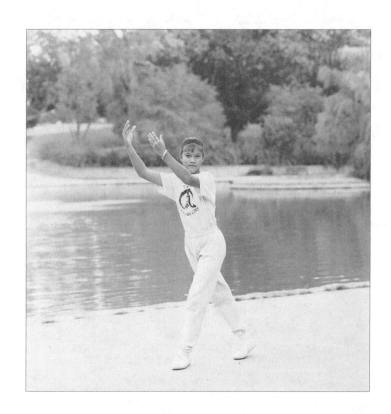

Sit on Golden Lotus

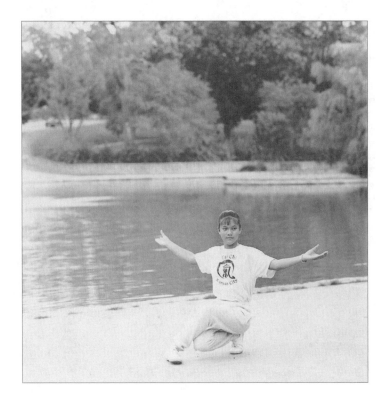

While promoting grace and balance, Sit on Golden Lotus works the thighs and legs. Some feel that the demands T'ai Chi puts on the thighs very effectively promotes circulation to the lower extremities, which allows the heart to work less hard to oxygenate the body.

Ride Wind to Dragon Flying

These motions promote a very subtle internal awareness of balance and movement. Every part of the body is worked and loosened in this series.

Ride with Wind and Waves

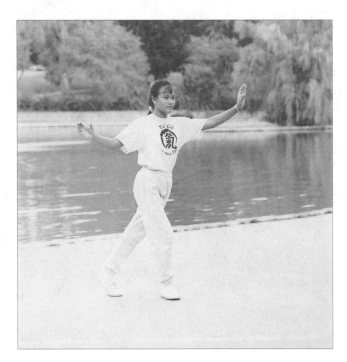

A very subtle shifting of the weight between the front and back legs exercises all the muscle groups in the lower body. The arm movements likewise loosen joints and tonify muscles throughout the upper body.

Dragon Flying Toward Wind

This movement is a very subtle internal motion that focuses awareness within.

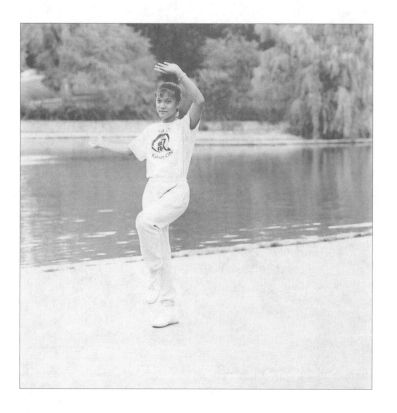

Purple Swan Tilts Its Wings

Nearly every muscle is loosened and strengthened by this move, but the abdominal muscles benefit especially. This series promotes spinal flexibility.

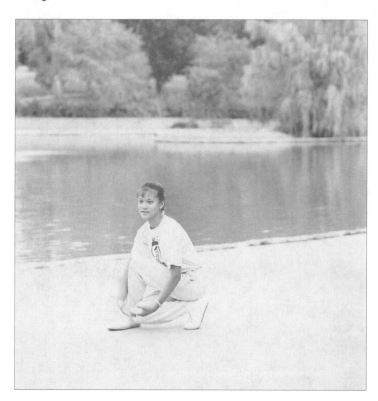

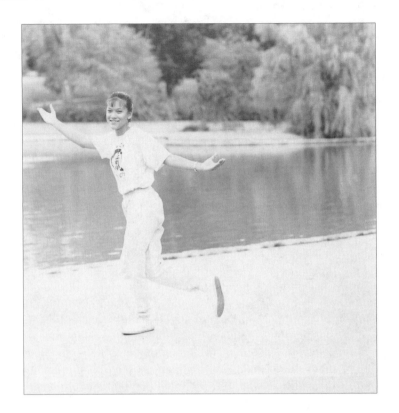

This exquisite movement is not only beautiful to the external eye but also promotes health, balance, and flexibility through the torso and spine.

The Least You Need to Know

- ◆ Mulan Quan movements promote elegance and balance.
- ◆ Mulan Quan promotes flexibility through the spine and extremities, which may keep you feeling young.
- ◆ Mulan Quan can tone muscles and especially strengthen the thighs, which may be very good news for your heart.

Chapter 17

Mulan Quan Fan Style

In This Chapter

- ◆ Discover the benefits of Mulan Quan
- ◆ Use Mulan Quan as emotional therapy
- ◆ Find the pearl within you through Mulan Quan

Mulan Quan is based in traditional T'ai Chi movement and *wushu* (which is Chinese for martial arts). However, it adds aspects of Chinese folk dance and gymnastics to provide a vessel of motion for the beauty of the practitioner to be poured into. Mulan Quan, therefore, reaches to the outward limits the practitioner can express, both with the wushu aspects and even as a spectacular sword form (which I'll introduce in Chapter 18, "Mulan Quan Sword Style"). Yet it also explores the softest, most delicate aspects of the user, which is most beautifully expressed in the Mulan Quan fan style.

There are two fan styles, the single fan and the double fan. This chapter introduces you to the basic single fan style. For information on video instruction resources, see the Appendix C, "Audio-Visual Resources." This chapter exposes you to how the forms look and elaborates on how they are performed and what benefits each provides. Again, the motion and multidimensional quality is best learned in a live class or at least with video instruction.

Mulan Quan styles are rapidly gaining popularity and have been involved in exhibitions and competitions from Beijing to Kansas City. Work is being done to eventually introduce Mulan Quan to Olympic competition.

Flying Bees Through Leaves

This section's movement works and stretches the entire body.

Notice here how this motion exercises the arm muscles and loosens the joints as you relax into the pose.

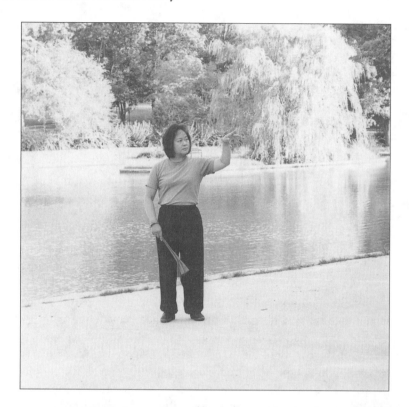

Flying Bees Through Leaves is quite graceful, but the movement is only a vessel through which to express yourself. Enjoy as you experience your own grace being poured into the vessel of your T'ai Chi. Furthermore, it tonifies the entire body from head to toe.

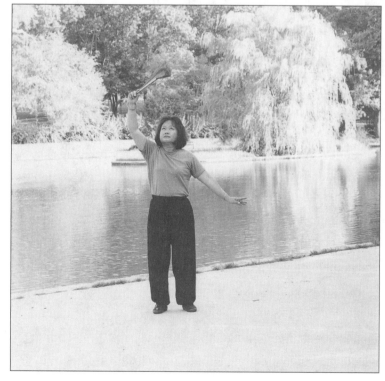

Stretching Cloud to Floating

Promoting equilibrium and refinement, this series is internal and subtle and yet externally strengthening to all muscles.

Stretching Left Foot

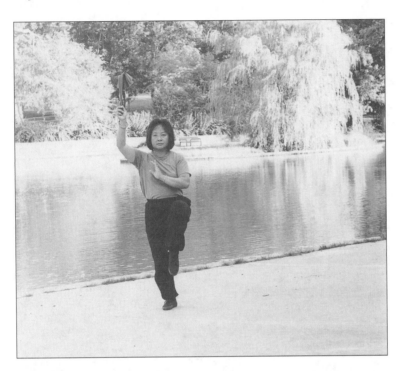

While strengthening the leg muscles, this movement fosters an internal awareness that improves your balance.

Cloud Lotus Floating

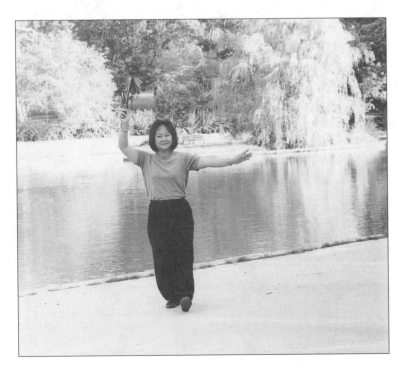

The external motion is refined by encouraging the practitioner to "feel elegant." Of course, besides that mental and spiritual benefit, it has a very practical purpose of working and loosening the arm's joints.

Miracle Touching Ocean

The beautiful names of this section are inspiring, but the movements hold even more. While creating very solid strengthening, these movements also affect the way we feel about ourselves. Mulan Quan can literally transform our self-esteem.

Know Your Chinese

In Chinese folklore, the **dragon** represents the *yang* (expressive) aspect of power and majesty, which may be why it is commonly used in T'ai Chi imagery to help practitioners access and evoke the limitless power of their dynamic nature.

Miracle Dragon Lifting Head

Miracle Dragon Lifting Head is actually well named because moving in a posture of head-lifted self-esteem (which T'ai Chi requires) actually transforms the practitioner over time in ways that may seem miraculous. Mulan Quan may be a powerful adjunct therapy for the many emotionally affected conditions, such as eating disorders, facing some young women today.

The Miracle Dragon Lifting Head encourages the practitioner to lengthen, enhancing and promoting good posture.

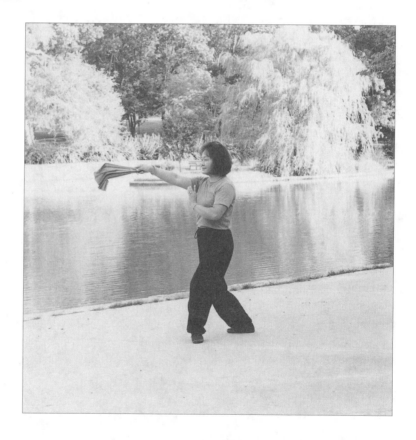

Swallow Touching Ocean

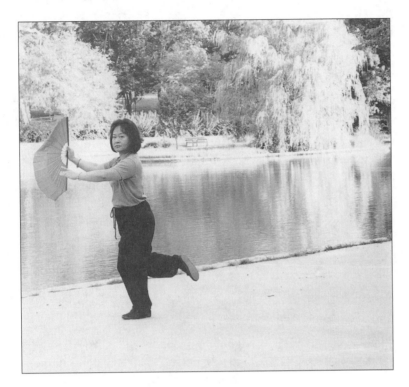

This movement powerfully strengthens the leg and back muscles, while promoting release of tension through the back.

Green Willow Twigs Dancing

This section offers great overall toning exercises, and its delicate footwork especially focuses toning in the leg.

Green Willow Twigs Swaying

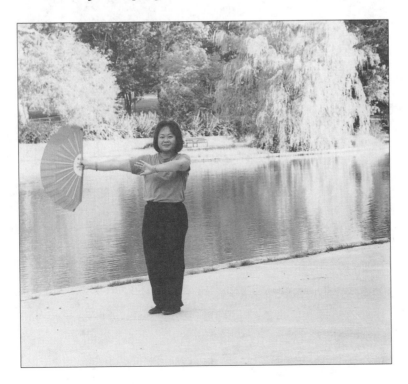

The deep rotation of the hip of Green Willow Twigs Swaying allows a subtle internal awareness of how the body shifts from its power point, or dan tien.

This posture works all the joints and muscles, offering great strengthening and toning throughout the entire frame.

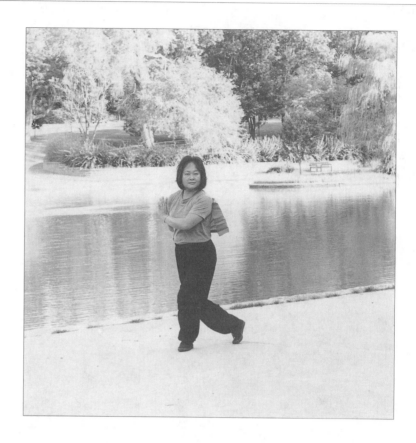

Dancing in Wind

The delicate footwork of Dancing in Wind is a great toning exercise for the legs, and its subtlety offers a meditative quality as it's performed.

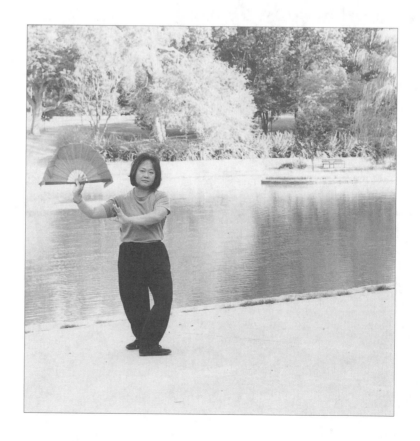

Dun Huang Flying Dance

While challenging the lower body to maintain balance, the upper body is rotated and flexed in a soothing, relaxed way.

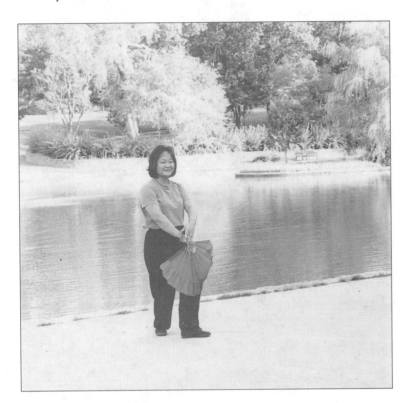

The shoulder and wrist rotations of this motion release stress and soothe your mind as you flow through its graceful ways.

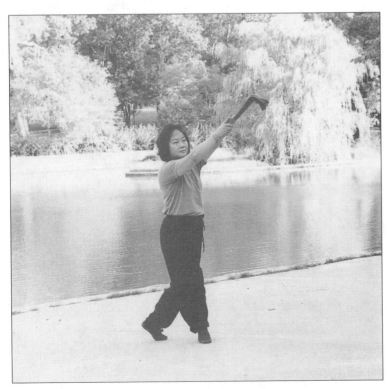

The spine and waist are flexed gently, promoting a litheness that is not only lovely but enhances all aspects of health, according to Traditional Chinese Medicine.

While the legs work and adjust to subtle posture changes, the upper body is gently stretched and loosened.

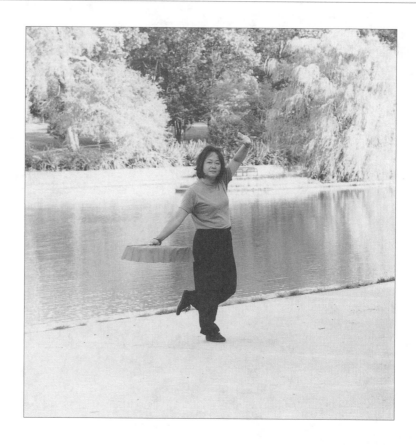

The Least You Need to Know

- Mulan Quan can change your self-image, which can positively change your physical appearance over time.
- Mulan Quan's self-esteem promotion may be a wonderful adjunct therapy to women facing emotional problems.
- The elegance Mulan Quan offers is really within you right now! Mulan Quan only helps you to express that part of yourself.

Chapter 18

Mulan Quan Sword Style

In This Chapter

- ◆ Developing internal power using the sword form
- ◆ Promoting balance and strength through elegance
- ◆ Balancing raw power and subtle beauty within your mind, heart and body

Mulan Quan is great for everyone, but again, women greatly benefit from the elegance and tender beauty it promotes. However, another profound benefit is its tremendous, yet subtle, power. The power of Mulan Quan is perhaps most dramatically observed in the performance of Mulan Quan Sword Style.

This chapter exposes you to some of the sword form postures, their benefits, and points to enrich your experience with them. It is recommended, however, that you use this book as a supplement to live classes or at least video instruction. The complexity of these lovely forms can be better comprehended when you can move, follow, and hear instructions at the same time.

Preparation to Eye on Sword

This section quietly prepares the mind and body before launching into the expansive motion of the Mulan Quan Sword Style.

Preparation Stance

The Preparation Stance is meant to focus and relax the mind, body, and heart.

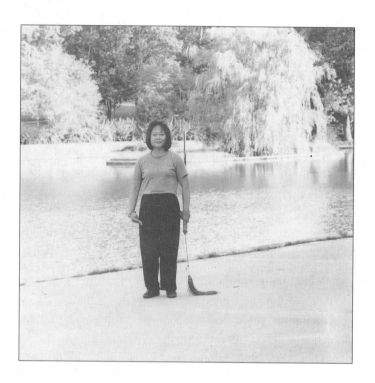

Left Foot Half Step with Eyes on Sword

Here is a full rotation of the shoulder and arm as the sword arm goes into a clockwise rotation.

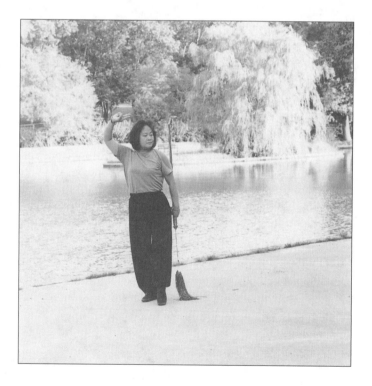

Forward Step to Low Jab

This series works the entire body, loosening and lengthening it from head to toe.

Forward Step, Holding Sword Under Elbow

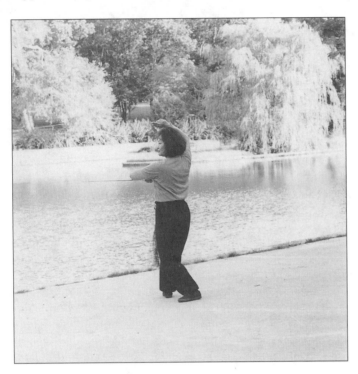

Your right foot steps right with weight shifting forward. Bring your sword-wielding arm straight out to the side, then around to the front and bent elbow. This movement helps to loosen the entire body as you breathe and allow your Qi to flow through all limbs, as well as through the sword hand.

Sword Exchange, Turn Body, and Low Jab

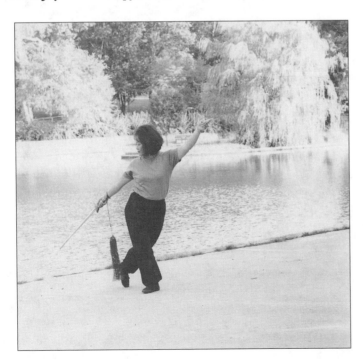

This movement fosters an elongation of the entire frame as the hips are rotated and the body loosens.

Sword Upright to Balance Body

In these motions, your entire body is strengthened with very desirable and select muscle toning.

Body Return, Step with Sword Upright

The abdominal muscles are toned in this movement as the back and legs are worked, as well.

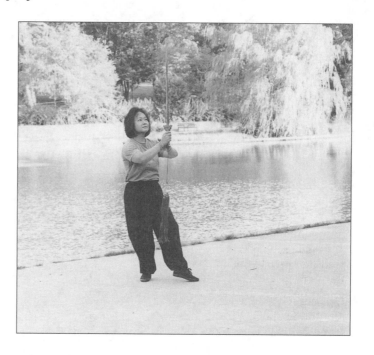

Vertical Sword and Balance Body

The shoulder and wrist joints are exercised here, which helps the practitioner to avoid calcium deposit buildup in joints that might negatively affect flexibility. Mulan Quan enables you to age while maintaining fluid, elegant flexibility.

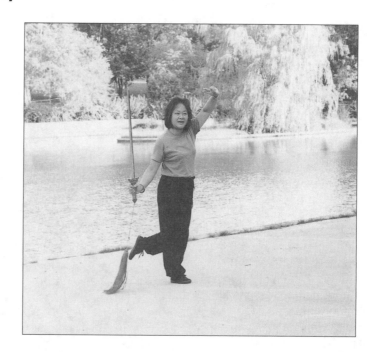

Turn Around to Up Jab

Balance, posture, and leg strength are found in this set of movements.

Turn Around, Lower to Sitting Position, Sword Upright

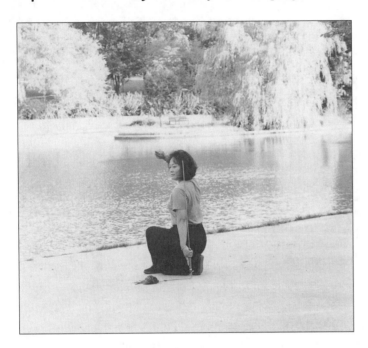

Leg muscles are both stretched and strengthened as you breathe and lengthen through this movement.

Step Up, Lower to Sitting Position, Sword Up Jab

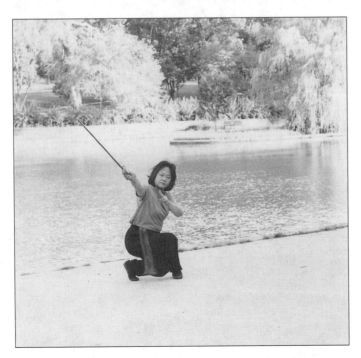

Practicing this movement with an attitude of "elegance and style" will have a wonderful impact on both your balance and your posture.

Level Sword to Lift Leg

The following set tonifies and beautifies your body in many ways.

Level Sword, Turn Body, and Lift Knee

While improving your balance, Level Sword, Turn Body, and Lift Knee also tones and strengthens.

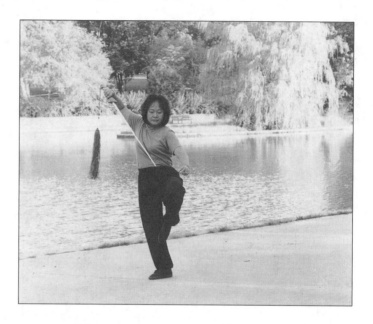

Lift Leg, Side Step, Side Chop with Sword

This may be the most beautiful of all Mulan Quan movements, yet it also works to loosen the body's muscles and joints.

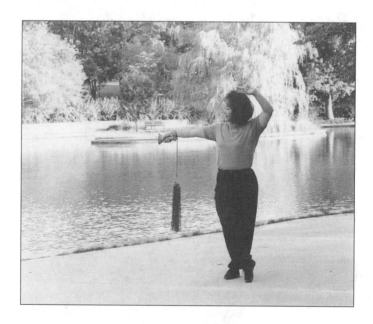

The Least You Need to Know

- ◆ The sword form promotes a sense of gentle power.
- ◆ Remember to make the forms fit your body.
- ◆ Let the thought of elegance elongate your form through the practice of these movements.

Chapter 19

Getting Gently Pushy with Push Hands

In This Chapter

◆ Learn the art of Push Hands

◆ Use Push Hands to learn about yourself

◆ Discover how masters resist many opponents effortlessly

Push Hands is a paradox. It is a sparring technique in a way, but it is also a quiet tool of self-awareness. The way you see Push Hands says as much about you as it does about Push Hands. To one person it may look like a delicate dance, while another may see a physical contest not unlike a sumo-wrestling match. Actually it is a tiny bit of both.

By moving your dan tien in toward your opponent, your weight shifts toward your front foot, and your Qi flows through the body exerting a very relaxed force (like the unbendable arm). So as your hand pushes toward your opponent, if the opponent is stiff, this will likely uproot their stance, causing them to lose their balance. If they are supple and yielding, they will absorb your attack and respond in kind.

The goal, however, is not to forcefully uproot your opponent. Instead, the purpose of Push Hands is to become accustomed to the ebb and flow of physical energy expressed in motion. If your opponent is pushy and abrupt, they will likely overextend themselves as they attack. This attack isn't violent; it's just their arm extending into your chest or heart area. When they overextend, they will come in off balance if you yield. When they retreat to try to catch their balance, they are vulnerable. A slight push can send a larger, more powerful opponent reeling when they are out of center.

When pushing hands you seek to maintain a delicate contact with your opponent, while remaining flexible and calmly aware of yourself. Push Hands is mainly about observing and responding with the most power and least effort. The expanded awareness and practice of experiencing different aspects of self that Push Hands promotes makes us more fluid and better able to become whatever is required and most useful at any given moment. Push Hands is training in being all things.

Notice that the pusher is focusing his energy toward the other by facing his palm toward the opponent as he pushes. The energy center, Lao Gong, on the Pericardium energy meridian is in the center of the palm of the hand. This is a highly sensitive point and also projects energy outward.

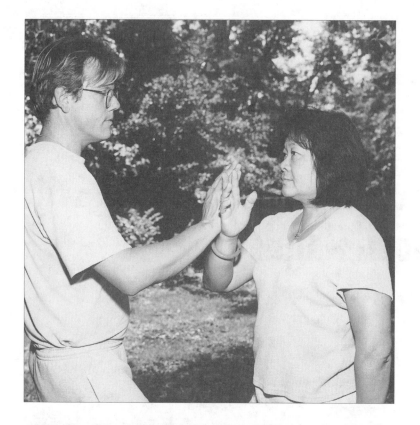

The goal of Push Hands is not to resist but to yield and deflect incoming power.

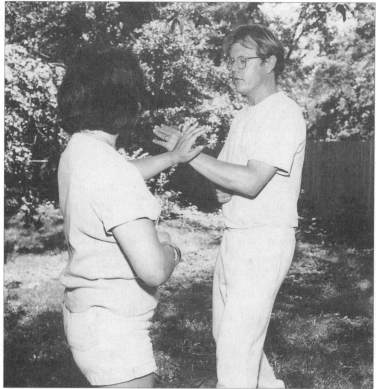

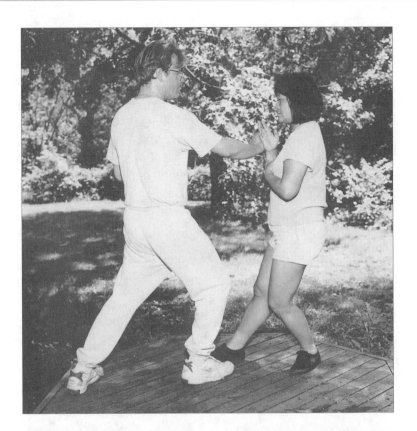

Remember the story of the snake yielding to the white crane's attacks.

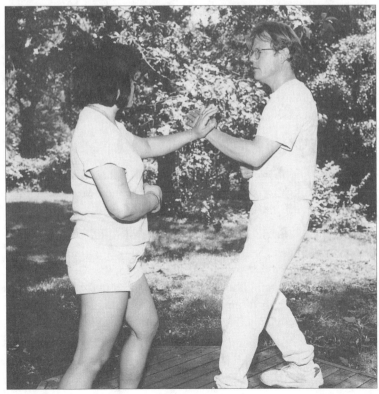

Think of a butterfly resting between the exchanging hands or wrists as you push or retreat from your opponent. Try to be sensitive enough to anticipate motions so that your advancing opponent does not crush the butterfly as you lithely retreat.

Realize that just as with all T'ai Chi, Push Hands is not physical force as we usually think of it.

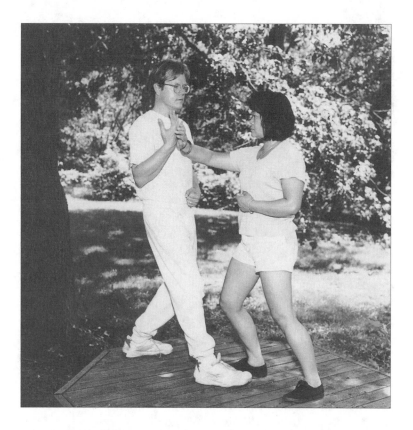

> **Sage Sifu Says**
>
> When pushing hands, envision a butterfly poised between your wrist and the wrist of your opponent. Try to have just enough pressure between them so the butterfly doesn't fly away, yet not so much that you crush it. Your goal is to maintain subtle contact, yielding when attacked, and advancing when the opponent yields.

Push Hands is done with the same effortless power as the Unbendable Arm presented in Chapter 4, "Expand the Mind and Lighten the Heart." Also, notice that in this exercise, the unused hand is a fist held at the ready near the chest. In T'ai Chi, as in all martial arts, nothing is done without reason. The resting hand is ever ready to spring into action. We don't think in fear, but in relaxed alertness.

The Psychology of Push Hands

Push Hands is about observing. As with all T'ai Chi, it is all-encompassing and has as much to teach us about our mind and heart as it does about our physical balance and dexterity.

If I am pushy and overpowering in life, this will show up in my Push Hands technique. I will often find myself overextending or overemphasizing the attack with little thought of staying centered. Likewise, if I am too timid, the dancing exchange of Push Hands will seem limp and lifeless—not much fun. The goal, as always, is to strike balance between both the raging bull and the shrinking violet that resides within us. Both aspects of self are perfect and absolutely necessary to making us a whole being, just as nature is perfect because it contains these extremes and everything between.

Practicing Push Hands can raise the raging bull from the shrinking violet and bloom delicate petals from the raging bull. As T'ai Chi expands your beingness, Push Hands can help by illustrating in an external social element the internal tendencies you may not have noticed about yourself or others.

Eventually, Push Hands may become a powerful business or marriage-counseling tool because it helps to illuminate how people interact. It's not about labeling one person's technique as good or bad, but rather about becoming aware of people's tendencies so that we can interact more effectively no matter where they are coming from.

Different Forms of Push Hands

There are several different forms of Push Hands. Some incorporate very directly applicable martial techniques that involve deflecting blows and tripping your opponent as they lose their balance. These are fun, but not necessary for most T'ai Chi training. If you are curious about these techniques, shop around for an instructor well versed in Push Hands. If your instructor does not do Push Hands, you may find weekend workshops that teach the techniques, or perhaps there may be someone who knows at T'ai Chi club gatherings. Contacting the T'ai Chi organizations listed in Appendix A, "The T'ai Chi and QiGong Yellow Pages," may help lead you to teachers or events that specialize in Push Hands.

> **CAUTION** **Ouch!**
>
> For those in a more frail physical condition using T'ai Chi as therapy, more martial Push Hands techniques are ill advised and really not necessary. You can play a basic Push Hands routine with a partner you can trust to be gentle enough. Or you can skip Push Hands altogether. As always, these tools are toys to play with. We only play with toys we enjoy and make us feel good, which is the point of toys in the first place.

Legends of the Masters

There are stories about T'ai Chi masters who exhibit almost superhuman strength when being pushed or when pushing others. Bill Moyer's documentary on the healing mind showed an old Chinese master who could withstand the onslaught of a half dozen pushing students without being budged and seemingly without really exerting himself. This same master also sent those students flying off across the lawn with hardly any indication of movement on his part.

There is an area of T'ai Chi that focuses on energy projection called "fa-jing," and it is claimed that some masters (like the one Bill Moyer met) can use the force of their Qi to withstand attacks and send opponents flying. However, there may be a physical element to this ability as well.

If the human body is a structure like a building, then engineering principles may explain some of this. If just the right structuring of materials in just the right way can build buildings that resist massive pressure in weight-bearing demands, can't the body likewise do so? If a T'ai Chi master were very attuned to how his body aligned bones and muscles with the support of the earth beneath, he may be able to resist great external force by using internal engineering principles. Also, as in Push Hands, if one was so self-aware of these principles, one could be subtly attuned to when this opponent offered the slightest break in their solidity. Then, the master would be able to uproot the opponents with the least bit of force. This would seem magical to the untrained eye, just as a remote control would seem magical to a cave man. However, it may really be just a matter of subtle awareness.

The Least You Need to Know

- Push Hands helps you become self-aware.
- Push Hands improves balance and power.
- For those rehabilitating from injuries or with balance problems, Push Hands may best be avoided.

Part  **6**

Life Applications

This part demonstrates how T'ai Chi can change your life and our world. T'ai Chi becomes a gateway to looking at life and health in a completely different way. By seeing our world and ourselves in a proactively empowered way, we can literally change the course of our lives and make our world a much better place.

This part details illnesses T'ai Chi can help treat. It also explains how corporations can support their employees' development of healthy lifestyles while maximizing profits by increasing productivity. You'll also learn how, in addition to business savings, society may save big on avoided social problems by incorporating T'ai Chi at all levels of society beginning with elementary public education.

Last, but not least, you'll discover how T'ai Chi and QiGong can help us literally change our world by enabling all of us to maximize our ability to be a healing force in this world.

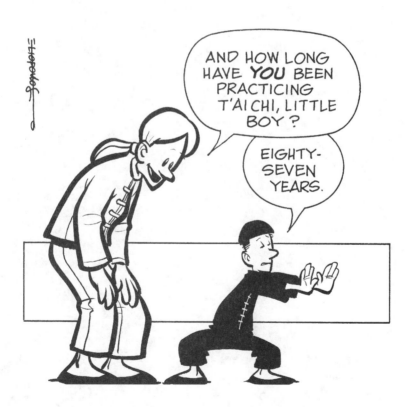

Chapter 20

T'ai Chi as Therapy for Young and Old

In This Chapter

- ◆ T'ai Chi for kids
- ◆ T'ai Chi for seniors
- ◆ T'ai Chi for women
- ◆ T'ai Chi for men
- ◆ T'ai Chi and sports
- ◆ T'ai Chi as a health therapy

T'ai Chi is for everyone. This chapter provides details on how T'ai Chi benefits specific people, their health conditions, and their athletic activities. In fact anyone, but especially health professionals and T'ai Chi/QiGong teachers, will find the last part of this chapter a powerful reference, listing maladies in alphabetical order, with details on how T'ai Chi or QiGong may help.

If you are treating a specific condition, you will find an introduction to how T'ai Chi may assist your ongoing therapy. For seniors, you will find out why T'ai Chi is the very best thing you can do for yourself. Specific reasons why children, men, and women should practice T'ai Chi are provided as well.

This chapter will also assist parents and/or T'ai Chi teachers who want to start a T'ai Chi class for kids. Kids are taught differently from adults, and this chapter will give teachers or parents some great insights into helping their kids make the most of T'ai Chi, and have fun doing it.

T'ai Chi for Kids

Kids are the embodiment of change, and change can be very stressful. Their minds and bodies grow at phenomenal rates, so they are constantly having to work with new and different bodies, making coordination and balance a big issue. T'ai Chi, with its emphasis on balance, is well suited to address all these challenges.

Preparing for Athletics and Life

T'ai Chi works to integrate the mind and body, skeletal and muscular systems, and left brain and right brain. In physical terms, this centering is built around an awareness of moving with good posture and from a low center of gravity, or the vertical axis and the dan tien.

Gifted athletes are people who are naturals at this kind of self-awareness and movement. Since most of our kids are not naturals, T'ai Chi can be a most effective way to help your child prepare for athletics and to simply be comfortable in their rapidly changing bodies.

Treating Attention Deficit Disorder (ADD)

ADD is a growing problem not only with children, but adults as well. T'ai Chi may be a wonderful adjunct therapy for treating ADD because it augments many of the mood management techniques recommended for ADD sufferers. A University of Miami School of Medicine study shows T'ai Chi is a powerful therapy for ADHD (Attention Deficit and Hyperactivity Disorder).

> **CAUTION**
>
> **Ouch!** _____
>
> Check with your child's therapist or physician before beginning T'ai Chi. Also, find an effective, understanding T'ai Chi instructor who has experience teaching children.

Drs. Edward M. Hallowell, M.D., and John J. Ratey, M.D., experts on the management of ADD wrote, "Exercise is positively one of the best treatments for ADD. It helps work off excess energy and aggression in a positive way, it allows for noise-reduction within the mind, it stimulates the hormonal and neurochemical systems in a most therapeutic way, and it soothes and calms the body."

The slow mindful movements of T'ai Chi have much to offer people who suffer from ADD. The following table explains why T'ai Chi may be a perfect ADD therapy.

T'ai Chi and ADD

What Experts Suggest	What T'ai Chi Offers
Set aside time for recharging batteries, something calm and restful, like meditation.	T'ai Chi is a mini-vacation.
Daily exercise that is readily available and needs little preparation can help with the blahs that occur and with overall outlook.	T'ai Chi is easy, requires no preparation, and is a daily mood elevator.
Observe mood swings; learn to accept them by realizing they will pass. Learn strategies that might help bad moods pass sooner.	T'ai Chi is a tool for self-observation of feelings and for letting those feelings go.
Use "time-outs" when you are upset or overstimulated; take a time-out; go away, calm down.	T'ai Chi can be performed in the bathroom at school or work, giving you a break from the stress.
Let go of the urgency to always finish things quickly by learning to enjoy the process.	T'ai Chi's slow flowing routine is about letting go of outcome and learning to love the process.
ADD usually includes a tendency to overfocus or hyperfocus at times, to obsess or ruminate over some imagined problem without being able to let it go.	T'ai Chi teaches the practice of letting go on a mental, emotional, and physical level with each exhale.

Teaching T'ai Chi to Kids

Not just kids with ADD, but all kids usually have difficulty with the slowness of T'ai Chi. Therefore, you simply speed it up. Teach each child at their own pace; some can go slower than others.

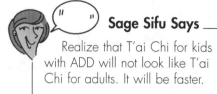

Sage Sifu Says

Realize that T'ai Chi for kids with ADD will not look like T'ai Chi for adults. It will be faster.

Give kids constant recognition for their T'ai Chi accomplishments. Ask each kid to demonstrate his or her new movements for the class at the end and have everyone applaud. If a kid forgets a move, jump in and do it with them. Over the weeks, they will look forward to the recognition and practice more.

T'ai Chi is a loose thing, not a rigid thing. It can work for everybody and can be taught in many fun ways. Keep a kid's T'ai Chi class moving and include stretching exercises from yoga or aggressive calisthenics to use up excess energy. Then, as the kids get more tired, ease them into slower movement.

Kids can do QiGong meditations, too. It isn't anything like adult meditations; there are more and different images that work. Try the children's meditation tape offered in the back of this book for examples.

T'ai Chi for Seniors

Seniors can find no better exercise in the world than T'ai Chi. *Prevention Magazine* reported that "T'ai Chi may be the best exercise for people over the age of 60 … providing cardio fitness, muscle strength, and flexibility all in one simple workout that is easy on the joints." T'ai Chi may help build bone mass and connective tissue, with zero joint damage, according to some studies. Other studies show that T'ai Chi is twice as good as any other balance exercise in the world. Since complications from falling injuries are the sixth largest cause of death among seniors, this is a very big deal. For seniors with chronic conditions, there are many maladies that T'ai Chi can help treat. For details see the section "The Therapeutic Powers of T'ai Chi and QiGong" at the end of this chapter.

Ouch!

Each condition is different, so check with your physician to discuss T'ai Chi's potential benefits to your case. T'ai Chi is extremely gentle and should not be confused with the harder martial arts, but consult your doctor before beginning the class.

If your mobility is limited in some way, that is no problem, even if you're in a wheelchair. There is a class for you, and if you are persistent, you'll find a teacher and a class that are perfect.

T'ai Chi for Women

There are many reasons why T'ai Chi is the ultimate exercise for women. Its ability to cultivate both elegance and power are two of these. In today's working environment where women are competing in the workforce with men and trying to break through the glass ceiling, T'ai Chi's ability to cultivate an inner sense of confident power can be very helpful. However, there are many biological reasons T'ai Chi can be helpful to women as well.

Halting Bone Loss

Bone loss is a big problem with many women. Studies indicate that stress may be a major factor contributing to the loss of bone mass in even relatively young women. The daily stress relief T'ai Chi promotes provides a powerful preventative therapy to help ensure a long active life for women.

For women, including those over 45, studies have shown that QiGong practice raises estrogen levels. This is highly desirable because reduced estrogen levels after menopause cause a loss of calcium from the bones and increase the risk of osteoporosis and heart disease.

Treating Eating Disorders

Women suffer from eating disorders ten times as often as men. Although often thought of as an adult problem, anorexia and bulimia most often start in the teenage years while the sufferer is still at home. Although I am unaware of any studies on the effectiveness of T'ai Chi as therapy for anorexia or bulimia, the underlying issues and symptomology seem to suggest that much of the treatment criteria are embodied in T'ai Chi practice.

> **CAUTION**
>
> **Ouch!** _____
>
> As always, do not attempt to self-treat any disorder, including an eating disorder. Suggest T'ai Chi and QiGong to your physician or therapist as an adjunct therapy. It may be a powerful addition to your ongoing treatment, but discuss it with your doctor.

For example, it is recommended that anorexia or bulimia sufferers strengthen their inner core of self and self-worth. The self-esteem that T'ai Chi practice builds and encourages can be a highly effective way to discover the power within one's self. The need for a restoration of biochemical and hormonal balance may be facilitated with T'ai Chi's ability to create a homeostatic effect throughout the body, not only physically, but also mentally and emotionally. T'ai Chi addresses the need to balance internal rhythms and needs with life's demands by those who practice it so they can become quietly mindful of subtle feelings and needs before they become a crisis born out in acute stress or panic.

Mood swings and depression are a part of bulimic bingeing, and feelings of lack of personal control are a part of many teenagers' anorexia or bulimia. Food, or denying ourselves food, provides us with a feeling of self-control over a world out of control. T'ai Chi's regular practice is designed to help us realize that we have a great deal of control over how we are impacted by the world. This centering enables us to feel more accepting of the fact that much of the world is beyond our control.

Preparing for Childbirth

T'ai Chi has much to offer a pregnant woman, if practiced very gently and with care. It is a slow and gentle exercise that can be performed by most pregnant women. Its gentleness and relaxed motion promote the circulation of energy and blood throughout the body, while its smooth abdominal breathing fully oxygenates the bodies of both mother and child. However, *only practice when it feels good* and *never strain yourself*. Rest whenever you need to and modify or forego any movement or exercise that doesn't feel right.

T'ai Chi breathing is a wonderful way to prepare for delivery. The famous Lamaze Technique is based on QiGong breathing techniques and pain-management tools. This aspect of T'ai Chi makes it perhaps the most effective exercise to prepare you for a safe, natural childbirth. Remember to breathe.

> **Sage Sifu Says** _____
>
> Although T'ai Chi is very gentle, some postures may be too low or somewhat strenuous for pregnant women. Do not practice these or adjust them so they are less strenuous. As your pregnancy progresses, change your T'ai Chi to make it less strenuous with each passing month. Always go slow and listen to your body. Do not do anything that doesn't feel good. Be sure your physician approves of T'ai Chi before beginning classes.

T'ai Chi for Men

Just as T'ai Chi can help women to develop their powerful dynamic side, T'ai Chi helps men develop their passive or receptive side as well, thereby helping men to become better homemakers and parents.

T'ai Chi's goal is to strike a balance between our dynamic (male/yang) side and our receptive (female/yin) side. Men and women have both qualities, and T'ai Chi helps us balance them.

T'ai Chi helps us let go of old self-concepts and prejudices, just as it teaches us to let go of tensions and fears. As our physical bodies relax and become more fluid, we become more flexible mentally and emotionally as well.

However, T'ai Chi can help you be that big strapping stud of an athlete as well. In fact, maybe it can help you keep up with the women who are advancing in every sport today.

T'ai Chi and Sports

T'ai Chi is the ultimate sports training tool because its goal is to cultivate balance, calm, and power, the basis for excelling in any physical activity. T'ai Chi can enhance any athletic performance. T'ai Chi's cultivation of awareness of the dan tien, or center of gravity, can be especially helpful for surfing, skateboarding, snow boarding, and skiing. In fact, a T'ai Chi instructor named Chris Luth conducts "T'ai Chi Skiing Workshops." However, the self-awareness, or biofeedback, element of T'ai Chi and QiGong can bring out the giant in any athlete. There are several very accomplished blind golfers. Yes, you read right, "blind" golfers. They will explain that golf (as are most sports at their core) is more of a game of "feeling" than sight. They explain that the sighted golfer is handicapped in a way because of their obsession with "outcome" rather than "process," or "feeling." T'ai Chi takes the awareness of the athlete internal to the nth degree, maximizing the power of any athlete in any sport, blind or sighted.

Weight Training

Gil Messenger, a student of Master Kuo Lien-ying, was a sports trainer as well as a T'ai Chi instructor. He often taught a form of QiGong meditation to weight trainers, who were surprised to discover that they could then lift more weight. We think when we are pumped and straining we are more powerful, but these weight lifters discovered that by allowing the body to let go, to fill with light, and to move from a calm center, they increased their physical power.

Golf

At an American QiGong Association conference in San Francisco, I had the pleasure to meet a golf coach who had worked with Tiger Woods, and in fact written a book about Tiger's incredible, almost super-human golf swing. His book theorized that the reason for Tiger's immense power was that as a young child he had practiced QiGong exercises with his dad. This introduced him to "feeling" his swing in a heightened way, and also taught him to swing from the dan tien at a very young age. You see the results, as Tiger has dominated professional golf for many years of his career. Another reason all children should be learning T'ai Chi and QiGong from kindergarten through university.

In golf, instructors encourage you to "swing with the belly button." This is another way of saying to swing with the dan tien. Many golfers discover that they can drive the ball much farther after practicing T'ai Chi for only a few months.

> **CAUTION Ouch!**
>
> The concept of swinging from the dan tien may also help reduce "golfer's back" problems. By thinking of swinging from below the navel (or dan tien) rather than from the navel, there is less twisting of the lower back.

Also, T'ai Chi's relaxed motion allows the limbs to be swung by the dan tien's motion with no muscle resistance. This in turn allows the entire force of the dan tien's turning to be projected outward through the hands and club into the ball.

Tennis and Racquetball

The same force used in golf is brought to bear in tennis and racquetball. If you play tennis or racquetball, you will also find an increased sense of control. Sometimes tennis players will describe a sense of slowing down, as if T'ai Chi practice made the game seem a bit slower than before.

Tennis players will also often discover less pressure in the knees after practicing T'ai Chi. Consciously moving from the dan tien can bring less pressure to bear on the knees when coming to an abrupt halt because when the head or upper body leads the movement, the knees must work harder to stop your momentum. T'ai Chi can also give you an off day exercise that is soothing to the joints, but still keeps the mind and body working together at a fine edge. You may be able to have fewer days on the court, while still improving your game, which may save your knees as well.

Baseball

The concept of swinging with the dan tien is exemplified in baseball's batting motion. Many batting coaches speak of "squashing the bug," which is another way of saying swing with the dan tien or body. An imaginary bug beneath the back foot is squashed as the body pulls the bat around and the back foot pivots. When performed correctly, the most powerful swings appear almost effortless. The mental calming and focus that T'ai Chi promotes can also improve the hit-to-strike ratio, as well as improving defensive reactions when fielding.

T'ai Chi's ability to improve balance is excellent for infielders, who must move on a dime and reach outward to make plays. However, pitchers are probably the greatest beneficiaries of T'ai Chi training. Just before going into a pitch, pitchers must for a moment hold their balance on one leg. This moment of balance is the most crucial point in a pitcher's windup and can determine both force and accuracy. Therefore, the amazing balance improvement T'ai Chi provides can be the most powerful weapon in a pitcher's arsenal.

The "Hard" Martial Arts

In the 1970s, the world was surprised to see a 19-year-old Canadian win the World Karate Championship. His secret was T'ai Chi. The centering, balance, looseness, and focus T'ai Chi promotes will greatly enhance the power and speed of any boxer or martial artist. More than any other exercise, T'ai Chi promotes increased reaction speed because it is therapy for not just external muscular performance, but for the mental and neural processes as well.

T'ai Chi as Therapy

The following subsections provide an introduction to how and why T'ai Chi and/or QiGong may be an effective therapy for your condition. If you or your doctor are interested in more in-depth explanations, refer to the end of this chapter for an alphabetical listing of maladies found to benefit from T'ai Chi or QiGong therapy. Master Ken Cohen's book, *The Way of QiGong: The Art and Science of Chinese Energy Healing*, may be very helpful as well (see Appendix B, "Suggested Readings"). Also the QiGong Institute's QiGong Computerized Database is a great resource, and www.smartaichi.com's resource library is as well.

Cancer Treatment

In Chinese hospitals, T'ai Chi and QiGong are often used in conjunction with chemo- or radiation therapies. QiGong and T'ai Chi therapies can lessen the side effects of radiation treatments, but T'ai Chi has many other benefits to offer. For example, a sense of hopelessness or helplessness can diminish the effectiveness of standard treatments. T'ai Chi, however, engages the patients in the healing process, giving them a sense of empowerment.

In China, QiGong may be a primary therapy for advanced, inoperable, and medically untreatable cancer. It can slow the progression of the disease, while maintaining appetite and helping with pain management. Beyond that, the emotional and mental clarifying aspects of T'ai Chi and QiGong can also help a patient prepare for their life transition in a more meaningful and spiritual way. By helping them to become more at peace in their lives, they may find the transition to death a less fearful event, thereby enabling them to make the most of their remaining days.

> **Sage Sifu Says**
>
> When you release a deep breath, think of the muscles letting go of the bones. On the next exhale, think of the brain, the mind, and the cranial muscles letting go of thoughts and worries. On the next release of breath, think of letting the heart and the muscles around it relax. Each release of breath becomes a deep cleansing and letting go on many different levels: physical, emotional, mental, and other levels we're not conscious of.

Cardiac Rehab and Prevention

Many cardiologists are prescribing T'ai Chi as an adjunct therapy for treatment of heart problems or as preventative therapy. T'ai Chi provides a gentle exercise that promotes circulation, but its meditative quality may offer even more benefits. T'ai Chi's stress-reduction qualities foster a feeling of self-acceptance and safety in the world, allowing practitioners to let go of the control issues that can make life seem like an endless state of panic.

Again, T'ai Chi gives us a daily dosage of homeostatic feelings of well-being. As we become familiar with this feeling of optimum health, we get more attuned with what foods, drinks, or activities promote or detract from that wonderful feeling. This biofeedback feature can be instrumental in helping people make lifestyle changes that may extend their lives by many years.

Stroke Recovery

Doctors now often recommend T'ai Chi for stroke recovery because T'ai Chi's soothing demands of left brain/right brain interaction and mind/body interaction can epitomize a physical therapy for stroke victims. T'ai Chi challenges patients to coordinate movement, but at the same time helps them feel at ease in the face of the frustration this challenge might cause. If balance is a severe problem, a spouse or friend can spot you to help maintain balance.

> **Ouch!**
>
> If you have a balance disorder and wish to use a climbing harness to prevent falls, discuss the exact purpose of the harness with a climbing expert. This will enable them to ensure the harness you use is appropriate to keep you from falling. This security will help you relax more, thereby allowing you to get more benefit from T'ai Chi. Ask the expert about the full-body harness, often used in caving as well as climbing.

In Kansas City, we are pioneering a new approach to T'ai Chi for stroke victims with balance problems. By securing a mountain climbing harness to the ceiling by a hook, a patient may perform T'ai Chi without fear of falling. One of the main balance benefits all T'ai Chi practitioners get comes from constantly testing the limits of their balance. As one drifts in and out of balance, the mind and body exchange data that effortlessly improves the balance, which often continues to improve for life. The figure below shows the harness approach. Note that the harness below is only illustrative and not sufficient to prevent falls; *a full-body harness, including a shoulder harness that secures in front of the upper chest, is required to prevent falling.*

Hospitals all over the world eventually will provide rooms filled with hooks for climbing harnesses so that stroke rehab or other balance-challenged patients can come and practice T'ai Chi without fear of falling. These same patients may wish to have harnesses installed in their homes by a qualified contractor. Contact your hospital and show them this section. Physical therapists can consult with mountain climbing supply stores to find the optimum full-body harnesses.

Do not use this harness to prevent falls.

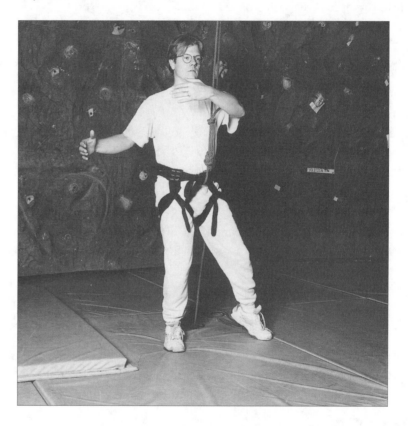

Addictions

T'ai Chi, as well as acupuncture, is being successfully used to help people break addictive patterns. A research program working with heroin addicts revealed that withdrawal symptoms decreased much more rapidly than non-QiGong control groups did. Furthermore, breaking an addiction, whether it's to cigarettes or heroin, is a very stressful endeavor. The body and mind crave and yearn constantly. This study also showed that the QiGong group had much lower anxiety and were able to find restful sleep five times faster than non-QiGong practicing addicts in recovery. The reason QiGong is so powerful lies in the essence of what an addict, or any of us stuck in unhealthy behaviors, craves.

What is it that they crave? Ultimately it is life energy. When a smoker gets a cigarette or an addict gets their fix, the first thing they do is sit back, enjoy the moment, and relax into the pleasure of their cigarette or fix. This moment of relaxed focused awareness opens their mind and body to an increased flow of Qi or energy. This is why a raging drunk can have so much energy, even when filled with alcohol. The problem is the cigarettes or drugs are destroying your body to open up to Qi, and when the drug wears off, the body clamps down, squeezing off the flow even more. So learning to open to Qi in a healthy, expansive way is one means for healing an addiction.

Note the pattern of addiction:

1. A prospective user is looking for access to Qi, or life energy, whether they realize it or not. When Qi is flowing through us we feel good, at peace, and capable.

2. When cigarettes, drugs, or alcohol are first used, the ritual of using them and/or the chemical they put in the body causes the user to relax and open to Qi flow. But this is a false and unhealthy way to open to it.

3. Since this is an artificial way to open up to the flow of Qi, the mind and body do not learn how to keep the flow open.

4. In fact, when the drug, whether it's nicotine or heroin, is gone, the body and mind tighten up even more than before. The chemicals and their reactions in the body are unhealthy and cause the mind and body to get tighter, squeezing off more Qi than ever before.

5. The user is then required to use more of the drug or to use it more and more often because now it takes a more forceful dose to open the mind's and body's gates to allow the Qi to flow through.

6. Eventually, the user's dosages, no matter how large, do not open the user to increased Qi flow or a feeling of "highness." Eventually even the largest dosages give the user only a lower-than-normal flow of Qi.

7. People who are heavily hooked on cigarettes or alcohol, and even more so with harder drugs, have a look of lacking life. They are becoming void of Qi. Their mind and body have become tight.

T'ai Chi and QiGong provide us with a healthy pattern of access to life energy, or Qi. This is what we all want. When we hug a loved one, we feel their Qi mingling with ours. When we pet our dog or cat, they revel in feeling our loving intention in our Qi flowing from our hand to their body. T'ai Chi and QiGong are tools to fill us with life, and they can be very effective tools for helping addicts find their way out of the maze they have stumbled into, finding a way back to being truly alive.

> **Sage Sifu Says**
>
> The more we can tap into ways to fill our bodies with life energy using tools like T'ai Chi, the less we will have to look outside ourselves for satisfaction. Our consumption level drops as our needs diminish. Therefore, T'ai Chi can also help the environment because less consumption means less trash.

The best drug program is preventative. T'ai Chi and QiGong will eventually be taught in schools worldwide. By teaching the mind/body awareness and powerful stress management tools these health sciences offer, many future drug, alcohol, or other addicts will avoid the desire for mood altering drugs or addictive behaviors or substances. Educating every student from kindergarten through university in mind/body internal awareness and health development techniques like T'ai Chi and QiGong, as a matter of standard education, makes perfect sense.

The Therapeutic Powers of T'ai Chi and QiGong

Although T'ai Chi and QiGong can play a positive role in many existing conditions, each condition is different, and you must discuss T'ai Chi as an adjunct therapy with your physician.

The following list contains some conditions T'ai Chi and/or QiGong may help. Realize that some of the research mentioned is sourced from research being done worldwide, with varying qualities of scientific method, and sometimes involving QiGong medical treatment by professional QiGong doctors or therapists using "emitted Qi." I refer you to the section on External QiGong in Chapter 10, "Introducing QiGong," to give you some idea of what emitted Qi is, but not necessarily fully reflecting the treatment used in the study. This section is meant to encourage a more expansive dialogue of treatment options between you and your physician and never meant to replace your standard care.

Many of the following listings are based on information provided by the QiGong Institute's Computerized QiGong Database, which contains 1,600 research abstracts. You, your teacher, your doctor, or anyone else can obtain this excellent research tool, at www.qigonginstitute.org. This QiGong Database is a must for every health professional/health reporter in the world today. Other research came from www.taichismart. com's resource library. You can visit the taichismart.com library to obtain article references for some of the T'ai Chi research referred to in the following list, and to keep abreast of new research on T'ai Chi and QiGong as it emerges from research centers worldwide.

- **ADD and ADHD.** Research at the University of Miami School of Medicine has shown that adolescents with ADHD (Attention Deficit and Hyperactivity Disorder) displayed less anxiety, daydreaming behaviors, inappropriate emotions and hyperactivity, and greater improved conduct, after a five week, two day per week class. T'ai Chi meets many of the criteria for mood management techniques recommended for ADD (see the "Treating Attention Deficit Disorder [ADD]" section earlier in this chapter).

- **Aging, slowing the aging process.** Research at Baylor Medical School has found that some cells from the bodies of long-term QiGong practitioners live *five times longer* than the same cells from ordinary test subjects.

  Other research from The Shanghai Institute of Hypertension looked at several aspects of aging. They determined that QiGong is an effective measure in preventing and treating geriatric diseases and delaying the aging process.

- **AIDS.** Studies indicate regular T'ai Chi practice may boost one's T-cell count, while improving outlook, and providing a soothing gentle exercise. The relaxed forms effectively oxygenate the body while moving blood and lymph throughout.

- **Allergies and asthma.** The stress-reduction benefits of T'ai Chi and QiGong help the body maintain elevated DHEA levels. Low DHEA levels have been directly linked to allergies. High stress levels are linked to the frequency and intensity of asthmatic reactions as well.

- **Angina.** Biofeedback aspects of T'ai Chi and QiGong can help students learn to regulate blood flow, by awareness of warmth in hands and feet. Evidence suggests this skill may alleviate some forms of angina.

- **Anorexia/bulimia.** See the "T'ai Chi for Women" section earlier in this chapter.

- **Anxiety, chronic.** The relaxed abdominal breathing that T'ai Chi and QiGong promote can be a beneficial adjunct to therapy.

- **Arthritis.** T'ai Chi's low impact causes no joint damage (unlike other higher impact exercises), while its weight-bearing aspect may encourage development of bone mass and connective tissue. Note: Those with arthritic knees may want to do modified T'ai Chi forms sharing weight on both legs rather than fully centering the weight over one knee.

- **Back pain.** *Prevention Magazine* reported a study where, after one year of T'ai Chi classes, a group of men and women ages 58 to 70 found increased strength and increased flexibility in their back, helping to reduce the odds of back pain.

- **Balance disorders.** T'ai Chi practitioners fall only half as much as those practicing other balance training, as reported by an Emory University study, and others.

- **Baldness, premature.** QiGong and T'ai Chi promote stress management and blood circulation. Some QiGong exercises, such as Carry the Moon, specifically promote circulation in the scalp.

- **Behcet's Disease.** Behcet's Disease is a kind of chronic recurrent disease. Neijing Central Hospital of Management claim to have cured five patients of Behcet's Disease. They believe this was due to QiGong's ability to build up immunological function and increase blood flow volume and by promoting saliva flow and increased oxygen intake.

- **Brittle bones/bone loss in women.** Research from the National Institute of Mental Health reports that the stress hormones found in depressed women caused bone loss that gave them bones of women nearly twice their age. T'ai Chi and QiGong are known to reduce depression and anxiety and provide weight-bearing exercises to encourage building bone mass and connective tissue.

- **Bronchitis/emphysema, chronic.** Sitting QiGong and/or T'ai Chi may show positive results over time in appetite, sleep, and energy levels, but also rather dramatically and healthfully in decreasing breaths per minute.

- **Burns, healing of.** Researchers at the Navy General Hospital of Beijing China studied emitted Qi on burnt rats. They noted that the QiGong treatment in some ways expedited the healing ability of burnt rats.

- **Cancer.** Several clinical studies reported that a combination therapy of drugs with personal practice of QiGong provided a better outcome than drug therapy alone.

- **Carcinoma.** The Guangzhou College of Traditional Chinese Medicine, Guangzhou, China, researched the effects of emitted Qi on carcinoma. They reported, "The emitted Qi may promote normal function of human immune cells while killing the tumor cells suggesting that QiGong is a feasible means to the treatment of carcinoma."

- **Cardiovascular benefit.** Research has shown that the extremely gentle low impact T'ai Chi exercise can provide the same cardiovascular benefit as moderate impact aerobic exercise. The Harvard Women's Health Watch reported, "studies support T'ai Chi [use] for heart-attack and cardiac-bypass patients, to improve cardiorespiratory function and reduce blood pressure."

- **Chronic Fatigue Syndrome (CFS).** Research in the *British Medical Journal* (February 2001) showed 84 percent of CFS patients adding exercise to their CFS standard care got "very much" or "much" better, as opposed to only 12 percent of patients receiving only standard care. CFS's chronic pain limitation may make T'ai Chi and QiGong's gentle motions and deep breathing (with its pain management benefits) an optimum exercise for CFS sufferers.

- **Chronic Fatigue and Immune Dysfunction Syndrome (CFIDS).** The Chronic Fatigue and Immune Dysfunction publication the *CFIDS Chronicle* (Summer 1999 Edition) had comments from a CFIDS sufferer on success using T'ai Chi as therapy. (You can contact CFIDS Association of America at 1-800-442-3437 or by visiting www.cfids.org online.)

- **Chronic pain.** Students often find anything between mild pain relief and complete alleviation of chronic pain by using T'ai Chi and/or QiGong, in some cases finding complete relief from long-term chronic pain conditions.

- **Circulation and nervous system disorders.** T'ai Chi promotes circulation and can have a very integrating effect on the mind and body.

- **Compulsive, obsessive disorders.** T'ai Chi and QiGong's mindful awareness of self and constant reassurance that we can breathe through and relax into any situation may be a helpful adjunct to therapy for OCD, which gently exposes patients to their fears. Again, introduce T'ai Chi and QiGong only with your therapist's approval.

- **Concentration/QiGong uses in education.** Although researchers in this study in Xinjiang China admit limitations in their research, they find encouraging signs that QiGong exercises could greatly enhance the educational experience for primary school children and beyond.

- **Coronary disease.** Ganshu College of TCM (Traditional Chinese Medicine) in China claimed to have found strong evidence that QiGong exercises may help with coronary disease.

- **Depression and mood disturbance.** Regular (daily) T'ai Chi practitioners usually find less incidence of depression and overall mood disturbance.

- **Diabetes.** T'ai Chi's stress management and increased circulation qualities make it ideal for diabetes. A Beijing University of Chinese Medicine and Pharmacology study found that blood sugar could be lowered successfully by doing QiGong exercises. 42.9 percent of patients in the study were able to take less medicine while having more staple foods.

- **Digestion, improving.** T'ai Chi's gentle massage of internal organs and stimulation of blood circulation and Qi promote healthy digestion.

- **Drug uptake.** The QiGong Institute reviewed voluminous studies done worldwide and concluded that QiGong and drug therapies are superior to drug therapy alone. The reason for this is believed to be found in QiGong's ability to enhance Qi and blood circulation to that area so that nutrients may more efficiently be delivered to the affected cells, and also waste products in the stressed tissue can be removed more readily.

- **Fibromyalgia.** Fibromyalgia is a modern epidemic, a chronic pain condition affecting 6 to 8 percent of the U.S. population. T'ai Chi has been recommended by some health professionals as a very desirable adjunct therapy for sufferers.

- **Flexibility enhancement.** Harvard Women's Health Watch reported an Emory University study showing that T'ai Chi may possibly improve elasticity in ligaments and tendons, create stronger knee flexors and extensors, and create better posture.

- **Gall stones.** The Navy General Hospital, Beijing China, did a study using emitted Qi to find if a particular emitted Qi therapy could help people pass gall stones. They found a positive treatment rate of 93.33 percent.

- **Gastritis.** Chronic atrophic gastritis (CAG) is a common yet difficult illness, according to researchers at the Institute for Industry Health in Xian China. Studying the effect of a combination of QiGong exercise with Tuina (Chinese therapeutic massage), they found that 97.1 percent of patients found some benefit.

- **Gastrointestinal malignant tumors.** The Department of Chinese Medicine, Second Affiliate Hospital with Jiangxi Medical College found that a group of patients using QiGong exercises with their standard chemotherapy, radiotherapy and Chinese medicine, had a significantly higher survival rate than those only getting standard medical therapy with no QiGong exercises.

- **Geriatric fitness.** *Prevention Magazine* reported that "T'ai Chi may be the best exercise for people over the age of 60 … providing cardio fitness, muscle strength, and flexibility all in one simple workout that is easy on the joints." Also, other studies show that T'ai Chi is by far the best balance conditioner. Research finding that T'ai Chi may also lessen tissue brittleness even further adds to the case that T'ai Chi is the best possible exercise for seniors.

- **Heart disease.** At the Institute of Psychology, Academia Sinica, a research study found that T'ai Chi and QiGong practice can positively affect the states of mind of subjects to lessen the incidence of Type-A behavior patterns, believed to increase the risk of heart disease.

- **Hemorrhoids.** Some QiGong breathing involves the sphincter muscles, which may directly alleviate hemorrhoid symptoms. T'ai Chi's ability to reduce constipation lessens the aggravation of hemorrhoid symptoms.

- **High blood pressure.** T'ai Chi can significantly lower high blood pressure in many cases.

- **Infections.** Regular T'ai Chi practice is believed to increase the T-cell count. T-cells are thought to consume viruses, bacteria, and even tumor cells.

- **Insomnia.** Students often remark of improved sleep and reduced insomnia after a few weeks of regular T'ai Chi and QiGong practice.

- **Leukemia.** The Immunology Research Center, Beijing, China, studied the effects of externally emitted Qi, to see how it affects Leukemia cells in mice. They found the mice treated with Qi emission had reduced numbers of L1210 cells (malignant tumor cells). However, researchers cautioned that the mechanism and the way emitted Qi does this needs to be further investigated.

◆ **Liver disease, hepatitis-B, and the like.** At Lixin County Hospital of TCM in Anhui province, China, they found that ten kinds of liver diseases, especially B Type Hepatitis, could be cured with the combination of drugs and QiGong.

◆ **Lou Gehrig's disease.** T'ai Chi is recommended by many support groups of neuromuscular diseases. Check with your doctor to discuss introducing T'ai Chi as an adjunct to your therapy.

◆ **Low blood pressure.** At Lixin County Hospital of TCM (Traditional Chinese Medicine) researchers believed QiGong combined with standard drug therapy to be good for low blood pressure.

◆ **Menopausal therapy.** The QiGong Institute reviewed voluminous studies done worldwide and concluded that QiGong and drug therapy is superior to drug therapy alone, including in the case of menopausal treatments. This mechanism of enhanced drug delivery suggests that QiGong could make possible smaller doses of drugs, which would cause less adverse side effects. For example, QiGong is reported to restore estradiol levels in hypertensive, menopausal women, leading to the possibility that estrogen replacement therapy might not be necessary or might be used at reduced levels.

◆ **Menstrual disorders.** Researchers at PLA General Hospital in Beijing, China, used acupressure, massage, and emitted Qi to treat 76 cases of various gynepathic diseases. The results were that 52 (68.42 percent) cases were nearly cured, 14 (18.42 percent) markedly effective, and 10 (13.16 percent) cases found the treatment to be effective.

◆ **Mental health.** The Institute of Psychology, Chinese Academy of Sciences, Beijing, China, conducted studies to see how QiGong practice would affect mental health. The result was that a group that had practiced QiGong for over two years had a curative rate on symptoms of psychosomatic disorders about *twice* as high as a QiGong group practicing less than two years.

◆ **Migraine.** Biofeedback aspects of T'ai Chi and QiGong can help students learn to regulate blood flow by increasing awareness of warmth in hands and feet. Evidence suggests this skill may alleviate some forms of migraines.

◆ **Multiple sclerosis.** MS support groups recommend T'ai Chi.

◆ **Muscle wasting** (and other tissue deterioration). Studies indicate that T'ai Chi may be an ideal exercise to help older people suffering muscle wasting.

◆ **Neurotransmitters** and QiGong's effect on them and how that impacts health. Researchers at Anhui College of TCM asserted that their research indicates that neurotransmitters are affected by QiGong practice in such a way to help regulate the function of the neuralgic system in such a way to prevent and help cure diseases.

◆ **Ovarian cyst.** Researchers at PLA General Hospital, Beijing, China, found a high success rate using a combination of acupressure, massage, and emitted Qi in curing or positively affecting the majority of cases of various gynepathic diseases, including ovarian cyst.

◆ **Paralysis.** Researchers at the PLA General Hospital of Beijing studied the effect of emitted Qi combined with QiGong exercises in treating paralysis. The effect of the treatment judged by the indexes of rehabilitation commonly used, was "excellent" in 23.25 percent of cases, "good" in 46.5 percent, "fine" in 23.25 percent, and "bad" in 6.99 percent of cases, with an overall effective rate of 93.01 percent.

◆ **Parkinson's disease/improving motor-skill control.** Parkinson's support groups recommend T'ai Chi, and many students claim significant reduction in tremors.

◆ **Posture problems.** T'ai Chi's gentle mindful awareness of postural adjustment make it a wonderful therapy for posture problems and for alleviating the pain or chronic tension associated with them.

◆ **Psychotherapy.** A German researcher points out that QiGong is gradually gaining prominence as a therapeutic tool in Germany, and pointed to positive effects of QiGong exercises for those dealing with neurosis, depression, anxiety, psychosomatic disorder, and psychosis. They caution that a wrong practice of the exercises, as pertains to specially sick people, can have bad effects and these subjects require competent guidance and assistance.

- **Respiratory diseases, chronic.** A collaborative study with the Research Institute of TCM, Tainjin College of TCM, and Tianjin Thorax Surgery Hospital was done on patients suffering from chronic bronchitis, asthma, pulmonary emphysema, and cor pulmonale. A group treated with QiGong exercise *and* drugs fared better than the one treated only with drugs.

- **Rheumatism.** *OT Week* magazine reported, "Areas where T'ai Chi has proven effective include rheumatism; weight management; treatment of back problems; management of high blood pressure; and stress reduction … and may speed recovery in postoperative patients …."

- **Sexual performance.** T'ai Chi's stress reduction and promotion of circulation can make it a very healthful way to improve sexual performance.

- **Stomach carcinoma.** The General Navy Hospital in Beijing studied the effects of emitted Qi on NK cells, which they believe play a role in cancer. They found a statistically remarkable effect of emitted Qi killing both adenocarcinoma cells of the stomach and the NK cells.

- **Strength enhancement.** After one year of T'ai Chi classes a group of men and women ages 58 to 70 found increased strength.

- **Tears, cleansing mechanisms and QiGong.** *Psychology Today* reported that the Tear Research Center has discovered crying may cleanse chemicals from the body that build up during emotional stress, including ACTH, a hormone that is considered the body's most reliable indicator of stress. Sitting QiGong's progressive relaxation therapy often leaves practitioners wiping away tears, perhaps explaining why we feel clearer and lighter after practice.

- **Thrombosis.** Department of Pathology, Weifang Medical College in Shandong, China, researchers claimed their research indicates "QiGong exercise could reduce thrombosis, RBC aggregability and blood viscosity, and could prevent and treat cardiovascular and cerebrovascular diseases."

- **Ulcers.** QiGong relaxation therapy coupled with reductions in external stress factors have shown substantial success, even with long term ulcer problems.

- **Weight loss.** *OT Week* magazine reports that T'ai Chi has been proven effective with weight loss. T'ai Chi promotes healthy weight loss in many ways. It burns calories, but also helps reduce stress levels. This stress reduction helps reduce nervous snacking. Furthermore, T'ai Chi's slow quiet mindfulness also helps us to get in touch with our *homeostatic* or healthful potential, and what that feels like. This steers us away from foods or activities that do not promote health and toward those that do.

> **Know Your Chinese**
>
> Modern psychologists refer to a state of mental and emotional well-being as **homeostasis** or a homeostatic state. T'ai Chi promotes this by smoothing our Qi, the life blood of our mental, emotional and physical being. T'ai Chi is the epitome of a homeostatic exercise.

The Least You Need to Know

- T'ai Chi helps kids with physical development and focus.
- Teach kids faster T'ai Chi and spice it up with harder exercises.
- T'ai Chi is perfect for kids, seniors, women, men, and athletes for many different reasons.
- If your physician or therapist is unfamiliar with T'ai Chi and QiGong, show them this book.
- No matter what ailment you have, T'ai Chi and/or QiGong can probably help.

Chapter 21

"Tie"-Chi: Corporate T'ai Chi

In This Chapter

- ◆ The benefits of starting a T'ai Chi program at work
- ◆ Why T'ai Chi's a natural for the office
- ◆ What T'ai Chi can accomplish at the workplace
- ◆ Ways to incorporate T'ai Chi into your office or workplace

Corporations all over America are integrating the powerful health and personal growth tools of T'ai Chi into the fabric of the workplace. Why? Because T'ai Chi can save companies big money, is very applicable to the office, can lessen workplace injury, reduce stress, and boost performance.

This chapter details how T'ai Chi accomplishes these goals, so you can speak with authority to your company's Wellness Director about it. Many companies will pay for a T'ai Chi program, making it well worth your time to suggest it to the Wellness Director.

A growing selection of T'ai Chi programs are now being offered in many cities by T'ai Chi, stress management, or wellness program consulting companies. To get more information on organizations or companies that offer them, check the World Wide Web or Yellow Pages under the previously mentioned headings. Also, contact information is provided in Appendix A, "The T'ai Chi and QiGong Yellow Pages," for Stress Management and Relaxation Technology (SMART), which offers such programs.

The Bottom Line on Stress Costs to Business

You can help your company understand how sponsoring T'ai Chi classes is in their best interest as well as yours. One of corporate America's highest unnecessary production costs is in lost productivity *due to employee stress*. U.S. businesses are losing $300 billion per year due to stress (that's over $7,500 per employee, per year), which may be why the Occupational Safety and Hazard Administration (OSHA) has declared stress a workplace hazard.

Using T'ai Chi as Stress and Pain Relief

Companies and corporations are increasingly turning to T'ai Chi as a solution to stress. Companies that have offered T'ai Chi to either their employees, clients, or executive staffs include Sprint, Hallmark, Inc., Black and Veatch Corp., Associated Wholesale Grocers, BMA (Financial), and Columbia Hospitals, to name a few.

Penthouse T'ai Chi at BMA's Headquarters has been a popular wellness program. Approximately 100 employees attended the introductory Stress Management workshop.

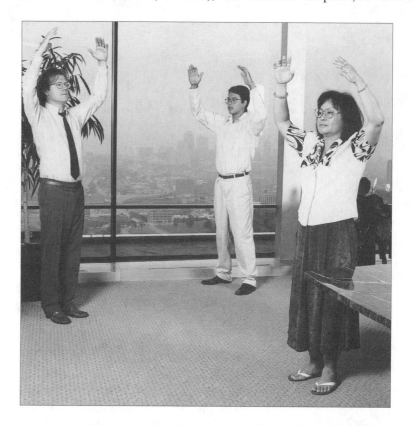

A community college near Kansas City provides T'ai Chi classes as a wellness program to their staff, and many participants are finding alleviation of chronic pain conditions, less stress, and fewer sick days. T'ai Chi is rapidly becoming the most popular wellness program for many companies. Isn't it great that companies are realizing that what is good for the employee is good for the company's profits as well?

Sage Sifu Says

Albert Einstein said, "Imagination is more important than knowledge." When T'ai Chi and QiGong help us let go of physical, emotional, and mental tension, it literally expands our "imagination muscle." As we let go of old patterns, we open up to new and exciting concepts that our old, tense bodies and minds couldn't comprehend. We learn more easily and are more creative in using what we learn.

Investing in Creative Potential

If T'ai Chi can help employees recover from illnesses and thereby reduce absenteeism, that can also mean major savings. But what about creativity? T'ai Chi's meditative quality enables practitioners to become more creative as they let go of being locked into old patterns. A popular corporate expression is to "think outside the box," which means to look beyond the established way of doing things, to try to find new and innovative approaches, capitalizing on constantly changing tools and technology. It's a useful concept, but how do you really think outside the box? You have to release the old ways of doing things. Again, T'ai Chi is about letting go of everything, mentally, emotionally, and physically which requires releasing prejudices and preconceptions, making you clearer and more open to new possibilities and potential. If T'ai Chi can help employees think outside the box, this will open them up to fresh innovative approaches and may boost profits more than anything you could begin to measure.

Helping with Lower Back Problems and Carpal Tunnel

Lower back problems are a large part of costly, unscheduled absenteeism. T'ai Chi is very effective at helping with chronic lower back pain, as well as other chronic pain problems.

Since T'ai Chi is the very best balance training in the world, causing participants to be half as likely to suffer falling injuries as others, T'ai Chi can reduce workplace injuries dramatically. Tell your company's Safety Director to look into the Emory University T'ai Chi study on balance. It will get his or her attention.

Some T'ai Chi exercises are very similar to exercises designed to prevent Repetitive Stress Injury, such as Carpal Tunnel Syndrome. Therefore, you may be hitting several birds with your well-thrown T'ai Chi stone.

T'ai Chi's a Natural for the Office

One thing that makes T'ai Chi uniquely ideal for the workplace is that it requires no special clothing or equipment. If you have 15 minutes and a quiet room, you are all set to experience some amazing stress reduction and energy boosting.

Since T'ai Chi is so slow and gentle, you often need not work up a sweat when taking a T'ai Chi break. By simply loosening your tie or kicking off your heels, you are all set. In fact, Sitting QiGong or simple Moving QiGong can be done right at your desk. As employees become more adept at these tools of breath and relaxation, they'll use them throughout the day to reduce stress and boost performance.

 Ouch!

Even though QiGong can be done at your desk, it is also good to take breaks away from the workstation, in a quiet board room or the rest room, where you can do T'ai Chi in relative silence. Then when you return to your workstation, the QiGong will be even more effective, as if you brought some of the silence with you.

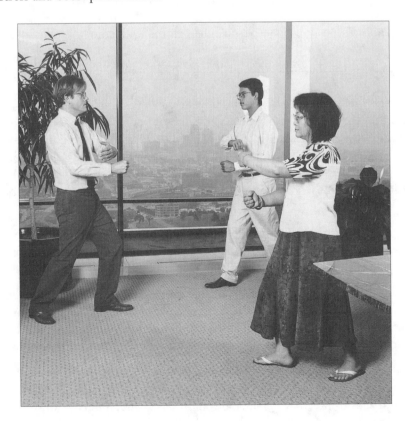

Notice that by simply kicking off your heels and loosening your tie, you are "suited" up for a T'ai Chi break.

What your co-workers and you will soon discover is that the more loose and flexible you are physically, the more flexible you will become in your social and business interactions.

We literally hold onto prejudices, grudges, and resistance to change in our body's tight muscles. We cannot open our minds if we don't allow our bodies to loosen up. T'ai Chi's promotion of deep loosening and relaxed motion promotes a letting go of the control issues we all have. It can facilitate a looser, yet more productive work environment as communication becomes easier between employees who less and less resemble walking, emotional land mines.

T'ai Chi diffuses the stress bombs that build up within us and can make the workplace not only less dangerous, *but more fun*. We can discover the "real person" in our co-workers as their rigid armor begins to fall away. Part of that "realness" is the fun part of ourselves we were in touch with as kids. A rigid workplace environment can hide that fun, more vulnerable part of us. Therefore, T'ai Chi may not only help us enjoy our work more, but the company of our co-workers as well. Again, the Chinese say T'ai Chi helps return us to that magical youthful state of mind, which is not childish but *childlike*.

Office Politics and the "Great Corporate Cosmos"

Most companies are painfully aware that the machinations of office politics are a severe drain on productivity. On a personal level, most of us are all too familiar with the energy drain that office politics can cause.

A T'ai Chi Punch Line

I worked as a human resources administrator for several years and came to realize that most employee problems are stress related. The more stress management tools like T'ai Chi HR departments can provide employees, the quieter things will be on the front lines of the HR office. Some employees have commented that when disagreements arise, whether they are between employees or between employees and management, T'ai Chi's calming influence made a constructive exchange of differing opinions possible.

The intra-office political maneuvering we often call office politics, which involves employees wasting time trying to alter office opinion of others through gossip or innuendo, is mostly rooted in fear and control issues. The more relaxed and at ease we are with ourselves, the more at ease we will be with co-workers, rather than reading our fear into office relationships. Again, T'ai Chi exercises not only help cleanse our mind and heart of rootless fears, but can help us let go of control issues. T'ai Chi's exercises, when done correctly, help us let go of attachment to outcome or destination, and just learn to flow through more effortless changes.

T'ai Chi helps us to break from unhealthy patterns of internal fear or stress responses, and this can resonate out to the office relationships, helping us and our co-workers be both calmer and more productive. Just as tension begets tension, calm can help beget calm in those around us.

Imagine if employees used their lunchtime not to gossip and politic themselves into a tension frenzy, but to take a break from it all. If you have an hour lunch, do T'ai Chi for half an hour before lunch or, if you have only half an hour, take 15 minutes. This will help your mind and body disconnect from whatever problems you may face at work, and could make the company and the world a vastly different place.

On the other hand, if you truly do not like your job, the quiet mindfulness that T'ai Chi offers can help you come to terms with it. Its focusing aspect may help you decide what you want, how to get it, and how to be calm and poised enough to perform a great interview for the job you do want. Then someone who really does want your job can come along and fill it, and the great flowing energy of the corporate cosmos can do its thing.

T'ai Chi, Inc.—Incorporating T'ai Chi into Your Workplace

T'ai Chi encourages us to let go of old ways and patterns while opening us to new, better ways of doing things. As discussed earlier, T'ai Chi can help us think outside the box, to be open to fresh, innovative approaches. This is how T'ai Chi is being introduced to the workplace. Companies are doing it in their own way, and finding out how to use T'ai Chi's tools to fit their needs. Below are several sections on the nuts and bolts of making T'ai Chi part of your company's wellness program. If you are not the Wellness Director, bring this section to him or her.

Considering Costs

Costs can vary widely. If you are a Wellness Director, the important thing to remember is that cheaper is not better. If you get a cut rate T'ai Chi program that few employees take advantage of, then you are not really saving your company any money. If absenteeism or disciplinary problems decline or pro-ductivity increases after the introduction of a T'ai Chi class at your company, then your company will profit in the long run. It is therefore in your best interest to find a good T'ai Chi instructor, one who is knowledgeable, approachable, and fun, and who can connect daily work stresses to her T'ai Chi instruction approach.

A T'ai Chi Punch Line

Many health insurance compa-nies are now subsidizing or covering the cost of T'ai Chi and/or QiGong classes. Contact your carrier to find out if they do or ask them to if they do not.

Investing in T'ai Chi Programs

There are several ways companies can invest in T'ai Chi. Some companies passively promote T'ai Chi, offer-ing a space for employees to practice during lunch or after work. Others do much more.

The best T'ai Chi and Stress Management seminars are optional. Provide employees with the option of working or attending the seminar, but do not make the seminar mandatory. Most people will opt for the seminar to get a break from work anyway, but the quality of the seminar is completely different if the employee has chosen to be there. This is the first step in an employee creating his own healthy lifestyle. If it's someone else's idea, we resist, but if we feel empowered to change ourselves, we have a vested interest in a positive outcome.

For example, company investment in a full stress management consulting program maximizes the benefits T'ai Chi offers. This usually involves a two-day program of about three hours per day, whereby the presenter gives an in-depth introduction to T'ai Chi and QiGong to prepare employees and the HR or Wellness Department to carry weekly classes.

This can lead to daily morning or afternoon T'ai Chi breaks, provided in a vacant boardroom, for example. Some companies may reward T'ai Chi practitioners with a 30-minute morning break, if instead of drinking coffee and sodas for 15 minutes, they use the 30-minute break to attend morning T'ai Chi classes in the area provided. This could be done in conjunction with a weekly one-hour video or live T'ai Chi class during lunch or after work.

For the daily T'ai Chi breaks, sign-in sheets could be used to document employee participation. This information may be helpful to acquire rebates or subsidies from company health insurance providers to cover the cost of T'ai Chi classes. Ask your carrier.

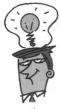

A T'ai Chi Punch Line

British dominance of the seas in the 1700s can, in part, be linked to the simple discovery that citrus fruits cure scurvy. Feeding British sailors limes, therefore, made it possible for British ships to stay at sea for much longer missions than enemy ships. Today's captains of industry who realize that stress is the greatest threat to *their* crews and who give their people tools like T'ai Chi to avoid illness and burnout will dominate in business.

Also, it is good to collect testimonials from employees from time to time, as these usually list a myriad of health benefits each person gets from T'ai Chi, which also could be passed on to health insurance providers.

Other ways to offer company classes:

◆ Company invests in T'ai Chi classes by local instructors

◆ Company splits cost of classes in varying ratios with employees

◆ Company provides space and contacts instructor, but leaves payment up to employees

◆ Company cosponsors one-time introductory seminar with instructor and then allows instructor to recruit for community classes off-site from company

◆ On-site company classes are usually held before work, during lunch, or immediately after work. Companies are wise to consider offering employees who participate a half-hour of paid time to participate in class.

For example, if employees attend a morning class, have half of the class start before work and half during paid work time. The potential savings in employee health, productivity, and attitude will more than make up for the minimal investment of the half hour of pay. Companies can thereby take the lead in encouraging employees to take up healthful habits that in turn promote decreased absenteeism, increased productivity, and diminished disciplinary problems.

The Least You Need to Know

◆ "Tie"-Chi can save companies big money.

◆ T'ai Chi can be done in work clothes in an office.

◆ T'ai Chi can help employees get along.

◆ Show this book to your Wellness Director, and you might get free classes at work.

◆ Companies can increase productivity by offering T'ai Chi classes to their employees.

T'ai Chi's Philosophy of Balance and Flow

In This Chapter

◆ A T'ai Chi diet plan

◆ Discover herbs and teas as medicine

◆ Increase health and prosperity by using Feng Shui

◆ Learn about yourself with the *I Ching*

◆ Use T'ai Chi to really enjoy life

T'ai Chi is not an end in itself. T'ai Chi is a passageway to a healthier lifestyle. Dietary changes, the inclusion of regular massage therapy, acupuncture tune ups, and the power of positive thinking can all catapult you forward into even greater rewards that T'ai Chi offers. This chapter exposes you to many interesting and wonderful tools to further your life adventure in self-awareness and limitless growth.

The Yin Yang of Diet

T'ai Chi's movements are a blend of hard and soft, exertion and relaxation, force and yielding. In fact, the T'ai Chi symbol is the yin/yang symbol—the symbol of balance. Just as T'ai Chi and QiGong are built upon the concepts of balance, so is every other aspect of healthy living. Chinese cooking adheres to these same principles.

In Chinese cooking, a good cook balances the use of yin foods and yang foods to create a meal that is not only delicious, but provides optimum health benefits. In a way, a good Chinese chef is almost like a pharmacist, blending nutrients, herbs, and Qi into a prescription that treats the eyes, palate, and health.

This ancient yin/yang symbol is actually called "T'ai Chi." It represents two things: that everything in the universe exists within each individual thing (even you), and that we should seek balance in all things.

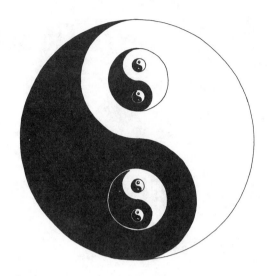

Sage Sifu Says

Many nutritionists see the Chinese diet as optimum, approximately 50 percent grain (rice), 30 percent vegetables, and 20 percent meat. Each person is unique, and our needs vary depending on our current health and activities. Ask your physician or a qualified dietician to discover your optimum diet.

Be aware that just eating Chinese food does not mean a healthy diet. There are healthy and unhealthy Chinese foods as well. Stick to stir-fried rather than batter-fried meats and vegetables. Steamed fish is excellent. Use your own good judgment.

Green vegetables are yin food. They are cool and easily digested and are helpful for certain parts and functions of the body. Meat is a yang food. Yang is power and provides great energy to the body, but is less easily digested. Chinese herbs are divided into cool and hot, dry and wet, each of which is good for certain conditions. There are many good books on Chinese herbs. Again, your food becomes not only a culinary treat, but also a prescription for optimum health.

Chinese Herbs and Teas for Health Conditions

Ginseng tea is made from ginseng root. The roots resemble a person's head and body. Ginseng has yang qualities. If a person's condition is overly yin, or cool and damp, an herbalist may suggest herbs promoting the yang qualities of dry and hot. For example, fresh ginger tea may be good to treat some early cold symptoms. Bitter melon soup, a yin food, may be used to treat an overactive yang condition like nosebleeds. Consult a qualified herbalist for more detailed information. Make sure your physician is aware of any herbal therapy you may engage in.

Ouch!

The Chinese health philosophy frowns on iced drinks because they introduce too much yin into the body too quickly. This shocks the body and upsets the balance. Hot or tepid drinks are preferred because the body is naturally warm.

Feng Shui: Architectural T'ai Chi

The Chinese believe that Qi, or life energy, not only flows through living things but through all things. According to this belief, we move in a great ocean of invisible energy that affects and interacts with energy from other beings, nature, and even buildings. In fact, the Chinese have developed an architectural system to affect the way energy flows through your home or business in order to maximize health, happiness, and prosperity—it's called *Feng Shui* (pronounced *fung-shway*) and is like architectural T'ai Chi, or T'ai Chi for your house.

Have you ever noticed how almost all Chinese restaurants have aquariums and many near the front door? This arrangement is based on Feng Shui. Running water is very good for the room's Qi.

Western architecture often uses running water for decorative purposes. However, science is now suggesting that the use of water in architecture is also functional. Many homes and geographical areas are bombarded by positive ions in the air. This can aggravate allergies or cause other physiological or mental discomforts. Some of this positive ion overload is because of modern electricity, but some is a natural phenomenon. Running water produces negative ions, which can balance the ions in a room, home, or business, making it more pleasant and more healthful. If a restaurant makes you feel more at ease, you will likely come back there more often, making the restaurant more prosperous. So, Feng Shui works on principles based on a subatomic understanding of the energy dynamics in a room, which in the end can lead to a happier, more prosperous existence.

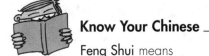

Know Your Chinese

Feng Shui means "wind" and "water." Wind represents universal forces, while water represents earth forces. Balancing the two creates optimum health and prosperity.

The *I Ching*

As you learned in Part 4, "Kuang Ping T'ai Chi: Walk on Life's Lighter Side," on the Kuang Ping Yang style of T'ai Chi, which has 64 forms, there are 64 possible combinations of hexagrams in the *I Ching*.

There are many ways to use the *I Ching*, and there is some debate about how or what it really does. Some think it is a fortune-telling device, while others see it as a tool for self-analysis or contemplation of self. There are 64 possible hexagrams, which represent all the possible ways life can transform.

Some modern analysts compare the hexagram system of the *I Ching* to the Rorschach test, where the person reading the hexagrams is really defined by how she sees them. To read your *I Ching*, you throw the hexagrams out, or shake yarrow sticks from a cup, and the way they fall tells you what to look up. There are books that list the hexagrams meanings. They are often just vague enough so that you must interpret for yourself the detailed meaning for your life. Therefore, when we use this method of divination we are compelled to introspection, to understand who we are, what we want, and where we want to go in life. Seen in this light, the *I Ching* can be a very healthful and potentially invaluable tool. Some bookstores will have books, or even kits, so that you can practice using the *I Ching* system yourself.

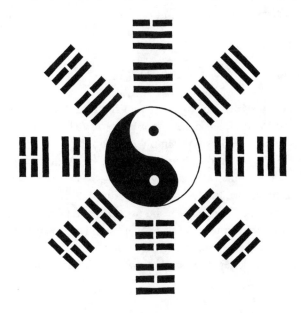

The 64 possible hexagram combinations represent all the possible forms of life's changes, just as styles of T'ai Chi with 64 movements represent possible physical changes we go through.

Rest and Rejuvenation

The yin and yang symbol of T'ai Chi symbolizes that we must balance our natures in our bodies and in the world around us. In our modern fast-paced lives, we are too reliant on busyness and constant noise. We consider television to be a form of relaxation. While a small amount can be, the amount of hours most Americans watch television is actually unhealthy. In fact, the American Medical Association has stated that more than two hours per day is unhealthy.

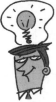

A T'ai Chi Punch Line

One day my wife and I went to a temple in Hong Kong, and while there had our fortunes forecast by a priest using the *I Ching*. After divining our fortune, the priest told my wife, "You are pregnant." We laughed because we knew that we had been careful. Two days later, my wife got dizzy, so we rushed her to a clinic where the doctor did blood tests. The doctor came back and announced, "You are pregnant."

Just as activity is important to our health, so is absolute rest. Most of us probably find it difficult just to sit, to simply be and serenely enjoy the absence of stimulation. At first, the slowness and quiet quality of T'ai Chi and QiGong drive many people a little nuts.

This is a cleansing process. The more anxiety we feel, breathe through, and let go of, the more we settle into a clarity and calmness that we eventually learn to enjoy. By sitting still we become aware of anxieties and tensions that we may have buried in our subconscious mind. These repressed feelings can manifest as muscle tension, asthma attacks, volatile emotions, and so on, unless we become aware of them, feel them, and then begin to breathe through them by physically letting the muscles let go and the mind relax. The cleansing pleasure of that "empty awareness" is perhaps the most healthful thing we can do for ourselves. It gives our mind a chance to rest, to heal, and to recharge. This also gives our spiritual nature an opportunity to come forth. We can get a new perspective on life, just by sitting. Just as a drug addict must go through a period of anxiety to let go of the craving for drugs, those of us that are addicted to "busyness" and constant stimulation (TV or whatever) must go through that anxiety period. But eventually we touch into the bliss of stillness of mind.

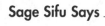

Sage Sifu Says

A famous Vietnamese monk once said that we are like glasses of dirty water. Each day the dirt gets shook up, and we become cloudy and unclear. If we take time to sit still, our stress settles down, and we again can see clearly.

T'ai Chi Teaches Mindful Living

T'ai Chi's slow process and seemingly endless progression from one movement to the next teaches us to let go of outcome and be in the moment. In the West, this is called "stopping to smell the roses." With T'ai Chi, we don't just think about stopping to smell the roses. We simply must do it. You cannot stand to perform a 20-minute slow-motion exercise like T'ai Chi and stay in a rush-rush-hurry-hurry mentality. It is impossible. Therefore T'ai Chi is like a magic formula that actually changes who you are. Its methodology forces us to love the act of living, just as we must love the feel, the sensation, the breath, and the motion of each T'ai Chi movement, so that we don't anxiously wait for it to be over. Life becomes a sacrament, every moment, and every person we touch becomes sacred and a miracle. As T'ai Chi's slow mindfulness causes us to subtly attune to the miracle of our own existence, we see the world around us as miraculous. On a physical level, as we daily immerse ourselves in Qi, or life's energy, we connect with that quality in all living things.

The mindful living that T'ai Chi teaches spills out into every aspect of our lives. The following is a list of exercises you can perform to bring forth that T'ai Chi mindfulness.

◆ **Savor the smell and taste of liquids.** When you take a sip of water with a lime twist or hot tea, really smell the rich odor as you drink. Let the aroma fill your awareness. As you swallow it, feel the heat or cold go down your throat. Experience its descent all the way into your stomach.

◆ **When you hold a hot cup of tea, watch the steam rise.** Get your face right up next to it. The steam is agitated atoms that burst free of the surface and scream outward into space, just like the huge bursts that erupt from the surface of the sun. Enjoy this fabulous display of erupting atoms.

◆ **Simplify your diet.** Drink more water with a lime twist and less soda or beer. Take the time to really taste and smell the lime. Lime is an exquisite gift we've been given. Usually we drink very sweet over-flavored things because we don't slow down enough to really taste them. So we need the shock value of 13 sugar cubes and the other sticky stuff that comes in most cans of soda.

◆ **Eat more fruits and vegetables.** Really stop and chew them. Feel their texture, their temperature, and savor their subtle flavor and smell.

◆ **When you cook, feel the food as you cut it up.** Listen to the sizzling as it cooks and really smell the richness of its aroma. Pretend for a moment that this was your last day on earth, and you would never be able to smell these smells, hear these sounds, or taste these tastes again.

◆ **Sit and watch nature.** Nature cannot be analyzed or fixed. Nature simply washes over you. Watch the clouds move, the trees sway, and the weather unfold. This world is a miracle placed here for your enjoyment. Don't take its beauty for granted.

◆ **Just listen** when your spouse (or children or friends) talks to you. Observe their faces, the excitement in their voices. Let the images of their day wash over your mind. Do not worry about how you are "supposed" to respond. Enjoy their presence.

◆ **Observe people, experience them.** Imagine for a moment that you were the only person on earth, and there was never ever going to be anyone else but you. You probably would be filled with desire to speak to others, to enjoy their existence. Here they are, enjoy.

◆ **Let life wash over you.** Do what needs to be done, whether it's washing dishes or paying bills with a sense of unhurried pleasure, like the way T'ai Chi movements are done. If we don't run from what we must do, it can be pleasant, and all things simply work out, as if we did nothing at all.

> **Sage Sifu Says**
>
> The T'ai Chi symbol, or yin/yang symbol, literally means the supreme ultimate point in the universe. When you follow the suggestions to allow T'ai Chi to weave its mindfulness into your life, you begin to feel more and more as though you are in the center of the universe.

The Least You Need to Know

◆ Balance your diet, like your life.

◆ Drink "fresh" ginger tea at the first sign of a cold.

◆ Open, flowing interior design does much more than just look good.

◆ *I Ching* games can help you understand yourself better.

◆ T'ai Chi teaches savoring life and smelling the roses.

Chapter 23

Do T'ai Chi: Change the World

In This Chapter

◆ Lowering unemployment and healthcare costs
◆ Helping schools
◆ Reducing crime and violence
◆ Cleaning up the environment and healing our world

T'ai Chi is widely misunderstood. Is it an exercise, a martial art, or a meditation *technique?* Actually, T'ai Chi is all those things, but it also offers so much more. T'ai Chi can be a key to discovering our personal empowerment. As we find that we can take control over our body's circulation, our blood pressure, and our stress responses, we are empowered. This empowerment begins to resonate out to every aspect of our lives—work, relationships, and society.

As we feel empowered and T'ai Chi works its clarifying magic, we find learning easier and more exciting. We become drawn to learning as the world becomes fresher and more magical because of our new attitude of well-being. T'ai Chi cultivates and supports our childlikeness, our curiosity, and our zest for life.

T'ai Chi also teaches us how precious and miraculous life can be. When we treasure each moment of our lives, we are much less likely to engage in acts that endanger our health or our freedom. When we feel at peace within ourselves, we are much less likely to hurt others. Much violence is the act of someone in personal pain who externalizes that pain on others. T'ai Chi can help heal that pain, thereby reducing much violence.

T'ai Chi and Unemployment

Since people who grew up in high-stress households have higher unemployment rates, T'ai Chi may help both parents and children change that pattern. Furthermore, because many people are increasingly required by the modern economy to change careers several times, T'ai Chi's promotion of letting go of the past and relaxing into change can be helpful to adults in today's job market.

England's Royal Academy of Pediatrics College released a study that concluded that "stressful" households caused problems for children that could last a lifetime. One thing they discovered was that children from such households endured higher unemployment levels than kids from more peaceful households. We know that stress limits our creativity and can affect our self-esteem. T'ai Chi's ability to provide children with a tool that can help them find a calm place within, even when home is "less than calm," can be of powerful help to them.

In today's modern workforce, it is estimated that most of us will change, not jobs, but careers over five times in our lifetime. For people who find change difficult, this can be excruciatingly stressful and even life threatening over time. In a world of constant and relentless change, T'ai Chi's ability to help us mentally, emotionally, and physically let go can be a great help.

By being able to let go of past employment and being open to new information and self-definitions, we can be ready to flow into our next occupation. This flowing can happen, not only less stressfully, but with an adventurous anticipation, just like when we were kids. This is what T'ai Chi can help us do as individuals and as a society.

When you catch yourself considering worst-case scenarios while engaged in a task or project, take a deep breath and let your entire body release thoughts, tensions, and fears. Then make a list or flow chart of what is required for success. This will let you realistically decide whether to proceed rather than resist change because of irrational fears. T'ai Chi promotes a sense of being in the moment, of dealing with the tasks at hand, and of letting go of fear-based projections of the future.

T'ai Chi and the Healthcare Crisis

Approximately 80 percent of the illnesses that send us to the doctor are due to stress. The six leading causes of death are stress related. Our health care crisis is literally due to stress. Stress can be managed, and there is perhaps no more effective stress management tool than daily T'ai Chi and QiGong meditations.

Hospitals and insurance carriers are beginning to incorporate T'ai Chi and QiGong into what they offer clients. Physicians, neurologists, cardiac and hypertension specialists, and mental health providers are prescribing T'ai Chi for a host of physical, emotional, and mental conditions. Medical university nursing programs are also introducing T'ai Chi to their students as part of their training. Others schools are considering offering it to all medical students.

T'ai Chi begins to show us that we have a healthcare crisis simply because we choose to have a healthcare crisis. Each of us has it within our own power to dramatically lower our dependence on general health care, pharmacology, and surgery. The fastest growing investment industry in the United States today is pharmaceuticals. The top three are ulcer, high blood pressure, and mood-altering medications. T'ai Chi and/or QiGong can have significantly positive effects on all three of these conditions in some cases.

T'ai Chi and QiGong are not at odds with modern Western health care. They can be partners with it. You don't decide between medication or surgery, and T'ai Chi. If you need medication or surgery, then use it. However, medication and surgery should not be our first line of defense. If we practice T'ai Chi, we may never develop the need for certain medications or for much heart surgery. Again, stress is the reason most of the physical conditions requiring medication or surgery develop in the first place. If we daily water our "T'ai Tree" roots with the soothing balm of life energy, we will be less likely to ever need that medication or surgery, saving ourselves pain and money, while saving our society a great financial burden. We cannot afford to ignore our body's signals and our health until we are in a crisis situation and then expect society to lavish money upon us for expensive surgery or medication. This isn't just about Medicare alone; *all* our health insurance premiums are skyrocketing due to a national need to become mindful of our health. T'ai Chi can save us all big money and help us feel good while doing it.

> **Sage Sifu Says**
>
> When going to the doctor, think less of expecting the doctor to "heal you." Rather, think in terms of you and the doctor in partnership. Ask the doctor what healthful habits or activities you can engage in to facilitate your healing. The question should be, "How can I heal me?"

T'ai Chi in Education

Studies show that change, even change for the better, is stressful. A good example is when you upgrade your computer. The newer program gives you new tools to make your work faster and more efficient, but letting go of the old ways and learning the new is often stressful.

So each day our children in many ways are learning new ways to do everything, both at home and at school. Kids today are under tremendous stress because the world is changing very fast, and they will see changes we never dreamed of in our lives. Therefore, the best tool they can be given to launch out upon the world with confidence and health is, you guessed it, T'ai Chi.

Helping Students Stay Current *in a Fast Current!*

Remember how T'ai Chi brings you back to the calm center no matter how fast life's carousel is spinning. In today's rapidly changing world, this is a very important tool to give our children. No matter how much math, science, and economic facts we give them, they will be lost if they don't know how to thrive healthfully in a world of change. Why? Because our understanding of math, science, and economics is changing on an almost daily basis. Of all the discoveries made since the inception of man, nearly all have been made in our lifetimes, and the world is only getting faster with the explosion of the information age. Therefore, children with mind/body training that can help them adapt to new ways easier and more healthfully will have a distinct advantage over kids *who only learn* the current ways things are done, or the current textbook facts.

If you refer back to the "Stress Is the Symptom" section in Chapter 3, "Medical T'ai Chi: The Prescription for the Future," you'll see that we too often respond to stressors (like change) in

> **A T'ai Chi Punch Line**
>
> If you look at many long-term T'ai Chi practitioners, Chinese or Western, you will find very vibrant people, often at the pinnacles of their professions. T'ai Chi practitioners do not fear and run from change, but find it essential to a full life.

an unhealthy way. When this happens chronically, it can even inhibit our thinking processes, literally shrinking parts of the brain. So by teaching T'ai Chi, we help children be calm, and provide them a physical model to relax through changes, which thereby can improve their mental function.

Studying Health from the Inside Out

Hopefully every school will eventually provide T'ai Chi instruction through all levels of education and to teachers as well. Teaching universities are beginning to incorporate it into their advanced credit offerings for teachers at all levels, and many teachers are finding T'ai Chi on their own to deal with personal stress from overcrowded classrooms and low education budgets. T'ai Chi is a cross between physical education and health science. It may eventually become a staple of health science. What better way for kids to learn about their body and health than by paying attention to the laboratory they walk around in every day, their own miraculous minds and bodies, through practicing T'ai Chi's mindful exercises.

Although most of the high school T'ai Chi classes I've taught have been in health science, instructors in physical education, art, and drama are considering T'ai Chi as an adjunct to their classes.

Helping Students Avoid Drugs

Some schools are already providing T'ai Chi to students. I have personally taught T'ai Chi and QiGong relaxation therapy to students in the elementary, junior high, high school, and university level through health science, college preparatory programs, and drug abuse prevention programs. Health science teachers have told me that students claim the main reason they begin smoking or using drugs and alcohol is to alleviate stress. Of course, those of us with more life experience know that in the end, drug abuse creates more stress, but it is not enough to simply tell kids to "just say no." We must take the next step and provide them with tools to manage the enormous stress they face in an increasingly complex world.

T'ai Chi and Crime and Law Enforcement

T'ai Chi is now being taught in prison, as well as in court-sponsored rehabilitation programs. T'ai Chi's ability to build self-esteem, heal childhood trauma, and manage potentially violent stress makes it an incredible coping tool for anyone trying to change. If we want to reduce crime, finding ways people can become productive parts of society is a cost-effective and just plain effective way to do it. It costs twice as much to send a child to prison as it does to send that child to Harvard. The United States has incarcerated more of its children than any nation in the world, per capita. It is time to find creative solutions like T'ai Chi and mind/body fitness training to heal the very roots of crime—*the potential criminals*. To do this before the crime occurs will save us all much pain and vast amounts of money.

> **A T'ai Chi Punch Line**
>
> Many people using T'ai Chi to rehabilitate from drug abuse problems like the fact that T'ai Chi gives them something to replace the old habits with. Rather than just denying themselves the high they loved, they are growing toward a new life as T'ai Chi helps them improve each and every day.

Law enforcement officers work in constant danger and often see only the worst sides of people. This can be very stressful. Historically, stress-related maladies like alcoholism, drug abuse, coronary heart disease, diabetes, and suicide have been problems within law enforcement, according to *Police Chief Magazine* and the U.S. Public Health Service. T'ai Chi may be an effective multipurpose way to help law enforcement officers deal with job-related stress. T'ai Chi's martial applications would be an added bonus to officers learning T'ai Chi's soothing stress-management tools. T'ai Chi can help in several ways. First, it can help officers dump job stress after work. Then if they do go out for a drink after T'ai Chi class, they will be doing it for pleasure, rather than for stress reduction. This can mean the difference between a couple of social drinks and a mind-numbing binge.

Second, if officers are less stressed on duty, they will likely see more options in any given situation. Problems can be diffused more easily when in a calmer, clearer state. Even in difficult situations, T'ai Chi's calming effects can resonate, especially if it helps the officers sleep better, which T'ai Chi is known to do. So T'ai Chi's calming aspects can help diffuse potentially dangerous situations, which leaves the officer with less stress to take off duty. Less stress begets less stress, and so on and so on.

Hopefully, departments will eventually provide officers with seven-hour shifts and use the last hour for T'ai Chi decompression time. This will make business sense for all the reasons listed in the chapter on corporate T'ai Chi, but these benefits are magnified since law enforcement's stress can be even higher.

T'ai Chi and Violence

This sounds strange, but most domestic violence is a very ineffective form of stress management. Domestic violence is a way that a very unhappy person takes out their personal stress on their loved ones. It's ineffective because as we tear down those around us, that eventually tears us down. We create a sanctuary of pain rather than a loving home.

T'ai Chi can change that from many angles. If children begin to use T'ai Chi's mind/body fitness stress-management tools to self-heal in school, the cycle of pain at home will be changed and diminished in some ways. Then if parents can be encouraged to learn these tools through community services, they will change the cycle even more effectively. There is a great spider web of connection in a community that will be affected as well. If one parent breaks a cycle of abuse and pain, his or her children will not spread that pain by being mean to the children around them at school. Or by growing up and passing it down to their kids by being violent to them.

> **A T'ai Chi Punch Line**
>
> Many T'ai Chi practitioners hear others tell them they have "changed," "are calmer," or "are easier to be around," before they even notice the changes in themselves. Even when you are feeling stress, others may see you as "mellow" in comparison to the rest of the world.

Alcohol or other substance abuses aggravate much domestic violence. The benefits of T'ai Chi for drug rehabilitation are discussed in Chapter 20, "T'ai Chi as Therapy for Young and Old."

Substance abuse and domestic violence all set a destructive dynamic in motion that reaches far beyond the home. There is a famous "kick the cat" story that shows how a community is affected by one person's calm or rage.

An executive gets a traffic ticket on the way to work and then fumes at his administrative assistant. She in turn snaps at the other executives and employees she deals with. They get ticked off and snap at their co-workers, who are testy with people in the other companies they deal with on the phone, and so on. Eventually thousands of people who have had a lousy day hit the freeway and begin to give the one-fingered salute to other motorists. And so it goes.

Finally all these seething people get home and yell at their spouses, who yell at the kids, who walk upstairs and kick the cat.

T'ai Chi can inverse this process ending up with thousands of family cats getting a loving caress by kids growing up in a more loving world, nurtured by parents who work at companies that provide health tools to them like T'ai Chi. Sound far-fetched? Not really. Stress is the source of much of our communal pain, and stress management like T'ai Chi is a balm that can dramatically heal it.

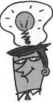

A T'ai Chi Punch Line

Once you learn T'ai Chi, you'll begin to notice people practicing everywhere you go, in any country in the world. T'ai Chi is an international language. My students have done T'ai Chi with people in England, France, Japan, Vietnam, Mexico, China, El Salvador, and Cuba, to name a few. As you travel, T'ai Chi will give you a pleasant vehicle to interact with and meet other people, even if you don't speak their language.

A study done by the Transcendental Meditation Foundation (which teaches an excellent form of stress management called TM) found that when a small percentage of the population of a community, school, or organization practiced TM, it had a positive impact on that entire social body.

Therefore, even though most people will never practice T'ai Chi, the few that do may change the entire community in positive ways.

T'ai Chi and the Environment

At first, it may not seem like T'ai Chi has anything to do with our world's environment, but it does. The word *T'ai Chi* means "the Supreme Ultimate Point in the Universe." This means that every single part of the entire world exists within each and every thing, even you and me. Modern physics demonstrates this by explaining that all things are made of energy, *the same energy*. You, I, the sun and moon, and Earth's oceans and mountains are all made of the same energy. We are connected. This is brought home even more as science explains that you and I and everyone on this planet has breathed an oxygen atom breathed by Jesus, Buddha, and Mohammed. The world gets smaller.

Sage Sifu Says

Each time you walk outside look up at the sky and at the trees or grass. Let the full breadth of nature's beauty wash over you. Think of opening your body to the universal energy as if you were an open airy sponge that could fill with the life around you, and likewise you can expand out to merge with it. If you make this a habit and take 30 or 60 seconds to do this each time you walk in or out of your home, it will change your life.

When you practice T'ai Chi and especially sitting QiGong, you often feel at peace, somehow connected to the world around you, as if you were the center of the universe. This experience leaves you feeling as though you matter, yet it also leaves you feeling as though every other person and every other thing in this world is of vast and profound importance as well.

T'ai Chi and QiGong reminds us that we are energy by immersing our mind and body in the experience of it each day. This constant immersion reminds us how closely we are linked to all things. This isn't an illusion. The illusion is that we think we are separate from the world. The rainforest and ocean are the Earth's lungs and thermostats. Without them we perish. So, to feel "connected" to the world is to become real. T'ai Chi and QiGong help us to become more and more real.

Our decisions about how to live in our world will be healthfully influenced by the "realness" T'ai Chi cultivates. This will be a powerful asset to building a cleaner, healthier world. As mentioned in Part 1, "T'ai Chi:

Relax into It," T'ai Chi promotes a feeling of optimum mental, emotional, and physical health therapists call *homeostasis*. By tuning into that healthful center everyday, we are more drawn to ingesting healthful foods, water, and air, and therefore more conscious of the state of our small planet because this is where our water, food, and air come from.

As with all things, the world's environmental health begins with our own state of health. Your heart beats to supply oxygen to the entire body. However, the first thing the heart feeds is itself because if it is healthier, stronger, and clearer, it is more useful to its world (your body). Therefore, by feeding yourself the healing force of life energy everyday, you enable yourself to be a healing force as you flow through the world *around you*.

The Least You Need to Know

- ◆ T'ai Chi helps heal our society, our world, and us.
- ◆ T'ai Chi saves money in healthcare and may lower crime and unemployment rates.
- ◆ T'ai Chi helps us all "just get along."
- ◆ T'ai Chi influences our environment in a positive way.

Chapter 24

Celebrate World T'ai Chi and QiGong Day

In This Chapter

◆ Unleashing the power to change the world

◆ Getting involved in T'ai Chi and QiGong day

If we want to make something truly spectacular of our world, there is nothing whatsoever that can stop us.

—Rainer Maria Rilke

Too often in our lives we underestimate and undervalue our power as human beings. T'ai Chi and QiGong practice are designed to unblock the rigid limitations we hold so that the greatest potential within us can flow up and out through our relaxed mind and body. This may sound like a grandiose ideal, until you realize that it is very true, and the first edition of this book *proved it to the world!*

In this chapter, I'll explain why it's actually very unhealthy for human beings to settle for less than their greatest potential, for *repression of enthusiasm and hope can diminish our health*. Studies reveal that when people give of themselves to make the world a better place it improves their physical and mental health personally. Kind of an "Instant Karma" if you will (kudos to John Lennon). And T'ai Chi and QiGong help energize and motivate us for "right action," as T'ai Chi philosophy extols us to aspire to. I'll close with ways you can expand your T'ai Chi and QiGong journey to include joining with tens of thousands worldwide each year to be part of a fun and beneficial global health and healing event, known as World T'ai Chi and QiGong Day. And this chapter will explain how your community activism may improve your health as well.

Unleash the World-Altering Power Within You!

Not only are *you* truly profound and unique, but you are holding a truly profound and unique book. Because the first edition of this book *actually launched a world event, changing the world in a healing way.* For World T'ai Chi and QiGong Day has educated millions about T'ai Chi and QiGong. Therefore, this book doesn't just "talk the talk"—it *walks the walk* of T'ai Chi's expansive personal power.

> **CAUTION**
>
> ### Ouch!
>
> When you catch your mind revolving around the negatives of "I can't do this," or "I can't change that," practice the QiGong breathing/energy exercise taught in Part 3, "Starting Down the QiGong Path to T'ai Chi." Let your mind and body *let go of everything.* Releasing negatives will fill you with hope as you fill with light."

> ### T'ai Sci
>
> Bill Joy, Chief Scientist for Sun Microsystems (a backbone of the Internet), explained that "the speed of technological change is doubling exponentially every few months." Psychological studies show modern change is stressful. By learning to breathe and relax through T'ai Chi's changing postures, we learn to relax into the changes of the stampeding future.

As we practice T'ai Chi, we realize it changes our lives, by showing us that most of what holds us back is not "out there" in the world, as much as it is *in our own mental and emotional limitations*, in the form of rigidity we've constrained ourselves with unconsciously. As earlier chapters explained, this mental constraint actually constrains circulation and health functions over time. But, it also holds back our lives. My T'ai Chi and QiGong practice enabled me to open to large expansive ideas like, for example, creating World T'ai Chi and QiGong Day, first by announcing it in this book's first edition. Then, these powerful tools gave me the stress-management techniques needed to endure the stress of actually fulfilling that dream.

This ability to open to new possibilities and manage the stress of seeing them to fruition, is increasingly needed by all of us in these modern times. This is because we all have much greater potential and also more stress due to the emerging information age. We are in an age where ideas are communicated globally in nanoseconds, meaning our thoughts and dreams can become not only personal realities, but global realities very quickly.

And the speed of change is about to go into hyper-speed, as we are on the verge of the creation of *tiny computers* only 10 atoms across that will compute in hours what today's computers *might take centuries to compute.* When ideas become reality at this speed, we are literally on the threshold of *living the lives of our dreams.* So T'ai Chi and QiGong's ability to help us clear our thought processes, relax into change by handling stress better, and find more inspiration and hope, changes the world. The end result is we will find ourselves getting healthier by feeling more empowered and less victimized by a rapidly changing world that often seems out of control, *surfing the waves of change rather than being beaten down by them.*

Embracing an Idea That Changes the World

The way T'ai Chi's personal empowerment changes the world is rooted in the T'ai Chi philosophy that *each of us contains aspects of the entire world.* Therefore, by becoming more attuned to our own health and life patterns we tap into the entire world's rhythms and patterns as well. Our example of personal growth and health heals the world the way cleaning drops of water eventually cleans an entire pool.

The physical benefits of T'ai Chi and QiGong actually change the world around us, as they teach you to breathe and relax through challenges and fears. This helps us discover the courage and power to change things in our lives and the world that don't work as well as they could, rather than just *tightening up* and complaining about what we don't like. From the quiet place in our backyard (and mind), when we do our T'ai Chi, great things can emerge through our loosening mind and body to permeate all aspects of our lives and world with calm and clarity. Enabling us to see life's "big picture."

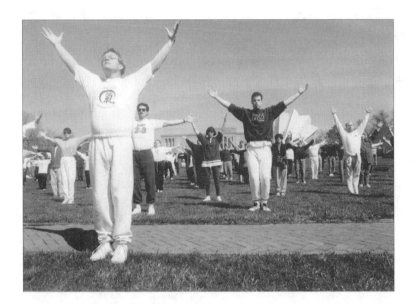

World T'ai Chi Day, inspired by the first edition of The Complete Idiot's Guide to T'ai Chi and QiGong, *was reported in* The New York Times, The South China Morning Post, FOX National News, CNN Headline News, *and hundreds of media worldwide.*

Learning the Essence of QiGong

When I first began organizing World T'ai Chi and QiGong Day, I was invited by the National QiGong Association to come and speak to their annual forum. While there, I met an extraordinary man named Master Li. He'd been perhaps the best Kung Fu coach in China's long martial arts history, but gave it all up to begin teaching QiGong for health. He stopped me in the hall one day and asked this, "Why are you organizing this World T'ai Chi and QiGong Day?" *"Are you doing it for love?"* he asked.

This caught me off guard, because I'd been doing it simply because it was proven to help people's health. But, Master Li insisted that it must be much more. He said the world's Qi, or life energy, was depleted of love in this age of hustle and bustle, no one taking the time to enjoy life or one another. This great QiGong master, and one of the world's greatest martial artists, gave me *the quintessential QiGong lesson* when he said, "Love is the essence of QiGong." I realized over time that he was right. Not just about World T'ai Chi and QiGong Day, or QiGong, but about everything we do in our lives. If we don't do it for love, it is meaningless, and will not last, or have any real consequence in the grander scheme of life. Even when battles must be fought, if we do it with the intention of our love of peace, we find greater victory. This seems to be what T'ai Chi philosophy has always been trying to suggest in extolling us to employ "right thinking" and "right action" as we flow through our lives, to be "nurturing to all things" as Taoist philosophy writes. As always, QiGong practice goes to the center of life, whether it be health issues, or ways of behaving.

> **Sage Sifu Says**
>
> Chinese philosophy explains how *all the universe* exists in *each of us.* So by learning how to heal ourselves and our community—*we heal the world.*
>
> When we are flowing in the Tao, using our lives to nurture and heal life, Taoist philosophy tells us that we have great unseen support for everything we do.

> **A T'ai Chi Punch Line**
>
> Some may begin using T'ai Chi or QiGong to get "special powers" to dominate others with. However, from my experience that doesn't work. To truly experience the deep benefits of T'ai Chi and QiGong, we have to let go of such trivial behaviors and desires. T'ai Chi and QiGong make us more caring, loving people. As Sun Tzu wrote in *The Art of War,* "the highest way is not to fight and win in every battle; the highest way is to win in every battle without fighting."

Allowing Our Greatest Potential to Emerge

When we hold on to fears, angers, or trivial obsessions, our mind tightens down, our health is diminished, and our vision squeezes to a tunnel vision, *cut off from the flow of life*. That's how we "hold on" to things physically, physical things like forks, spoons, or baseballs, and so on, by *squeezing them*. And this is also how we hold on to thoughts and emotions—*by tightening our consciousness around them*. This in turn tightens our physical atoms of our body and being, which can translate into "pinched" nerves and high blood "pressure" as the mind tightens down the body. When we hold onto *old stagnant images* of ourselves, others, or the world, there is no room for new *inspired* images of reality to flow through us. Even though there is always a *new, better reality* wanting to emerge through our minds into the world all the time, this gripping of old reality keeps us tight. T'ai Chi and QiGong are designed to teach us to breathe…and *to let go*…of everything our mind and heart hold on to, so fresh creative and *inspired* thoughts can continually flow through us. Just as that same *loosening* unlocks physical power.

T'ai Sci

The "spir" in "inspired" means to breathe, as in breathing new life into reality. When we squeeze onto old realities in our heart and mind, we suppress our inspiration, and this damages our health. Doctor Andrew Weil, the great author and Harvard educated physician, explains that many of our health problems are rooted in poor breathing habits. It may be that our "life" problems are rooted there, too.

Sage Sifu Says

Feelings are important. When we feel irritation or upset, that is information that our lives, or our world, are in need of change. This is the purpose of feelings, to communicate a need for change. T'ai Chi and QiGong enable us to breathe into those feelings, hearing their purpose without being overwhelmed by them. In this way we become very adaptive to challenges.

Fear is often what keeps us *locked down and rigid*. This is because breaking out of old patterns can make us feel unusual and lonely, and this is "frightening." The fear of that alienation causes us to freeze up, squeeze down, and suffer increased stress damage, as well as denying the world our precious inspired thoughts and feelings. So you see fear often causes us to limit ourselves, rather than expanding outward and upward toward limitless visions of possibility. Both T'ai Chi and QiGong offer great therapies to work through fear, and in a way, make the energy behind fears *our ally*. Not running from fear, but *being with it*.

Making the feeling of fear an ally can help us deal with problems rather than running from them. Each of us in our own way often expends huge resources running away from fear rather than feeling it. My dad suffered from delayed stress syndrome from World War II, and when his mind would begin to fill with fear, he always wanted to drive, as if he could drive away from who he was and what he was feeling. He wasn't alone, as much of the world thinks it can "drive away" from problems. We burn more and more CO_2-producing fossil fuels even as scientists warn that we may be dangerously elevating the global temperatures by creating "green house gasses." Yet we still drive and drive away from our fears. By being with our fear, and doing our T'ai Chi everyday, we may save much more than our health.

In summary, T'ai Chi and QiGong can …

◆ Help us get healthier, which means we think more clearly.

◆ Help us learn to be with our fears, so that we don't have to run from them.

◆ Help us use the energy of fear as a catalyst to help us take on the tasks of change that evolving modern life throws at us.

◆ Provide that "wakeful rest" state that can allow the truly "great ideas" that exist within all of us to come out. Great ideas like World T'ai Chi and QiGong Day.

Becoming Involved in World T'ai Chi and QiGong Day

World T'ai Chi and QiGong Day begins on the Saturday of the week of United Nations World Health Day each year at 10 A.M. local time, worldwide. Visit www.worldtaichiday.org for exact dates each year. It begins at the earliest time zones with mass events in Australia, where Australians come out in public and do T'ai Chi and QiGong together. Then as the Earth turns, T'ai Chi and QiGong players in Asia, Africa, Europe, and the Americas join in and eventually this healing global T'ai Chi movement ends with the final events in Hawaii. We even had an event on the North Pole one year!

T'ai Sci
Research shows that when we "care" about others in the world, it actually makes us healthier. Getting involved in a healing event like World T'ai Chi and QiGong Day, to help *others* learn how to get healthier, *may actually make us healthier.*
Lili Feng, Associate Professor at Baylor College of Medicine is working to prove how truthfulness, tolerance, and compassion may directly affect the physical function of the immune system.

As an individual, you can *get involved* and hopefully *get healthier* by helping with this global healing event. Teachers and schools can get involved as well and meet new students, grow their class size, and expand public health. Visit www.worldtaichiday.org and find events in your area, or list your event if you're a teacher or school, and print out Free Organizing Kits.

If you do T'ai Chi and QiGong, publish articles or letters to the editor about how you've benefited from it in your life. Encourage local hospitals, bookstores, and media to do educational specials around T'ai Chi and QiGong and other natural health modalities, like airing *QiGong: Ancient Chinese Healing for the 21st Century.* Encourage your workplace wellness director to have a T'ai Chi, QiGong, or other stress-management program (see Chapter 21, "'Tie'-Chi: Corporate T'ai Chi").

Go to the Internet and contact every T'ai Chi and QiGong group and refer them to www.worldtaichiday.org.

We are entering an extraordinary time in human history with access to modern *and ancient wonders* to make life better and better. We are learning that by healing ourselves we heal the world, and vice versa. And today we have access to the best of both modern and ancient sciences. By marrying the dynamic power of our modern Western technological world's information age with the inner peace and clarity that ancient Eastern wisdom has cultivated and refined for us over the last 2,000 years, we may be at the beginning of a wondrous human renaissance where health and clarity merge with limitless potential to *create the world of our dreams.*

The Least You Need to Know

- You have the seeds for wondrous change *in you.*
- Fear limits our ability to expand our mind and world to open to hopeful visions.
- T'ai Chi and QiGong can help you breathe, and relax open to limitless possibility.
- Joining in World T'ai Chi and QiGong Day can help change the world.
- Your world and our world become limitless as we practice life tools enabling us to relax into the future.

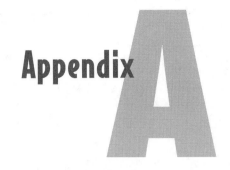

The T'ai Chi and QiGong Yellow Pages

This appendix provides an extensive listing of T'ai Chi and QiGong organizations, schools, publications, web resources, and natural health centers worldwide, including the United States, Australia, Canada, New Zealand, South Africa, and the United Kingdom. For contacts in nearly 50 other countries visit www.worldtaichiday.org. Due to the volume of listings the veracity of each listing cannot be verified, and it is listed as clearinghouse information to assist in your search for a school near you, and not an endorsement. You are your best judge of what school or teacher is right for you. Always use your own good judgment and discretion when contacting and choosing a school or teacher.

To find even more information on the following contacts, visit www.worldtaichiday.org to find website links and continually updated information for all the following listings. The following listings are arranged by city, school, and telephone, when possible. Note: For purposes of this directory all "Tai Chi," "Taiji," or "T'ai Chi" references will be abbreviated as "TC." All "QiGong" (or Chi Kung) references will be abbreviated as "QG." All "Martial Arts" will be seen as "MA." "Kung Fu" or "Gung Fu" is "KF."

National T'ai Chi (TC) and QiGong (QG) Organizations and Schools

National Registries

National QG Assn.
Nationwide and Int'l.
www.nqa.org

Int'l. Taoist TC
Society—worldwide
www.taoist.org/

Registries by State

Alabama

Birmingham, AL
Blue Dragon Academy
205-824-3777

Guntersville, AL
Blue Dragon Dojo
256-582-5211

Alaska

Anchorage, AK
Touch of Tao
907-279-0135

Anchorage, AK
Sifu Ray's Studios
907-248-0349

Anchorage, AK
Touch of Tao
907-351-6072

Anchorage, AK
Inst. of Med. QG
907-351-6072

Anchorage, AK
Taoist Retreate
907-263-8178

Anchorage, AK
Dao Dancing
907-245-4205

Anchorage, AK
Jade Lady Meditation
907-562-2863

Anchorage, AK
Mountain, Wind, Water
907-279-5484

Anchorage, AK
AK Taoist Arts
907-248-5192

Kenai, AK
Seven Stars TC
907-776-8810

Arizona

Flagstaff, AZ
Inner Way Healing
928-213-7247

Fountain Hills, AZ
Body in Harmony
480-816-4843

Glendale, AZ
Essence of Essence
623-773-0176

Phoenix, AZ
Two Fishes Swimming
602-973-8693

Phoenix, AZ
Deanne Hodgson
602-789-7415

Rio Rico, AZ
White Birch TC
520-281-8458

Sierra Vista, AZ
Acdy. of Fitness
520-458-8082

Sun City, AZ
Adelantein, Inc.
623-977-9790

Tucson, AZ
TC Chuan Dragon
520-326-9046

Tucson, AZ
Dr. Zee's Inst.
Chinese Healing Arts
520-297-2470

Arkansas

Little Rock, AR
Four Winds TC
501-614-9225

California

Albany, CA
Warrior-Sage Exec. Prog.
510-524-4940

Albany, CA
Walking Your Talk
510-917-7503

Alhambra, CA
Tai Ji Club
Sun Anuang
626-576-2319

Arcadia, CA
Draco Arts
Marvin Quon
626-254-9393

Baldwin Park, CA
B. Pk. Adult and Cmty. Ed.
626-939-4456

Benicia, CA
Daoist MA
707-246-0331

Berkeley, CA
Bay TC Wu Style
510-237-7196

Berkeley, CA
Cal Taiji
William Dere
510-642-3268

Berkeley, CA
Bodymind Healing Ctr.
510-849-2878

Burbank, CA
Jian Mei
Int'l., MA Assn.
M. Wen Mei Yu
818-563-1878

Burbank, CA
Armenian
Black Belt Acy.
818-260-9191

Carmel Valley, CA
Jing Shen Chi
831-659-0234

Cardiff by the Sea, CA
Enhancing Tech. Unltd.
1-800-546-4061

Cerritos, CA
Cerritos Clg.
(Mick Branch)
310-467-5050, ext. 2528

Corona, CA
Sifu Mullen—Corona Parks
909-736-2241

Costa Mesa, CA
Hsing Chen Hlg. and MA
949-642-5511

Costa Mesa, CA
O.C. College/Phys. Ed.
949-432-5123

Duarte, CA
Dan Lee Acdmy. of TC
626-358-1469

El Segundo, CA
AEA TC Club
310-336-2268

Fairfax, CA
Energy Arts, Inc.
415-454-5243

Guadalupe/Santa Maria, CA
Tai Qi Qi Gung
(Rama Ananda Das)
805-343-1344

Idyllwild, CA
Shaolin QG
909-659-6238

Irvine, CA
Just TC Prod.
949-494-7110

Laguna Beach, CA
Kuang Ping TC
949-460-9654

La Mesa, CA
Hsing-I MA Inst.
619-698-6389

Loma Linda, CA
L. L. Univ./Drayson Ctr. TC
(Sifu Kurland)
909-558-4975

Lomita, CA
Manuel Marquez—Shaolin
310-539-1374

Los Angeles and Malibu, CA
Nat'l. TC Ch'uan Assn.
(Doria Cook-Nelson/Dan Paik)
310-659-5600

Los Angeles, CA
Nat'l TC Chuan Assn.
213-484-8378

Los Angeles, CA
Nine Dragon Baguazhang
310-935-2412

Los Angeles, CA
Healing Tao of Los Angeles
310-455-1936

Los Angeles, CA
Chew Pao Wo TC
323-664-9639

Los Angeles and Santa Monica, CA
Peaceful Way TC
310-479-3646

Malibu/Studio City, CA
Doria Cook-Nelson
310-659-5600

Menifee, CA
Mt. San Jacinto College
909-487-6752, ext. 1701 and 1702

Mill Valley, CA
TC for Seniors
(Mark Johnson)
1-800-497-4244

Mission Viejo, CA
Saddleback Clg. East Arts
949-582-4900, ext. 3432

Monterey Park, CA
QG Int'l.
(Sifu Jason Tsou)
818-753-3200

North Hollywood, CA
QG Int'l.
818-753-3200

North Hollywood, CA
Wrights KF Fitness Acy.
5126 Lankershim Blvd.
91601

Oakland, CA
TC Chih/QG
510-540-8062

Orange County and Southern California
Warrior of Light
714-957-9346

Orinda, CA
Bodymind Healing Ctr.
510-849-2878

Palo Alto, CA
TC Chih w/Dona Marriott
650-948-1827

Pasadena, CA
TC for Now
626-798-7948

Perris, Menifee, CA
Perris Bethel AME Church
909-657-5705

Pico Rivera, CA
TC for Seniors
(Bill Ferrel)
562-801-5009 (office)
562-696-8462 (home)

Poway, CA
Poway Kenpo Karate
858-486-1003

Riverside/Corona/
Norco/Moreno Valley, CA
RCC Young At Heart TC
Sifu Villalobos/Kurland
909-222-8090

Riverside, CA
UCR-Sifu Harvey Kurland
909-787-5801, ext. 1600

Riverside, CA
SoCal NWTC Chuan Assn.
(Sifu Ruth Villalobos)
909-657-5705

Riverside, CA
Myra Allen—NWTCCA
909-789-1738

Riverside, CA
UCR Student Rec. Ctr. TC
909-787-5731

Riverside, CA
UC Riverside, Phys. Ed.
909-787-5432

Running Springs, CA
Tension Masters and QG
909-867-6227

Sacramento, CA
Jujitsu-Do MA Center
916-728-2237

Sacramento, CA
Tara Stiles
916-454-5526

Sacramento, CA
Judy Tretheway
916-921-9184

San Bernardino, CA
Ctr.—Spirit Enrichment
909-885-1290 or 909-384-0061

San Diego, CA
Hsing I MA Inst.
619-698-6389

San Diego, CA
SD Taiji and QG Assn.
619-463-8260

San Diego, CA
Taoist Sancty. of San Diego
619-692-1155

San Diego, CA
The Chi Garden
760-749-9345

San Diego, CA
T'ai Chi Chih/QG
858-272-5067

San Diego, CA
TC/QG Healthways
858-793-8939

San Diego, CA
Golden Leopard Kempo
www.goldenleopard.org

San Diego, CA
N. Clairmont Rec. Ctr
858-581-9926

San Francisco, CA
East/West Acdmy. Hlg. Arts
415-788-2227

San Francisco, CA
Int'l Tibetan QG Assn.
415-982-5303

San Francisco, Bay Area, CA
Donald/Cheryl Lynne Rubbo
415-456-9095

San Francisco, CA
American QG Assn.
415-788-2227

SF East Bay Area, CA
TC Chih/QG School
925-253-9723

San Francisco, CA
Mountain Wind QG
415-282-4896

SF/Berkeley, CA
UCSF and UC Berkeley
415-221-7422 (phone/fax)

San Francisco, CA
TC with heartLove!
510-237-7196

San Francisco, CA (SF and S. Bay)
Bay Area Chen TC
415-378-8661

San Francisco, CA
World QG Fed.
415-788-2227

San Jose, CA
The Longevity Center
408-295-5911

San Jose, CA
Quang Ping Tai-Chi
408-287-6346

Sanger, CA
TC Club of Sanger
556-875-5930

San Jacinto, CA
Mt. San Jacinto Clg.
909-487-67-6752, ext. 1701 and 1702

San Leandro, CA
TC, SL Adult School
(Rosalind L. Braga)
510-667-6089

Santa Barbara, CA
SB Clg. of Oriental Med.
805-898-1180

Santa Cruz, CA
TC Natural Health Club
831-423-2037 or 831-429-0166

Santa Cruz, CA
TC Ch'uan
Catalyst Assoc.
831-427-1467

Santa Monica, CA
Shaolin QG/Emperor's
College of TCM
909-659-6238

Santa Monica/Los Angeles, CA
Peaceful Way TC Chuan
310-479-3646

Santa Monica, CA
SMTC Chuan/QG
(Joe Lopez)
310-394-1458

Santa Rosa/Occidental, CA
Jane Golden's TC/QG
707-874-2042

Sebastopol, CA
Integrative Body Works
707-824-9630

Sebastopol, CA
Taolist Med. QG Center
707-829-1855

Silicon Valley, CA
The Longevity Center
408-295-5911

Templeton, CA
Templeton Healing Arts
805-434-5177

Temple City, CAQG
QG Int'l/Kungfu
818-753-3200

Ventura County, CA
TC Chih
1-877-982-4244 (1-877-9TAICHI)

Ventura, CA
Dr. of Oriental Medicine
(Fred Siciliano)
805-654-8776

Walnut Creek, CA
TC Chih/QG
925-254-3368

Watsonville, CA
Cass Redmon
831-684-1876

West Los Angeles, CA
Peter Asco Tai-Chi
310-474-4959

Westminster, CA
Bone Marrow QG
714-890-0809

Colorado

Boulder, CO
Healing Tao QG Ctr.
303-545-0983

Boulder, CO
Human Performance Assn.
dgdelaney@aol.com

Colorado Springs, CO
KF Acy. and Hlg. Arts Ctr
719-641-6572

Colorado Springs, CO
Mvmt. for Well-Being
(JudyAnne Light)
719-444-8414

Denver, CO
TC Chih at Earth Spirit
303-239-9638

Grand Junction, CO
Colorado TC
970-245-7468

Lafayette, CO
Rocky Mnt. Body/Mind Institute
303-499-2755

Lakewood, CO
Green Mtn. Rec. Ctr.
303-987-7830

Nederland, CO
QG Research/Practice Ctr.
303-258-0971

Pagosa Springs, CO
Yung-Sen Chen, D.O.M.
970-264-6471

Parker, CO
Omega MA
303-680-3567

Pueblo, CO
Gaia Inst. Wellness Ctr.
719-545-8440

Woodland Park, CO
KF Acy. and Hlg. Arts Ctr.
719-686-1830

Connecticut

Weston, CT
Dynamic Peace
Taiji (Myles MacVane)
203-221-7839

Branford/West Haven, CT
Silent Dragon Schools
203-488-8558

Chaplin, CT
Starfarm TC
860-455-0353

Colchester/Norwich, CT
Peaceful Wolf TC
860-873-1409

Elmwood, CT
White Lotus MA
860-232-0109

Greenwich, CT
Greenwich Hospital
203-863-4277

Killingworth, CT
Eagle's Quest TC
(David Chandler)
1-800-4TAICHI
(1-800-482-4244)

Manchester, CT
Malee's School of TC/KF
860-646-6818

Manchester, CT
Ju Nan Shin
MA Acdmy.
860-643-JUDO, ext. 5836

Meriden, CT
Central CT TC
203-235-5703

New Haven, CT
Silent Dragon-KF/TC
203-937-0402

Newington, CT
Dragonfly TC
860-665-9034

North Westchester, NY
Red Lion TC (also in CT)
(Linda Schneiderman)
914-242-0778

Norwalk, CT
Waterwheel TC
203-852-0522

Shelton, CT
Dynamic Defense Systems
(Hassan Z Sailed)
203-922-9343

Stamford, CT
HealthGain.org
203-637-3417

Unionville, CT
Chi-Lel QG
860-675-8484

Waterford, CT
C. C. Chen's
Yang Style TC
860-444-0355

West Hartford, CT
White Lotus MA/
Reiki Center
860-232-0109

West Haven, CT
Silent Dragon TC KF
203-937-0402

Woodbury, CT
USA MA
203-266-9172

Delaware

Newark, DE
Chinese MA and TC Inst.
302-731-5992

Wilmington/Newark, DE
Sun KF School
302-731-5992 or 302-764-2284

Wilmington, DE
Ming Tao TC
302-636-0706

Wilmington, DE
TC for Life
302-354-0435

Florida

Boca Raton, FL
KF Cnsrvtry.
561-367-7788

Bonita Springs, FL
Dragon's Gate, Inc., QG/TC
941-435-6641

Bradenton, FL-Lee's
White Leopard KF
941-795-6986

Deland, FL
Golden Phoenix TC/QG
386-734-4020

Dunedin, FL
Chinese MA Ctr.
727-734-8222

Fort Lauderdale, FL
TC/QG at the Tennis Club

Fort Lauderdale, FL
QG Wellness Ctr.
(Stacy Kropp)
954-476-6654

Hollywood/Fort Lauderdale, FL
Chung TC Ctr.
954-229-9580

Hollywood, FL
Healing Tao of S. FL.
954-927-2836

Hollywood, FL
East Coast TC/QG
954-925-6654

Jacksonville, FL
Ctr. for Ntr'l. Health
904-396-3896

Jacksonville, FL
Cobalt Moon Hlg. Ctr.
904-246-2131

Jacksonville, FL
TC Foundation/School
904-723-6080

Lake Worth, FL
SNI—Massage and Therapies
561-582-5349

Longwood, FL
White Dragon KF/TC
407-924-7686

Miami, FL
Wing Lung KF/TC Assn.
305-253-7162

Miami, FL
Chinese Internal MAs
305-218-5229

Miami, FL
WITHIN Wellness Ctr.
305-668-0570

Naples, FL
Maria Okie Baum
941-514-4764

New Smyrna Beach, FL
TC by the Sea
904-423-0083

Orlando, FL
Life-Align
407-699-5444

Orlando, FL
Falun Gong
407-673-1255

Orlando, FL
Life-Align
407-699-5444

Plantation, FL
White Crane Natural Living Ed. Ctr.
954-474-5404

Pompano Beach, FL
Qi Gong Care
954-782-6281

Sarasota, FL
3 Treasures School
941-488-7384

Siesta Key/Sarasota, FL
Tantra TC/TC Chih
941-346-1024

Stuart, FL
Chinese MA, Long yu Feng
561-521-4447/220-2552

Tampa, FL
Golden Golden Dragon QG Inst.
813-361-5862

Tampa, FL
Univ. of S. Florida's TC
rtabler@hsc.usf.edu

Venice, FL
TC/KF Alliance
941-492-2167

Vero Beach, FL
VBTC/KF Club
561-778-8877

Georgia

Athens, GA
Shaoming School of TC
706-548-6252

Atlanta, GA
TC Chuan
404-881-0030

Atlanta, GA
Relief Enterprises
770-987-3983

Carrollton, GA
Tallapoosa Center
770-214-8077

College Park, GA
TC Health Scty.
770-996-5622

Decatur, GA
Tai-Chi Assn., Inc.
404-289-5652

Roswell, GA
Christopher Gresov, Ph.D.
770-552-1232

Hawaii

Big Island, HI
TC Assn.
(Sifu Howard James)
808-965-7622

Hilo, HI
Peter Tam Hoy's Scl. of TC
808-982-5403

Honolulu, HI
Limin QG TC Ctr.
808-941-9707

Honolulu, HI
East West QG Int'l.
808-941-9707

Honolulu, HI
Tse QG Centre
808-528-8501
866-Tse-Tse-8

Honolulu, HI
Dong Family Int'l
TC Assn.
808-949-5774

Kailua, HI
Joe Bright's TC
808-247-0679

Kaua'i, HI
Kaua'I School of TC
808-828-1139

Kihei, HI
Tiger and Dragon
(Cory Williams)
808-879-7067

Lihue, HI (Kauai)
dba Ke ala T'ai Chi
(Nii and Bailey, LLC)
808-245-7318/822-2447

Makawao, Maui, HI
HI TC Ch'uan Assn.
808-572-6994

Idaho

Boise, ID
Dancing Bear
TC/QG School
208-424-9528

Illinois

Arlington Heights, IL
Forest View Ed. Ctr.
847-718-7700

Carpentersville, IL
Martin Miller
847-426-5158

Chicago, IL
Wai Lun Choi's Chinese MA
773-472-3331

Chicago, IL
Freedom Acdmy. 3001
1-800-864-2133

Chicago, IL
The Admiral
773-561-2900

Chicago, IL
Chicago TC quan Assn.
773-973-1684

Chicago, IL
Integrative Wellness
773-769-3169

Chicago, IL
The Human Process, Inc.
773-769-0993

Effingham, IL
Champions Martial Arts
217-342-5425

Joliet, IL
TC and Massage
(Jeff Lindstrom)
815-722-1029

Kankakee, IL
Stress Mngmt. Workshops, Inc.
815-474-8388

Lake Zurich, IL
LZ Park District
847-438-5146

Niles, IL
World Qi-Gong Ctr.
847-581-9090

Northbrook, IL
Ching Ying TC/KF
847-679-3113

Oak Park, IL
TC and QG classes/Oak Park
708-848-7050

Peoria, IL
Tai Ji for Life
309-692-4209

Plainfield, IL
Greg Mucci Ten Lives TC
815-722-1029

Springfield, IL
Wellness Institute
217-629-9897

St. Charles, IL
TC Shaolin Chuan Assn.
630-443-0070

Waukegan, IL
Juhua Shan Yangsheng Gong
(S. E. Alleyne)
847-599-8886

Indiana

Bloomington, IN
New School TC
812-332-9741 or 812-339-2219

Bloomington, IN
IN Univ. Taiji
(Madeleine Gonin)
812-323-0197

Bloomington, IN
The Arana Center
812-336-5009

Highland, IN
Krucek QG Acdmy.
219-923-1788

Indianapolis, IN
Tigerlily TC/Aikido
317-579-9055

Indianapolis, IN
TC of Indianapolis
317-887-3430

Milan, IN
Kissell Shaolindo
812-654-2165

Seymour, IN
Middle Way TC
812-522-7482

Whiting, IN
Arts of Wisdom KF/TC
219-659-8513

Iowa

Des Moines, IA
Chinese MA Acdmy.
515-274-1065

Kansas

Kansas City, KS
Stress Free Living
(Dan Baxley)
913-334-6676

Lawrence, KS
Lunaria Holistic Hlth.
785-841-1587

Mission, KS
Compltry./Alt. Med. Ctr.
913-432-3966 (phone/fax)

Overland Park, KS
TC/QG
913-648-2256

Kentucky

Murray, KY
TC Assn. of Murray
270-753-9371

Salyersville, KY
Wayne Hall TC/Chi QG
606-886-9450

Versailles, KY
KY TC Assn.
859-879-9434
or 502-222-5277

Louisiana

New Orleans, LA
Acdmy. of MA
504-466-4060

New Orleans, LA
School of Ntr'l. Living
504-949-8876

New Orleans, LA
Chen Pan-ling Inst.
504-861-4283

Shreveport, LA
Lee's KF/TC Ctr.
318-869-1122

Maine

Brunswick, ME
N. Chi MA Ctr.
207-721-0299

Portland, ME
Full Circle Synergy TC
207-780-9581

Rockland, ME
Mussel Bch. Hlth. Club
207-594-1957

Turner, ME
Yeung Style TC
abyss@megalink.net

Wallagrass, ME
Laughing Dragon Tao TC
207-834-6986

Wiscasset, ME
Wiscasset Rec. Ctr.
207-882-8230

Maryland

Annapolis, MD
QG with Kimberly
410-626-7557

Annapolis/Severna Pk, MD
Peaceable Dragon
410-626-8951

Baltimore, MD
Com. Health/Network, Inc.
410-235-9194

Baltimore, MD
LifeQuest MD TC Assn.
410-654-6793

Baltimore, MD
TC in Baltimore
410-296-4946

Bethesda, MD
Cloud Hands TC
301-562-0992

Camp Springs, MD
Skyvalley Tai Ji
301-379-4370

Ellicott City, MD
Ohashiatsu
410-313-8501

Frederick, MD
Scott Acdmy. of MA
301-694-4714

Gaithersburg, MD
Dancing Mtn. TaijiQuan
301-565-3320

Laurel, MD
School of TC of MD, Inc.
301-953-3115

Rockville, MD
WuWei TC w/David Chen
301-460-6575

Silver Spring, MD
Wu Shen Tao Hlth./MA Ctr.
301-565-0665

Silver Spring, MD
MD Dance of Phoenix QG
301-622-6328

Takoma Park, MD
Chan's QiGong
301-270-8416

Sykesville, MD
Three Treasures Health
410-549-0156

Massachusetts

Boston, MA
Bow Sim Mark TC
617-426-0958

Boston, MA
Guang Ping Yang TC Assn.
508-362-0079

Boston, MA
Boston Healing Tao
617-628-6570

Boston, MA
Pa Kua KF School
603-595-8257

Boston, MA
AndyG.com
617-713-3840

Boston, MA
Yang's MA Assn.
617-524-8892

Boston, MA
Asian-Amer. Cultural Ctr.
781-532-2259

Chelmsford, MA
Oriental Culture Instit.
508-572-1246

Dedham, MA
Dedham Commty. House
508-362 0079

Duxbury, MA
Moving Meditations
781-834-4343

Franklin/North Attleboro, MA
KF Academy
508-520-3717 or 508-699-2233

Hanover, MA
Harmony Wellness Ctr. TC
781-829-4300

Holliston, MA
Chinese Med. and TC Ctr.
508-429-3895

South Yarmouth, MA
Midcape Racquet and Hlth.
508-394-3511

Millbury, MA
Wah Lum KF and TC Inst.
508-752-3534

Northampton, MA
Deer Mountain TC Academy
413-584-4615

Norwood, MA
In the Moment Wllns. Ctr.
508-362-0079

Norwood, MA
Guang Ping Yang TC Assn.
781-762-9281

Plymouth, MA
Dragon Gate Int'l. Arts
508-833-8852

Salem, MA
North Shore Healing Tao
978-744-5685

Somerville, MA
Boston Healing Tao
(Dir. Marie Favorito)
617-628-6570

South Yarmouth, MA
Midcape Racquet and Hlth.
508-362-0079

Watertown, MA
Pooled Resources
(Judith Poole)
617-923-8856

Wayland, MA
Longfellow Club, QG
617-923-8856

West Newton, MA
European Health Spa, QG
617-923-8856

Yarmouthport, MA
Guang Ping Yang TC Assn.
508-362-0079

Michigan

Ann Arbor, MI
Peaceful Dragon TC and KF
734-741-0695

Birch Rung, MI
Cloud Hands
517-624-5548

Holt, MI
Eight Willows KF Group
517-694-5851

Lansing, MI
Moving Stillness
517-229-4208

Livonia, MI
Traditional Arts—Orient
734-425-3741

Mt. Pleasant, MI
Pat's TAI JI FUN
517-773-3553

Saginaw, MI
Cloud Hands
517-752-0362

Troy, MI
Yang Cheng Fu TC Center
248-680-8938

Minnesota

Duluth, MN
Healing Tao
(Kate Pearson)
218-722-0881

Duluth, MN
Duluth TC Study Group
218-723-6476

Ely/Isabella, MN
School—Herbest Ridge
218-365-2420

Minneapolis/St.Paul, MN
Dragon Door QG
651-645-0517

Rochester, MN
The Rochester TC Club
507-289-7777

St. Paul, MN
Three Rivers Crossing QG
651-291-7772

St. Paul, MN
World Inst. for Self-Hlg.
612-998-8811 or 651-645-2985

St Paul, MN
Wendy Howard—TC Chih
651-489-3775

St. Cloud, MN
St. Cloud Karate/TC Inst.
320-252-0144

Mississipi

Ocean Springs, MS
Teoul Moon KF
228-209-6277

Sandhill, MS
Medical QG America
601-291-4930

Missouri

Hartsburg, MO
Synature
573-556-6716

Joplin, MO
School of TC
417-624-2466

KC Metro, MO
Stress Mngt. TC/QG
913-648-2256

KC Metro, MO
TC w/Linda Bowers
816-931-2193 or 913-631-9470

Milan, MO
Chin Tao Dojo—TC
660-265-3855

Springfield, MO
Springfield TC
417-836-8567

Springfield, MO
TC for ME!
417-888-0479

St. Louis, MO
Chinese Internal Arts
(Justin Meehan)
314-772-9494

St. Louis, MO
Turtlehawk Studio
314-776-1729

St. Louis, MO
Olivette Chai Chi/QG
314-567-6443

St. Louis, MO
Wu Hsing Chuan 5-Animal
314-721-6003

St. Louis, MO
U. City TC and QG Assn.
314-567-6443 (phone/fax)

St. Louis, MO
Feng Zhiqiang TC USA
(Sifu Herb Parran)
314-432-6152 (home)

St. Louis, MO
Learn TC with Anna Lum
314-567-5384

Montana

Clancy, MT
MountainSpirit QG
406-933-5390

Eureka, MT
Dancing Dreamers Ctr. QG
406-889-3966

Helena, MT
Sacred Mountain School TC
406-449-4759

Nebraska

Hastings, NE
South Central Taekwondo
402-463-2262

Lincoln, NE
TC Fitness
402-310-5990 or 402-474-0897

Omaha, NE
Omaha TC Assn.
402-292-6745

New Hampshire

Barrington, NH
Quest MA Academy
603-664-8938

Dover, NH
TC and QG Health w/Maya
603-749-1575

Londonderry, NH
Path of Harmony TC and QG
603-434-0655

Londonderry, NH
Alt. Health Collaborative
(Daniel L. Sayer)
603-624-1307

Manchester, NH
Yang Chengfu TC Ctrs.
(Michael Coulon)
603-663-3181

Nashua, NH
Healing Arts in Motion
603-881-3189

Nashua, NH
MA Ctr. for Personal Dev.
603-598-4200

New Jersey

Brick, NJ
China Hand KF Academy
732-920-0605

Cedar Grove, NJ
TC Chih
973-857-5981

Cedar Knolls, NJ
Hanover Taichi Club
973-538-9434

Clifton, NJ
TC Chih
973-777-6722

East Brunswick, NJ
Andy Lee Yang Chengfu TC
732-238-1414

Edison, NJ
World Inst.—Self-Hlg.
732-548-6534

Franklin Lk./Mntclr., NJ
Joanne Kornoelje
973-783-2972

Hackettstown, NJ
TC Now
1-800-366-3311

Hamilton, NJ
Phoenix Academy of MA
609-585-9366

Harrisburg, NJ
Penn. Chen TC quan Assoc.
1-888-625-1097

Irvington, NJ
Nat'l. Hlth. Inst.
QG and Tc
973-372-0700

Jersey City, NJ
Heaven and Earth Soc. TC
646-295-5090 or 201-725-4761

Medford, NJ
Harmony TC
856-797-0406

Metuchen, NJ
Black Belt Institute
732-205-9797

Middlesex, NJ
World Inst.—Self-Hlg.
732-563-4884

Middletown, NJ
Kum Sung TC MA
732-706-0900

Mt. Laurel, NJ
QG Research Society
856-234-3056

Mt. Laurel, NJ
Silver Tiger TC
856-778-4209

North Plainfield, NJ
TCC
908-757-3050

Oceanview, NJ
American Eagle TC/QG
609-390-0200

Oceanview, NJ
Teacher Training TC/QG Systems
PO Box 368
Oceanview, NJ 08230

Piscataway, NJ
Brian O'Connor's TC Group
732-699-0571

Short Hills, NJ
Aloha Holistic Health
973-376-4669

Tinton Falls, NJ
Red Bank Acupnctr./Wellns.
732-758-1800

Voorhees, NJ
Mind-Gym
1-888-VIRTUA-3 (1-888-847-8823)

New Mexico

Las Vegas, NM
Peter Stege, D.O.M.—QG
505-454-0003

Santa Fe, NM
White Crane Healing Arts
505-473-3063

New York

Albany, NY
TC and KF Assn.
518-459-6869

Athens, NY
Sleepy Hollow TC Assn.
518-945-1596

Beacon, NY
Homestyle QG
845-838-3165

Buffalo, NY
Shaolin Wahnam—Phil
716-308-4774

Buffalo, NY
Yang Chengfu TC Centers
(James Fox)
716-652-5221

Carmel, NY
Yang Chengfu TC Centers
(Bill Walsh)
914-225-0662

Congers, NY
Gongopeh TC and QG
914-267-2083

Croton-on-Hudson, NY
School of TC Chuan
1-800-446-6228

Depew, NY
Bill Adams's MA and Fitness
716-668-5004

Farmingdale, NY
Sun Tao TC
(John Page)
516-756-9129

Glens Falls, NY
Mark Tolstrup TC and QG
518-798-3023

Great Neck, NYC, NY
Har-Tzion
516-466-0605

Hampton Bays, NY
TC Center
(Tina Curran)
631-723-1923

High Falls, NY
Marbletown School of TC
914-378-5380

Hudson, NY
Human Performance Assn.
212-969-0552

Huntington, NY
Inner Way-Roger Sencer
631-423 4171

Long Beach, NY
Toburan Wholistic Health
www/toburan.com

Long Island and Sound Beach, NY
Long Island School of TC-Chuan
1-888-9TAICHI (1-888-982-4244)

Monticello, NY
Cheng Man-Ching TC, HTM
845-794-6847

Morrisville, NY
Wu Style TC
(David Dolbear)
315-662-7727

NYC, NY
TC Chih/TC
(Carolyn Perkins)
212-371-0133

NYC, NY
TC Chuan for Living
212-243-3172

NYC, NY
Lawrence Galante's TC
212-414-1266

NYC, NY
Taoist Yoga
(Sharon Smith)
212-243-6771

NYC, NY
H Won TC Inst.—Soon TC
212-594-3860

NYC, NY
Mark Sabin TC quan/92nd St. Y
212-677-0649

NYC, NY
H. Won T'ai-chi Inst.
212-594-3860

NYC, NY
The Universal Tao
212-243-6771

NYC, NY
Chen Style—TC Rsrch. Ctr.
212-928-3049

NYC, NY
William CC Chen TC, Inc.
212-675-2816

NYC, NY
Taoist Arts Center
212-477-7055

NYC, NY
Yang TC
(Richard Jesaitis)
646-698-3375

NYC, NY
The Seed, Ctr. QG Dept.
212-343-1541

NYC, NY (Queens)
Forest Hills TC Assn.
(Michael Ferstendig)
718-544-3656

NYC, NY
Ancient Fitness Academy
212-658-9891

NYC, NY
School of TC, Inc.
212-502-4112

NYC, NY
Heaven and Earth Soc. of TC
646-295-5090 or 201-725-4761

NYC, NY
Ancient Fitness Academy
718-774-9489

NYC, NY
Ahn TC—Studios
212-481-2553

Nyack, NY
Nyack KF/TC Academy
914-353-7800

Patchogue, NY
Water Tiger TC in Park
(Laurince D. McElroy)
631-475-5730

Petersburgh, NY
Yang Chengfu TC
(Beth Bacon)
518-658-3929

Pulaski, NY
Sequoia Spiritual Retrt.
315-298-5277

Rochester, NY
Wu Xing Institute
716-392-5141

Rochester, NY
Northeastern MA
716-889-7330

Rochester, NY
Rochester TC Ch'uan Center
716-461-0130

Sparkill, NY
Dominican Center, TC Chih
914-359-6400, ext. 215

Staten Island, NY
Rick Barrett TC
718-720-0367

Syracuse, NY
Central NY TC and QG Center
315-427-0098

Syracuse, NY
Syracuse TC Chuan Academy
315-455-3888

Tarrytown/Manhattan, NY
EverSpring Center
914-631-2773

Warwick, NY
Hudson Valley TC
1-888-727-6929

Warwick, NY
Warwick TC
914-988-9781

West Hempstead, NY
Chen Dottie School
516-292-1757

White Plains, NY
TaiJiWS
914-206-7627

Woodstock/Catskill Mnt., NY
Healing Tao Summer Retrt.
1-888-432-5826

Yonkers, NY
Chinese Rsrch. Inst.
914-965-9196

Yorktown Heights, NY
Nat Costanzo's KF/TC Ctr.
914-243-5646

North Carolina

Asheville, NC
Mountain Dragon TC/KF
828-285-0564

Asheville, NC
Ctr. for Personal Mastery
1-800-274-8197

Chapel Hill, NC
Magic Tortoise TC School
919-968-3936

Charlotte, NC
The Peaceful Dragon
704-544-1012

Forest City, NC
Indominable Spirit TC
(Ray Rice)
828-288-1049

Gibsonville, NC
Silk Tiger School of TC
336-449-3284

Greensboro, NC
East Gate Acpnctr. Ctr.
336-370-4399

Greensboro, NC
EarthStar TC Ctr.
336-272-7127

Raleigh, NC
Inner Mtn. Jrny. TC Chih
919-821-1172

Vandemere, NC
Dragon Gate Taijiquan
252-745-7840

Winston-Salem, NC
Golden Flower TC Schools
337-768 1260

North Dakota

Fargo, ND
The Spirit Room—TC and QG
701-237-0230

Ohio

Ashtabula, OH
Wellness/Total Lrng. Ctr.
440-997-5353

Bayview, OH
TC Wu Style/Horn's MA
419-684-9179

Bedford Heights, OH
Golden Pyramid MA Ctr.
440-232-4694

Bowling Green, OH
School-Herbest Ridge
419-833-3526

Cincinnati, OH
White Willow School of TC
513-791-9428

Cincinnati, OH
Essence in Movement
513-792-2302

Cincinnati, OH
Soaring Crane QG and TC
513-674-1179

Cincinnati, OH
Mighty Vine Wellness Club
513-241-9355

Cleveland, OH
Susana Weingarten QG
216-289-4144

Cleveland, OH
Healthy Hm., Healthy Body
440-845-7357

Cleveland, OH
QG Academy
216-749-9811

Dover, OH
Chinese TC
330-343-7648

Lakewood, OH
Tao's Healing Way
216-521-9779 or 216-226-5161

Mansfield, OH
Purple Bamboo Int. Arts.
(Laurie Brady)
419-525-0407

Mentor, OH
Karate Kajukenpo Assn.
440-951-0463

Middletown, OH
Miami University Club
(Dr. Michael Steward Sr.)
513-422-1735

Monroe, OH
Quisno Wellness Ctr. Club
(Dr. Michael Steward Sr.)
513-422-1735

Oxford, OH
Oxford Club. Univ. Campus
(Dr. Michael Steward Sr.)
513-422-1735

Pomeroy, OH
Ramona Compton
740-992-5208

Stow, OH
White Birch Traditional MA
330-329-5990

Toledo, OH
Dragon Tai-Chi Players
419-578-1067

Toledo, OH
Toledo TC
(Carl Holas)
419-474-8736

West Chester, OH
School
(Susan Evans)
513-779-4757

Kirtland/Lake County, OH
Prisma Ctr. QG/Wholstc.
440-256-2273 or 1-888-729-2273

Youngstown, OH
TC Step One
330-746-5933

Oklahoma

Tulsa, OK
Nutri-Chi QG
918-437-3949

Oregon

Ashland, OR
Shaolin Wahnam QG/KF
541-552-0346

Bend, OR
CenterPoint Health Inst.
eorem@hotmail.com

Corvallis, OR
QG Assn. of America
541-752-6599

Eugene, OR
Tranquility Thru Movement
541-484-1680

Eugene, OR
Abode of the Eternal Tao
541-345-8854

Eugene, OR
Strawberry Gatts School
sgatts@hotmail.com

Eugene, OR
The School of TC Chuan
(Bill Faust)
541-345-3389

Forest Grove, OR
Yang ChengFu TC Ctr.
(Dave Barrett)
503-357-8917

Lake Oswego/Portland, OR
Pat Fisher—TC Chih
503-635-4336

Portland, OR
CloudWater TC
503-640-4892

Portland, OR
Wu Dao Jing She—Int'l. QG
503-252-8589

Portland, OR
School of TC Chuan
503-222-2289

Pennsylvania

Allentown, PA
Little Tiger TC and Therapy
610-432-5001

Belle Vernon, PA
Chon's Korean Karate TC
724-929-3822 or 724-929-3128

Bethlehem, PA
School Thomas Ardizzone
610-758-9596

Blue Bell, PA
Greater Philly. Karate/QG
610-2879-3686

Bristol, PA
Dragon Moon MA Assn.
215-788-3313

Brodheadsville, PA
Gentle Strength QG Group
570-992-3448

Bucks County/Levittown, PA
Three Dragon Flame
215-364-5350

Doylestown, PA
Rolly Brown's TC
215-862-1924

Erie, PA
Body Awareness—TC quan
814-456-9084

Fairless Hills, PA
Core Essence/QG Training
215-547-1655

Hanover, PA
Margery Erickson/TC Chih
717-632-4358

Kingston, PA
Chinese Health Institute
570-822-1988

Kingston, PA
Sakura MA Ctr./TC
570-288-7865

Lancaster, PA
Central PA QG Assn.
717-295-2423 or 717-295-1246

Lansdowne, PA
Tiger Mountain Taijiquan
610-623-1525

Lansdowne, PA
Trinity Untd. Mthdst.
610-623-1525 (leave message)

Lebanon, PA
Bow Sim Mark's TC Arts
717-274-2961

Leechburg, PA
Inner Strength, Inc.
724-845-1041

Lehigh Valley, PA
Manawa Universal Arts
manawatc@aol.com
610-944-0072

Meadville/Franklin, PA
Cootie Harris School—TC
jrhoople@netscape.net

Palmyra, PA
Judy Bayliss' Chi Lel QG
717-832-0982

Philadelphia, PA
TC and Bodymind Empwrmnt.
215-886-7363

Philadelphia, PA
Holistic Hands
215-248-4716

Philadelphia, PA
Chen Taijiquan Assn.
1-888-625-1097

Philadelphia, PA
QG Research Society
856-234-3056

Philadelphia, PA
Ba Z TC/KF (Wu Tang Sys.)
215-882-2804

Philadelphia, PA
Goldenlight Ctr.
215-695-0870

Philadelphia, PA
Penna. Chen TC Quan Assn.
1-877-762-6521

Pittsburgh, PA
Yin Cheng Gong Fa Assn.
724-940-1818

Uniontown, PA
White Dragon TC/Wlns. Ctr.
724-434-1140

West Chester, PA
Peter Herman's TC
610-696-4664

Westtown, PA
TC at the Concept School
610-696-4664

York, PA
TC Chih
(Cathy Lehman)
717-755-6119

Rhode Island

Harrisville, RI
Dalant Studio—Yang TC/QG
401-568-9835

South Carolina

Charleston, SC
The School of TC Chuan
(Kathleen Post)
843-883-9626

Columbia, SC
Circle's Ctr. TC and QG
803-254-5487

Columbia, SC
Columbia School of TC
803-783-2494

Spartanburg, SC
Nine Star Healing Arts
864-582-8779 or 864-621-0831

Tennessee

Cookeville, TN
TC Instruction
931-839-6539

Knoxville, TN
Flying Dragon Chinese MA
865-219-0303

Knoxville, TN
5 Elements TC School
865-690-6490

Nashville, TN
TC Chuan Assn., Nashville
615-429-0840

Nashville, TN
YMCA
(Tom Williams)
615-834-1300

Texas

Arlington, TX
John P. Painter, Ph.D., N.D.
817-860-0129

Austin, TX
Tom Gohring's TC
512-422-4245

Austin, TX
TaiChi People
512-236-1503

Austin TX
Heloise Gold—TC/QG
512-444-6139

Dallas, TX
Lee's White Leopard KF/TC
972-991-1088

Deer Park, TX
Hassan Z. Saijyid/Judy Covin/Tandy Robinson
281-476-1742

El Paso, TX
Texas TC
Sifu Ray Abeyta
915-584-8758

EL Paso, TX
Center for Internal Arts
915-584-4730

Fort Worth, TX
Taijiquan, QG, Chi-Lel
817-454 6888

Fort Worth, TX
North Texas Kinematics
817-498-5023

Georgetown, TX
TC Chih/TC (Jo Trautmann)
512-868-2583

Grapevine/Ft. Worth, TX
Chi-Works
817-808-8990

Houston, TX
Wu Shu KF Fed., Inc.
713-464-3128

Houston, TX
EastWest Wellness Center
281-480-2425

Lago Vista, TX
Dr. Olaf Haug's TC and QG
512-267-9784

League City (Houston), TX
Al Garza's MA America
281-332-5425

Lubbock, TX
Larry Sava—HealthPoint
806-722-3162

San Antonio, TX
Yang Chengfu TC Centers
(Horacio Lopez)
210-225-2743

Wichita Falls, TX
TC/KF Club-Wichita Falls
940-322-7184 or 940-322-8898

Wichita Falls, TX
D.S.I. TC KF Club
940-322-8898

Utah

Provo, UT
TC Group
801-361-1883

Salt Lake City, UT
Dao-yin Taiji Study Grp.
801-295-7266

Virginia

Accotink/Alexandria/Burke/
Arlington/Oakton, VA
Peaceable Dragon
703-455-4858

Annandale, VA
TC/Kali/Silat Orgz.
703-941-7406

Arlington, VA
White Birch School—KF/TC
703-920-9746

Arlington, VA
Skyvalley Tai Ji
301-379-4370

Charlottesville, VA
Blue Ridge Chi (TC)
434-293-8983 (voicemail)

Chesapeake, VA
Great Bridge Rec. Ctr. TC
757-548-9971

Williamsburg/
Hampton Roads, VA
Starr Natural Hlth.—QG/TC
757-599-9168 or 757-713-6699

Herndon, VA
Qi Elements School—TC/KF
703-435-4400

Richmond, VA
Pa Kua KF School
804-794-8384

Richmond, VA
Oriental Med. Spclst., PC
804-350-7767

Springfield, VA
Sheng Zhen QG
703-455-4858

Troutville, VA
Toan Chau Nguyen TC Ctr.
540-977-3925 or 540-977-3750

Winchester, VA
Pat Rice-Yang Chengfu TC
540-667-7595

Washington

Anderson Island, WA
TC Chih-Rita Jacobsen
solucid@yahoo.com

Bellingham, WA
Bellingham KF/TC Club
360-714-0264

Kirkland, WA
Judy Jones, TC Chih
425-899-2264

Oak Harbor, WA
TC
(Jill Vulcano Reed)
360-675-1464

Port Orchard, WA
American Shaolin MA
360-895-7819

Port Orchard, WA
Shoayin Body Work, Inc.
360-874-1209

Seattle, WA
Chinese Wushu and TC Acdmy.
(Master Yijiao Hong)
206-749-9513

Seattle, WA
Embrace the Moon TC and QG
206-789-0993

Seattle, WA
Yin Yang Arts Center
206-935-2315

Seattle Area, WA
Wu Dang Internal Arts
206-550-4908 or 425-883-1883

Seattle, WA
QG Longevity Assn.
206-547-2435 or 425-883-1883

Seattle, WA
Yang Jun-Yang Chengfu TC
206-447-2759

Shelton, WA
Dong Family Int'l. TC
360-432-9477

Spokane, WA
School of TC Chuan
509-747-3715

Spokane, WA
Northwest TC Assn.
jhspok@yahoo.com

Vashon, WA
Island Internal MA
206-463-6309

Walla Walla, WA
Wen Wu School of TC
509-529-7501

Washington, D.C.

DC Metro Area
The TC Ch'uan Study Ctr.
703-759-9141

Washington, DC
TC Chih w/Dale Buchanan
703-736-5543

Washington, DC
Skyvalley Tai Ji
301-379-4370

West Virginia

Huntington, WV
Eight-Treasures TC and QG
kelliott@foothills.net

Wheeling, WV
Appalachian TC and QG Assn.
304-845-3662 or 304-242-1979

Wisconsin

Appleton, WI
QG Life Enhancement Ctr.
920-738-6628

Brookfield WI
Quest Int'l., Self-Defense
262-783-2273

Hudson, WI
Wind and Water QG
715-381-5630

La Crosse, WI
Univ. of Wisconsin
608-785-8166

Lake Geneva, WI
WMB Training
(Walter Brown)
262-249-8802

Madison, WI
Silver Dragon TC/QG
608-233-9446

Manitowoc, WI
Bruckner's MA Academy
920-682-1001

Menomonie, WI
YamaMizu Ryui WI School MA
715-235-7711

Milwaukee, WI
Milwaukee TC—Yang
414-454-9445

Milwaukee, WI
Inst. Holistic Med.
414-438-9488

Milwaukee, WI
TC Studies
414-328-9064

Milwaukee, WI
Quest Int'l. Self Defense
262-783-2273

Milwaukee, WI
White Crane
262-784-5297

Waukesha, WI
Shao Lin Boxing, KF Inst.
262-548-8824

Wausau, WI
WI Wen Wu School of TC
715-845-8767

International Organizations and Schools

In this section you will find some detailed contact information for Australia, Canada, New Zealand, South Africa, and the United Kingdom. For T'ai Chi and QiGong contact information for nearly 50 other nations worldwide, visit www.worldtaichiday.org, where you will also find constantly updated and more expansive information for many of the following listings.

Australia

New South Wales

Bega, NSW
Gippsland/SCTC and QG Acdmy.
02-64941240

Fernmount, NSW
Black Eagle Boxing/Hlth.
02-66559249

Liverpool, NSW
Liverpool TC
(John Mills)
02-98250397

Miranda, NSW
Australian Clg. of TC/QG
(Sam Li)
02-95401044
(Rachel Addison)
02-95404045

Sydney, NSW
1 Better Health TC Chuan
2 TC Assn. of Australia
02-98250397

Sydney, NSW
Sydney Vision TC/QG Health
02-47586460

Sydney, NSW
Australia TC Vacations
taichismrt@aol.com

Sydney, NSW
Sydney TC and QG Ctr.
02-98188229 or 02-98100162

Queensland

Gold Coast, Queensland
Gold Coast TC Academy
07-55245238

Qld Ntrl. Therapies Clgs.
Mstr. Linage E. Montaigue
07-55920210

South Australia

Adelaide, SA
Moving Meditation/QG
08-83817969

Victoria

Bairnsdale/Gippsland/South Coast, Victoria
TC and QG Academy
03-51521870

Berwick, Victoria
Golden Lion Academy
03-97961066

Churchill/Morwell/Traralgon, Victoria
TC—Adv. Students and Health
03-51222588 or 04-19106469 (cell)

Melbourne, Victoria
Middle Park TC
03-96902238

Traralgon/Newborough,
Gippland, Victoria
TC and QG Acdmy.
02-64941240 or 03-51521870

Western Australia

Perth, WA
The Healing Chi Assn.
08-94051476

Canada

Alberta

Edmonton, Alberta
Chai Holistic Health Svc.
780-467-8701

Fort McMurray, Alberta
Fort McMurray Study Grp.
780-790-2055

Sherwood Park, Alberta
Chai Holistic Health Svc.
780-467-8701

British Columbia

Duncan, BC
100th Monkey QG House
250-748-2931

Duncan, BC
Long Life Qi Center
250-701-2266

Kelowna, BC
Dancing Dragon School
250-762-5982

Kelowna, BC
Yang TC Chuan Club
250-862-9327

Parksville, BC
Madrona Point TC
250-468-9950

Quesnel, BC
Rivers TC Studio
250-992-8024

Terrace, BC
Terrace TC Chuan
250-638-1594 (phone/fax)

Vancouver, BC
Chinese TC Assn. of Canada
604-421-6398

New Brunswick

Miramichi City
Miramichi TC and Aikido
506-633-7124

Nova Scotia

Halifax, Nova Scotia
NV School of KF and TC
902-443-5500

Ontario

Almonte, Ontario
Healing Tao/Chi Nei Tsang
613-256-4786

Brantford, Ontario
Yellow River TC School
519-759-8827

Cambridge, Ontario
Goshin Dojo
519-653-9185

Kitchener, Ontario
Cold Mtn. Internal Arts
519-576-3206

London, Ontario.
Phoenix TC Ctr.
519-439-8875

Ottawa, Ontario
World Institute for Self-Hlg., Inc.
613-591-9751

Ottawa, Ontario
Chow QG Ottawa
613-234-6369

Peterborough, Ontario
Peterborough TC Assn.
705-743-9161

Toronto, Ontario
Rising Sun School of TC
416-533-3352

Toronto, Ontario
Shaolin Wahnam—Jean
416-979-0238

Toronto, Ontario
Int'l. Inst.—Zhi Neng
416-497-9632

Toronto, Ontario
High Park MA Academy
416-769-9222

Toronto, Ontario
TC Ch'uan Study Group
416-975-5087

Toronto, Ontario
Mo's Society of TC
416-370 2987

Toronto, Ontario
East/West Acy.—Hlg. Arts
416-920-4008

Toronto, Ontario
Chow QG Scarborough East
416-284-1994

Toronto, Ontario
Chow QG N. Scarborough
416-297-6990

Toronto, Ontario
Chow QG Toronto
416-920-4008

Toronto, Ontario
Chow QG Etobicoke
416-231-2731

Quebec

Montreal, Quebec
Ecole de TC Quan
514-274-2513

Montreal, Quebec
Seven Stars TC School
514-286-0786

Pierrefonds, Montreal
Yang Chengfu TC
(Sergio Arione)
514-624-9264

Saint-Jean-sur-Richelieu
Yang Chengfu TC
(Michel Tremblay)
450-359-0388

Salaberry de Valleyfield
La Voie du TC Chuan
(Gilles D'Anjou)
450-371-1690

Ulverton, Quebec
Centre Pierre Boogaerts
1-888-922-1146

New Zealand

Auckland, and all NZ
Sing Ong TC
0-96258833

Wellington
Silum Fut Gar KuneAncient QG/Yang TC
64-43896633

Wellington
Wu Tao Academy—TC/QG/KF
64-44711818

South Africa

European Assn. for Trad'l.
Wu TC—Robert Rudniak
27-214235192

Countrywide
World TC Boxing Assn. (WTBA)
27-119432654

Cape Town
Leslie James Reed—Shaolin
27-214391373

Cape Town (HQ)
(US and UK) Int'l. TC/Shaolin Wushu
0-214391373

Johannesburg
Shaolin MA Ctr.
27-117872790

Johannesburg
Intr'l. Arts Resrch. Ctr. of SA
27-117626417

Johannesburg
Living Tao S.A.
7866410

Johannesburg [4 Locs.]
TC Quan Institution S.A.
27-825721919

United Kingdom

TC Quan and QG Fed. for
Europe—UK Hdqrtrs.
secretary@taichiunion.com

European Assn. for Trad'l.
Wu TC
(Daniel McGiff)
01-818889294

London/Manchester/Torquay
Birmingham/Huddersfield
Zhong Ding Assn.
02-088411054

Cambridgeshire

Peterborough
San Chai TC Agcy.
01-733270072

Channel Islands

Channel Islands
East-West Taoist Assn.
01-723354072 (UK number)

Coventry

Exhall Bedworth Nr
Healing Tao TC Class
07-803378856

County Durham

Newcastle TC with Me
British School of TC
01-913886520

Derbyshire

Chesterfield, Derbyshire
Lamas QG Assn. (Sifu Box)
01-246279515

Devon

Devon—QG Southwest
01-803863552

Hampshire

Portsmouth
University TC Club
02-392842568

Island of Anglesey

Amlwch/Llangefni/Llanerchymedd
"Health Through TC and QG"
Philip Mansfield on 01248 470231

Isle of Man

Sulby
Wu's TC Chuan Academy
01-624897041, 816069

Jersey

Jersey
East-West Taoist Assn.
01-723354072

Kent

Sidcup, Kent
Taoist Arts Org. (TAO)
01-813096717

Deal, Kent
Red Dragon Retreats
01-304362563

London

Crouch End, London
European Assn. for Trad'l. Wu Tai
02-088889294

Croydon, London
Master Khan Lamas QG Assn.
0-411261418

London, London
TC UK/Zenon Wudang TC
02-074074775

London, London
Tse QG Ctr.
01-619294485

Victoria
Master Khan Lamas QG Assn.
0-411261418

Manchester

Manchester
Tse QG Ctr.
01-619294485

Norfolk

Norwich
Norwich Tse TC and QG Club
01-603465189

North Yorkshire

Harrogate, N. Yorkshire
Lamas QG Assn.
(Mr. Jakobs)
01-423506788

Babworth, Nottinghamshire
Lamas QG Assn.
(Mr. Clarke)
01-777818822

Nottinghamshire

Easingwold, North Yorkshire
Lamas QG Assn.—Sifu Box
01-246279515

Lg. Eaton, Nottinghmshr.
White Cloud TC
01-158490048

Mansfield, Nottinghmshr.
Lamas QG Assn.—Sf Edwards
01-623646914

Newark, Nottinghamshire
Lamas QG Assn.
07-941154331 (Sifu Corroon)

Ranby, Nottinghamshire
Lamas QG Assn.
01-777860468 (Sifu Bailey)

Retford, Nottinghamshire
Lamas QG Assn.—Sijung Lowe
01-909 482190 or 01-777706808

Retford, Nottinghamshire
National QiGong College
01-777700055

Worksop, Nottinghamshire
Lamas QG Assn.—Sf Walker
01-909733892

Oxfordshire

Abingdon, Oxfordshire
Lamas QG Assn.
(Mr. Williams)
01-235532891

Headington, Oxfordshire
Lamas QG Assn.
01-235532891

Leys, Oxfordshire
Lamas QG Assn.
(Mr. Williams)
01-235532891

Oxford U, Oxfordshire
Lamas QG Assn.
(Mr. Williams)
01-235532891

Scarborough

Scarborough
East—West Taoist Assn.
01-723354072

Shropshire

Wellington, Shropshire
Arthritis Care
01-952242313

South Yorkshire

Doncaster, S. Yorkshire
LamasQG Assn.—Sf Sham
01-302538859

Doncaster, S. Yorkshire
Lamas QG Assn.—Mr. Browne
01-302721626

Whitby, S. Yorkshire
Lamas QG Assn.—Sf Sham
01-302538859

Surrey

Long Ditton
Jean Anderson, TC Teacher
02-083983029

Warwickshire

Town Bedworth, NR Nuneaton
Warwickshire, CV13 6 AY
Exhall TC Class

West Midlands

Birmingham
Kai Ming Assn.
(Mark Peters)
07831743737
01-214530500 (cell)

Yorkshire

Bradford, Yorkshire
Lamas QG Assn.—Sf Wharton.
01-274688642

Cleckheaton, Yorkshire
Lee Family Arts (LFA)
01-274879156

T'ai Chi/QiGong Associations and Actualism Centers

Actualism centers offer in-depth training in energy work, which is rooted in the same ancient truths as QiGong and Yogic energy healing, however Actualism is designed for the modern student and can make these sometimes esoteric concepts much more tangible and more immediately useful to the modern student. Visit www.actualism.org for details on what each Actualism Center offers. You'll find centers in several cities.

World T'ai Chi and QiGong Day
www.worldtaichiday.org
World T'ai Chi and QiGong Day works to recognize T'ai Chi and Qigong teachers for the tremendously valuable assets to society that they are. Thank you. Visit this site to find T'ai Chi and Qigong contact info worldwide. Any schools not listed in the following directory should visit the website and list, and for individuals, you should visit there regularly for new listings and updated information, research, etc., on T'ai Chi and QiGong worldwide.

National QiGong Assn. (NQA)
www.nqa.org
The NQA is an umbrella organization representing QiGong and T'ai Chi schools of all styles. It holds annual meetings to educate both novices and teachers in various forms of QiGong and T'ai Chi by coordinating teaching sessions with some of the world's top experts in the field and provides an organizing forum for schools to strategize how to bring these powerful health tools out to the larger national and global community.

American QiGong Association/World QiGong Federation
www.eastwestqi.com
The American QiGong Association and World QiGong Federation both work to bring QiGong researchers, teachers, and practitioners together to facilitate the expansion of QiGong usage for the betterment of world health and healing. A personal thanks to Effie Chow for her pioneering work with AQA.

Web Sources and Publications

www.qi-journal.com
Qi—*Journal of Traditional Eastern Health and Fitness*—Traditional Chinese Medicine. A powerful web resource!
Also the publisher of *Qi Journal* magazine, available at Border's bookstores and other major outlets.

www.worldhealingday.org
World Healing Day. This site brings together natural health proponents, like T'ai Chi and QiGong practitioners, with environmental health educators and natural, safe, and humane organic growers and livestock producers to advocate and envision ways to create a healthier, cleaner, and more humane world.

www.smartaichi.com
Smartaichi.com provides T'ai Chi and QiGong videos, audios, and other health and mind expansion products, including the Zen Alarm Clock. There you'll also find a research library on emerging T'ai Chi and QiGong medical and health research. (Web design by Astrachan Communications.)

www.QiGonginstitute.org
The QiGong Institute Promotes QiGong through research and education and is the producer of the QiGong Computerized Database, which provides over 1,600 references to QiGong medical and scientific research being done worldwide.

www.abodetao.com
Publisher of *The Empty Vessel*, a journal of contemporary Taoism. An acclaimed publication dedicated to the exploration and dissemination of nonreligious Taoist philosophy and practice.

groups.yahoo.com/group/qiresearch
This International Forum on QiGong Research enables researchers worldwide to share and compare ongoing research into the many aspects and benefits of QiGong.

www.FindTaiChi.com
Find contact info for T'ai Chi and QiGong schools worldwide.

www.tcfe.org
Find T'ai Chi in Europe through the European T'ai Chi and QiGong Federation, with over 500 member organizations throughout Europe and national organizations within most European countries.

www.taoist.org/
The International Taoist Tai Chi Society has members worldwide.

www.greenpartyusa.org
National Green Party USA Alternative Health Platform Plank—The Green Party USA's national convention is expected to provide considerable support for an Alternative Health Platform Plank, to encourage greater public awareness and use of natural health/preventative health maintenance techniques like T'ai Chi and QiGong. Learn more by contacting them at:

> **www.spiritofchange.org**
> *The Spirit of Change Magazine* is one of New England's premier holistic magazines.

> **www.visionmagazine.com**
> Provides articles and updates on many issues regarding holistic living.

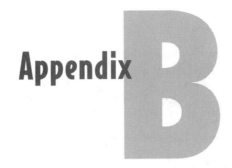

Appendix B

Suggested Readings

Bach, Richard. *Jonathan Livingston Seagull*. New York: The Macmillan Company, 1970.

Badgley, Laurence, M.D. *Healing AIDS Naturally*. Foster City, CA: Human Energy Press, 1987.

Batmanghelidj, F., M.D. *The Body's Many Cries for Water*. Falls Church, VA: Global Health Solutions, Inc., 1997.

Behr, Thomas E., Ph.D. *The Tao of Sales*. Rockport, MA: Element Books, Inc., 1997.

Benson, Herbert, M.D. *The Relaxation Response*. New York: Avon Books, 1975.

Booth, Jennifer. *Wind Blowing Lotus Leaf—the Way of Enlightened Action*. Warrior of Light Publications, 1999.

Borysenko, Joan, Ph.D., and Miroslav Borysenko, Ph.D. *The Power of the Mind to Heal*. Carlsbad, CA: Hay House, Inc., 1994.

Capra, Fritjof (author of *The Tao of Physics*). *The Web of Life*. New York: Doubleday, 1996.

Chen Pan Ling. *Chen Pan Ling's Original Tai Chi Chuan Textbook*. Blitz! Design, New Orleans, 1998.

Chopra, Deepak. *Ageless Body, Timeless Mind*. New York: Harmony Books, 1993.

Cohen, Kenneth S. *The Way of QiGong: The Art and Science of Chinese Energy Healing*. New York: Ballantine Books, 1997.

Diller, Lawrence H., M.D. *Running on Ritalin—a Physician Reflects on Children, Society, and Performance in a Pill*. New York: Bantam Books, 1998.

Gerber, Richard, M.D. *Vibrational Medicine*. Santa Fe, New Mexico: Bear and Company, 1988.

Greene, Brian. *The Elegant Universe—Superstrings, Hidden Dimensions, and the Quest for the Ultimate Theory*. New York, London: W.W. Norton and Company, 1999.

Lasorso, Vincent J. Jr. *Immortal's Gift—A Parable for the Soul*. White Willow School of Tai Chi, 2000.

Lee, Martin, Ph.D., with Melinda Emily and Joyce Lee. *The Healing Art of T'ai Chi*. New York: Sterling Publishing Co. Inc., 1996.

Leight, Michelle Dominique. *The New Beauty: East-West Teachings in the Beauty of Body and Soul*. New York: Kodansha America Inc., 1995.

Luk, Charles. *Taoist Yoga, Alchemy and Immortality*. York Beach, Maine: Samuel Weisner, Inc., 1973.

Mann, Felix, MB, LMCC. *Acupuncture: The Ancient Chinese Art of Healing*. New York: Random House, 1978.

McGaa, Ed (Eagle Man). *Mother Earth Spirituality—Native American Paths to Healing Ourselves and Our World*. San Francisco: Harper, 1990.

Rothstein, Larry, Ed.D., Lyle H. Miller, Ph.D., and Alma Dell Smith, Ph.D. *The Stress Solution*. New York: Pocket Books, a Division of Simon & Schuster, Inc., 1993.

Moyers, Bill. *Healing and the Mind*. New York: Doubleday, 1993.

Sandifer, Jon. *Acupressure for Health, Vitality and First Aid*. Rockport, MA: Element Books Limited, 1997.

Sang, Larry. *The Principles of Feng Shui*. Monterey Park, CA: The American Feng Shui Institute, 1994.

Shanor, Karen Nesbitt, Ph.D. *The Emerging Mind—New Research into the Meaning of Consciousness, Based on the Smithsonian Institution Lecture Series*. Los Angeles: Renaissance Books, 1999.

Sheldrake, Rupert. *A New Science of Life—Morphic Resonance*. Rochester, VT: Park Street Press, 1995.

Star, Jonathan, trans. *Rumi—in the Arms of the Beloved*. New York: Jeremy P. Tarcher/Putnam, 1997.

Talbot, Michael. *The Holographic Universe*. New York: HarperCollins Publishers, Inc., 1991.

Watts, Alan. *The Way of Zen*. New York: Vintage Books, A Division of Random House, Inc., 1985.

Weil, Andrew, M.D. *Spontaneous Healing*. New York: Ballantine Books, a Division of Random House, Inc., 1995.

Williams, Tom, Ph.D. *The Complete Illustrated Guide to Chinese Medicine*. Rockport, MA: Element Books, Inc., 1996.

Yu-Cheng Huang. *Change the Picture*. Yu-Cheng Huang, 1998.

Yutang, Lin. *The Wisdom of Laotse*. New York: The Modern Library, 1948.

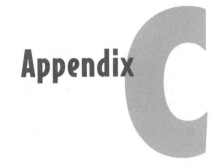

Audio-Visual Resources

Video instruction adds a powerful expansion to book instruction. Because with an instructor talking you through the movements, your analytical mind can "let go" more and *flow through it*, plus you can get a better feel for the timing of both motion and breath. The overall effect of video instruction is more relaxing and meditative.

Beyond video's advantages, DVD format is even better, because it enables viewers to go *directly to* the lesson of the day, and some DVD players allow you to "loop" video sections so you can make individual video Tai Chi lessons as long as you like, without the rewinding required by VHS video.

This appendix provides details on instructional videos for two of the T'ai Chi styles taught in this book, the T'ai Chi Long Form (see Chapter 15, "Out in Style: Right Style, That Is"), and the Mulan Short Form (see Chapter 16, "Mulan Quan Basic Short Form"), followed by order information.

Video and DVD Resources

T'ai Chi and QiGong: The Prescription for the Future Series

This acclaimed video series, by author Bill Douglas, was rated "Excellent" by *Book List Magazine*. It provides easy-to-follow guidance on the T'ai Chi long form illustrated in Chapter 15. The series is available as a set with three VHS videos or on DVD-ROM. The VHS set totals nearly four hours of viewing time. The DVD includes additional 20 minutes of bonus scenes, including exhibition of the entire Left Style (mirror-image style of the standard Right Style) of the Kuang Ping Yang long form.

Mulan Style Video

This video beautifully demonstrates and teaches the nuances of the Mulan Basic Short Form introduced in Chapter 16. The video is approximately 100 minutes.

Audio Resources

QiGong: Relaxation Therapy is a highly effective introduction to basic Sitting QiGong, or relaxation therapy, and this program has been used in major corporations and health network programs.

QiGong: Expanding Awareness takes the basic relaxation therapy to an entirely different level, giving the user a way to cleanse and clear their entire field of awareness of the daily loads of stress and anxiety.

QiGong: Earth Cleansing is what the author calls "The Meditation Tape for Those Who Can't Meditate!" It combines very tactile muscle tension and breath techniques to enable both mind and body to release their grip on the rat race and to find that calm center *no matter how intense life is.*

QiGong: For Children's Health and Relaxation is a fanciful journey of awareness that teaches children (and teachers/parents) breathing techniques to manage stress while enjoying a fanciful flying adventure of the mind.

Instructors or retailers are offered wholesale discounts when ordering five or more of any product item. Call 913-648-2256.

Where to Order

You can order these instructional videos and audio tapes online, by phone, or by mail.

To order online, go to www.smartaichi.com or www.taichismart.com. You can also send e-mail inquiries to the author at wtcqd2000@aol.com or wtcqd2000@yahoo.com.

To order by phone, call (toll-free) 1-877-482-4241 (U.S.) or 913-648-2256 (international; this is a toll call). To order by mail, complete the following form and send it together with your check or money order to:

> Stress Management and Relaxation Technology
> PO Box 7786
> Shawnee Mission, KS 66207-0786

Allow two to three weeks for delivery.

Deliver to:

Name: _____

Address: _____

City/State/Zip: _____

Phone number (with area code): _____

E-mail: _____

Item	Quantity	Unit Price	Total
DVD			
T'ai Chi and QiGong: The Prescription for the Future Series (four hours)	_____	$69.88	_____
Video (VHS)			
T'ai Chi and QiGong: The Prescription for the Future Series (three-video set)	_____	$65.95	_____
Mulan Style Video	_____	$27.95	_____
Audio Tapes			
QiGong: Relaxation Therapy	_____	$12.00	_____
QiGong: Expanding Awareness	_____	$12.00	_____
QiGong: Earth Cleansing	_____	$12.00	_____
QiGong: For Children's Health and Relaxation	_____	$12.00	_____
Add $4.50 for the first item; $1.50 for each additional		Shipping	_____
(Kansas residents add 7 percent sales tax.)		Tax	_____
		TOTAL	_____

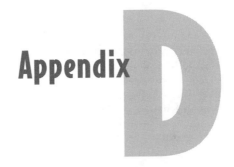

Appendix D

Glossary

abdominal breathing   The QiGong breathing technique, whereby the abdominal area, or lower lungs, fills first, then the upper chest, fully inflating the lungs. On the exhale, the upper chest relaxes inward as the lungs deflate, followed by the abdominal muscles relaxing inward allowing the lower lungs to deflate, fully expending the air from the lungs.

acupressure   A massage technique of stimulating the acupuncture points without the use of acupuncture needles.

acupuncture   A medical science that manipulates the flow of Qi, or life energy, through the body to maximize the body's health systems.

acupuncture maps   Diagrams or models to help acupuncturists locate the acupuncture points on the body.

aura   The sometimes visible aspect of life energy, whether through Kirlian photography or with the naked eye.

biofeedback   A computer program often used to train people to relax under stress, by showing their blood pressure, heart rate, and so on, while the participant uses relaxation techniques to normalize those indicators.

Bone Marrow Cleansing   Moving QiGong exercise designed to cleanse the bone marrow of stress that might inhibit the immune system.

Carry the Moon   Moving QiGong exercise designed to help the spine stay supple, support kidney function, and promote flexibility throughout the frame.

center   The physical, mental, emotional, and spiritual clarity that T'ai Chi and QiGong are designed to cultivate. Modern psychologists call this "homeostasis."

Chen style   An ancient T'ai Chi style and the basis of the Yang style.

Chinese Drum, The   A QiGong warm-up for T'ai Chi preparation.

Chinese Medica   The bible of Traditional Chinese Medicine, encompassing all known knowledge on acupuncture, herbal medicine, and QiGong.

crisis   The Chinese character for "crisis" is made of two characters, the character for "danger" plus the one for "opportunity."

dan tien   The physical center of your body. An energy center approximately 1½ to 3 inches below the navel near the center of the body.

DHEA   Adequate dehydroepiandrosterone levels are related to youthfulness and a more functional immune system. QiGong practice is believed to elevate DHEA levels.

Dong Gong   Moving QiGong.

energy meridians   In Chinese *jing luo*, or channel network. Modern acupuncturists may refer to them as "bioenergetic circuits." These are the paths that Qi moves through to circulate within the body, although they are not physical vessels like veins or arteries. They are energy channels where energy appears to flow more easily through the body's tissue. There are 14 main meridians, and 12 of those are directly associated with bodily organs, for example, heart, liver, and so on.

External QiGong   A Traditional Chinese Medical practice, whereby the provider allows his/her Qi, cultivated through internal QiGong practice, to flow, usually from their hands, out into the patient to help their healing process.

fan lao huan tong   In Chinese this means "reverse old age and return to youthfulness"; the goal of T'ai Chi and QiGong.

Feng Shui   The Chinese design art for creating flow and balance of energy within homes and other structures.

fight or flight response   The body's reflex response to stress that involves elevated blood pressure, heart rate, and feelings of subdued panic.

free radicals   Atoms with an extra electron, believed to contribute to the aging process. Regular T'ai Chi practice may reduce the cell damage that these cause.

Grand Terminus   The yin-yang symbol, and also the final movement of the Kuang Ping Yang style of T'ai Chi.

holistic   Chinese philosophy that sees the entire universe within each individual part, in much the same way that our body's building blocks of DNA coding is contained within each individual cell of our bodies.

homeostasis   Modern therapists use this term to describe a chemical, emotional, and mental sense of health and well-being. This is what T'ai Chi is designed to promote.

horary clock   Traditional Chinese Medicine's understanding of the ebb and flow of life energy patterns within the body. This understanding is used to treat various conditions using acupuncture, herbal, or QiGong therapy for optimum results.

Horse Stance   The basic stance for T'ai Chi, QiGong, and most martial arts.

hypertension   High blood pressure caused most often by unmanaged stress. High blood pressure is the cause of most heart disease.

I Ching   Also known as *The Book of Changes;* an ancient Chinese book of divination. The book is used to tell fortunes or to inspire people to look more deeply into themselves and their lives before making life decisions.

Jing Gong   *See* Sitting QiGong.

Kirlian photography   A photography method that appears to capture images of Qi or life energy.

Kuang Ping Yang style   The 64 movement long form of T'ai Chi brought to the West by master Kuo Lien Ying.

Lao-Tzu   The founder of Taoist philosophy.

master   One who cultivates a clarity in life enabling her to be a nurturing force to herself and the world.

Moving QiGong   Moving exercises, like T'ai Chi, that stimulate the flow of Qi through the body.

Mulan Quan style   A relatively modern form, yet rooted in a more ancient style. This may be the most elegant form of T'ai Chi, incorporating both dance and martial arts forms.

post-birth breathing   Normal abdominal T'ai Chi breathing.

pre-birth breathing   A form of breathing that requires the abdominal muscles to draw in on an in-breath, and relax out on an exhale.

psychoneuroimmunology   The modern science of studying how the mind's attitudes and beliefs affect our physical health.

Push Hands   A sparring tool and/or a subtle tool for self awareness, whereby two partners (or opponents) engage in a dancelike exchange, becoming aware of one another's posture and balance. This can be carried to an extreme of pushing the opponent down when they are vulnerable, or merely becoming gently conscious of when they are vulnerable without actually pushing them down.

Qi   Life energy. The Chinese character for Qi is also the character for air, as in breath.

QiGong   "Breath work" or "energy exercise." There are about 7,000 QiGong exercises in the Chinese Medica (the bible of Chinese medicine).

Sensei   A teacher; a term of respect often used in martial arts circles.

Sifu   Chinese for "one who has mastered an art." This term applies not only to martial arts, as a master chef or artist might be a Sifu as well.

sinking Qi   Settling the weight of the body into the leg you are shifting onto.

Sitting QiGong   Meditative exercises to promote the flow of Qi throughout the body.

Soong Yi-Dien   Loosen up. A T'ai Chi instruction to loosen the body, mind, and heart, encouraging the student to be more flexible and adaptable to all changes.

spirit   The Latin root of "spirit" is *spir*, to breathe, similar to the Chinese Qi, or life energy, expressed by the same word as "air."

stress   In Traditional Chinese Medicine the result of unmanaged stress is blocked energy and is the source of most physical, mental, emotional, and social problems.

T'ai Chi   A moving form of QiGong. Most Moving QiGong forms have only a few simple movements, and lack the continuous flow of the many multiple movements that T'ai Chi forms weave together.

T'ai Chi Ch'uan   "Supreme ultimate fist" or highest martial art.

Taoism   An ancient Chinese philosophy of life, which holds that the "Tao," the way of life, or the invisible force of nature's laws, can be accessed in states of alert calm. Regular immersion in the effortless power of life energy (through QiGong meditation) is believed to access the Tao for our lives, leading us to the most effortless and meaningful way to live.

Taoist Cannon   An ancient book that held all the early writing on QiGong, although at that time QiGong was called Tao-yin.

Taoist philosophy   Often thought of as T'ai Chi philosophy, because the subtle awareness of self and life energy is so directly applicable to Taoism's goal of getting in touch with the Tao's natural laws and quiet power.

Tao-yin   Leading or guiding the energy, another ancient name for QiGong.

T-cells   Cells that are believed to support our immune system by consuming virus, bacteria, and even tumor cells. T'ai Chi practice is believed to boost the body's production of T-cells.

To gu na xin   Expelling the old energy, absorbing the new, which was another name for QiGong.

Traditional Chinese Medicine (TCM)   The Chinese health sciences that see the body and mind as a holistic entity united by the flow of life energy or Qi. The three main branches of TCM are acupuncture, herbal medicine, and exercises such as T'ai Chi and QiGong, often used in combination.

vertical axis   The postural alignment for T'ai Chi.

Wan Yang-Ming   Philosopher who fused the physical motions of T'ai Chi Ch'uan with the philosophy of Taoism.

Wu style   A formidable martial art form of T'ai Chi popular in many countries.

Yang Lu-Chan   The great grand master of Kuang Ping Yang Style, who created it after studying the Chen family style.

Yang style   A form of T'ai Chi very popular in the United States and China.

Yellow Emperor's Classic of Chinese Medicine, The   The bible of Chinese Medicine in 200 B.C.E. It stressed that "true medicine" is curing disease before it develops.

yin and yang   The Chinese concepts of universal forces. All things are an eternally flowing interaction of two opposites; the ideal is healthy balance in all things. Yin is internal, dark, feminine, receptive. Yang is external, light, masculine, dynamic.

za-zen   The Zen art of meditation. Directly translated, it means "just sitting."

Zang Fu   In Chinese, "solid-hollow." A system that indicates how Qi, life energy, flows throughout and between organs. It is the model of how the entire body is interlinked by that flow, and shows how treating associated organs or energy meridians can improve others.

Zen   An oriental art of being here and now, allowing the mind and heart to let go of past and future attachments so that one can be fully immersed in the moment.

Index

L

Z

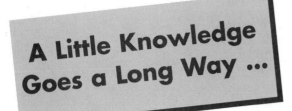
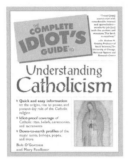
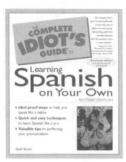
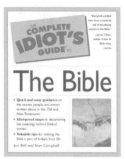
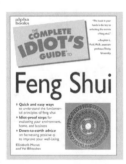
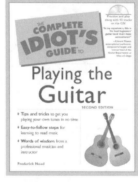
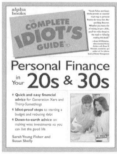
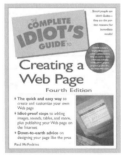
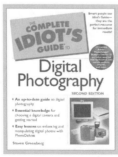
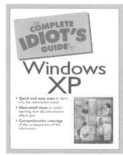
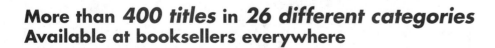